EXERCISE AND CHRONIC DISEASE

It is now widely accepted that there are important links between inactivity and chronic lifestyle-related diseases, and that exercise can bring tangible therapeutic benefits to people with chronic disease. *Exercise and Chronic Disease: an evidence-based approach* offers the most up-to-date survey currently available of the scientific and clinical evidence underlying the effects of exercise in relation to functional outcomes, disease-specific health-related outcomes and quality of life in patients with chronic disease conditions.

Drawing on data from randomized controlled trials and observational evidence, and written by a team of leading international researchers and medical and health practitioners, the book explores the evidence across a wide range of chronic diseases, including:

- cancer
- diabetes
- stroke
- Parkinson disease
- heart disease
- multiple sclerosis
- asthma

Each chapter addresses the frequency, intensity, duration and modality of exercise that might be employed as an intervention for each condition and, importantly, assesses those interventions in relation to outcomes that reflect tangible benefits to patients. No other book on this subject places the patient and the evidence directly at the heart of the study, and therefore this book will be essential reading for all exercise scientists, health scientists and medical professionals looking to develop their knowledge and professional practice.

John M. Saxton is Professor of Clinical Exercise Physiology at the University of East Anglia, Norwich. His research interests are focused on the effects of exercise and lifestyle interventions on wide-ranging health outcomes in clinical populations (including cancer and cardiovascular disease) and individuals at risk of developing lifestyle-related chronic conditions.

EXERCISE AND CHRONIC DISEASE

An evidence-based approach

EDITED BY JOHN M. SAXTON

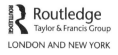

Routledge
Taylor & Francis Group

LONDON AND NEW YORK

First published 2011
by Routledge
2 Park Square, Milton Park, Abingdon, Oxon OX14 4RN

Simultaneously published in the USA and Canada
by Routledge
711 Third Avenue, New York, NY 10017

Routledge is an imprint of the Taylor & Francis Group

British Library Cataloguing in Publication Data
A catalogue record for this book is available from the British Library

Library of Congress Cataloging in Publication Data
Exercise and chronic disease: an evidence-based approach / edited by
John M. Saxton.
p. ; cm.
Includes bibliographical references.
1. Chronic diseases--Exercise therapy. 2. Exercise--Physiological
aspects. I. Saxton, John M., Prof.
[DNLM: 1. Chronic Disease--therapy. 2. Evidence-Based Medicine.
3. Exercise Therapy. 4. Exercise. WT 500]
RB156.E94 2011
616'.044--dc22   2010038188

ISBN 13: 978-0-415-49860-9 hbk
ISBN 13: 978-0-415-49861-6 pbk
ISBN 13: 978-0-203-87704-3 ebook

Typeset in Times New Roman
by Greengate Publishing Services, Tonbridge, Kent

CONTENTS

CONTRIBUTORS

Chapter 1: Introduction
John M. Saxton
School of Allied Health Professions
Faculty of Health
Queen's Building
University of East Anglia
Norwich, NR4 7TJ, UK
Tel: +44 (0)1603 593098
Email: john.saxton@uea.ac.uk

Chapter 2: Coronary heart disease
Gavin Sandercock
Department of Biological Sciences
University of Essex
Wivenhoe Park
Colchester, CO4 3SQ, UK
Tel: +44 (0)1206 872043
Email: gavins@essex.ac.uk

Chapter 3: Hypertension
V. A. Cornelissen and R. H. Fagard
UZ Gasthuisberg – IG Hypertensie
Herestraat 49
3000 Leuven, Belgium
Tel: +32 (0)16348707
Email: veronique.cornelissen@med.
kuleuven

Chapter 4: Stroke
Frederick M. Ivey, Alice S. Ryan, Charlene
E. Hafer-Macko and
Richard F. Macko
Baltimore VA Medical Center
Geriatrics Service/GRECC BT (18) GR
10 N. Greene St.
Baltimore MD 21201-1524, USA
Tel: +1 410 605 7297
Email: ssinglet@grecc.umaryland.edu

**Chapter 5: Peripheral arterial disease/
intermittent claudication**
Garry Tew and Irena Zwierska
Garry Tew
Centre for Sport and Exercise Science
Sheffield Hallam University
Collegiate Crescent Campus
Sheffield, S10 2BP, UK
Tel: +44 (0)114 225 2358
Email: g.tew@shu.ac.uk

Irena Zwierska
Keele University
Primary Care Musculoskeletal Research
Centre, Keele
Newcastle, Staffordshire, ST5 5BG, UK
Tel: +44 (0)1782 733972
Email: i.zwierska@cphc.keele.ac.uk

Chapter 6: Chronic obstructive pulmonary disease

Rachel Garrod and Fábio Pitta

Rachel Garrod
Consultant Respiratory Physiotherapist
Kings College Hospital NHS Foundation Trust
Pulmonary rehabilitation
Dulwich Community Hospital
East Dulwich Grove, SE22 8PT, UK
Tel: +44 (0)208 725 0377
Email: rachel.garrod@nhs.net

Fábio Pitta
Departamento de Fisioterapia
Universidade Estadual de Londrina
Av. Robert Koch, 60, Vila Operária
CEP 86038-440
Londrina, PR, Brasil
Tel: +55 43 3371 2477
Email: fabiopitta@uol.com.br

Chapter 7: Asthma

Felix S. F. Ram and Elissa M. McDonald
Massey University-Auckland
Private Bag 102 904
North Shore Mail Centre
Auckland, New Zealand
Tel: +64 9 414 9066
Email: fsfram@yahoo.co.uk

Chapter 8: Osteoarthritis

Marlene Fransen
Faculty of Health Sciences
Clinical and Rehabilitation Sciences
Research Group
University of Sydney, Australia
Tel: +61 2 93519829
Email: m.fransen@usyd.edu.au

Chapter 9: Osteoporosis

J. Y. Tsauo
School and Graduate Institute of Physical Therapy
College of Medicine
National Taiwan University and
Department of Physical Therapy

Hungkuang University, Taipei, Taiwan
Tel: +886 2 33668130
Email: jytsauo@ntu.edu.tw

Chapter 10: Rheumatoid arthritis

C. H. M. van den Ende
Department of Rheumatology
Sint Maartenskliniek
Hengstdal 3, 6522 JV Nijmegen, Netherlands
Tel: +31 (0)24 365 94 09
Email: e.vandenende@upcmail.nl

Chapter 11: Ankylosing spondylitis

Hanne Dagfinrud[1,2], Silje Halvorsen[1,2] and Nina K. Vøllestad[2]
[1] National Resource Centre for Rehabilitation in Rheumatology
Diakonhjemmet Hospital, Norway
[2] Institute of Health and Society
University of Oslo, Norway

Hanne Dagfinrud
Section for Health Science
University of Oslo
P.O.box 1153
Blindern
Gydas vei 8
Oslo, 0316, Norway
Tel: +47 22 45 48 41
Email: h.s.dagfinrud@medisin.uio.no

Chapter 12: Multiple sclerosis

Ulrik Dalgas
Department of Sport Science
University of Aarhus
Dalgas Avenue 4
8000 Aarhus N, Denmark
Tel: +45 27 11 91 21
Email: dalgas@sport.au.dk

Chapter 13: Parkinson disease

Gammon M. Earhart
Anatomy & Neurobiology, and Neurology
Washington University School of Medicine
Program in Physical Therapy
Campus Box 8502

4444 Forest Park Blvd.
St. Louis, MO 63108, USA
Tel: +1 314 286 1425
Email: earhartg@wusm.wustl.edu

Chapter 14: Type 2 diabetes

Stephan F. E. Praet[1], Robert Rozenberg[1]
and Luc J. C. Van Loon[2]
[1] Department of Rehabilitation Medicine &
Physical Therapy
Subdivision of Sports Medicine
Erasmus University Medical Center
P.O.Box 2040
NL-3000 CA Rotterdam, Netherlands
Tel: +31 (0)10 703 1887
[2] Department of Human Movement
Sciences
Faculty of Health Medicine and Life
Sciences
Maastricht University Medical Centre
Maastricht, Netherlands
Tel: +31 (0)10 703 18 87
Email: s.praet@erasmusmc.nl

Chapter 15: Obesity

Pedro J. Teixeira, R. James Stubbs, Neil A.
King, Stephen Whybrow and
John E. Blundell
Exercise and Health Department
Faculty of Human Movement
Technical University of Lisbon
Estrada da Costa
1495-688 Cruz Quebrada, Portugal
Tel: +351 21 414 9134
Email: pteixeira@fmh.utl.pt

Chapter 16: Chronic fatigue syndrome

Jo Nijs[2-4], Karen Wallman[1] and Lorna Paul[5]
[1] School of Sport Science, Exercise
and Health, The University of Western
Australia, Crawely, Western Australia
[2] Division of Musculoskeletal
Physiotherapy, Department of Health
Care Sciences, Artesis University College
Antwerp, Belgium
[3] Department of Human Physiology,
Faculty of Physical Education &
Physiotherapy, Vrije Universiteit Brussel,
Belgium
[4] Department of Physical Medicine and
Physiotherapy, University Hospital
Brussels, Belgium
[5] Nursing and Health Care, Faculty
of Medicine, University of Glasgow,
Glasgow, UK

Karen Wallman
School of Sport Science
Exercise and Health
The University of Western Australia
Stirling Highway
Crawely, Western Australia
Tel: +61 8 9387 1280
Email: kwallman@cyllene.uwa.edu.au

Chapter 17: Fibromyalgia syndrome

Borja Sañudo Corrales
Department of Physical Education
and Sport
Faculty of Educational Sciences
University of Seville
Avenida Ciudad Jardin, 20-22
E – 41005 Seville, Spain
Tel: +34 954556209
Email: bsancor@us.es

Chapter 18: Colorectal, breast and prostate cancer

Liam Bourke and John M. Saxton
Liam Bourke
Centre for Sport and Exercise Science
Sheffield Hallam University
Collegiate Crescent Campus
Sheffield, S10 2BP, UK
Tel: +44 (0)114 225 5628
Email: l.bourke@shu.ac.uk

John M. Saxton
School of Allied Health Professions
Faculty of Health
Queen's Building
University of East Anglia
Norwich, NR4 7TJ, UK
Tel: +44 (0)1603 593098
Email: john.saxton@uea.ac.uk

ACKNOWLEDGEMENTS

I would like to acknowledge several outstanding people who inspired me at different stages of my life. My parents and grandparents for their support and trust in the choices that I made, and for the lessons I learned from them. Aidan Trimble, Chris Hallam and Ken Johnson were early role models, who showed me what remarkable achievements could be made through dedication. Alan Donnelly and Priscilla Clarkson were magnificent supervisors and mentors during my doctoral studies – and 'Amherst 1993' was a truly exceptional experience! Tom Cochrane gave me a great opportunity for further personal and professional development at an early stage in my career and two excellent career mentors, Graham Pockley and Mike Smith, guided my path and provided me with lots of 'food for thought' during my time in Sheffield. I would also like to acknowledge my students, who have shown tremendous dedication and innovation in applying their skills as exercise scientists within the realms of health and disease and in doing so, have 'pushed the boundaries'. Finally, I would like to thank all contributors to this volume for taking time out of their busy schedules to produce a chapter which is based on the solid foundation of their own experience and innovative thinking in this field of research and extensive knowledge of the literature.

I dedicate this book to my wife Paula, my children John and Mary, and my family for their understanding and support.

1

INTRODUCTION

John M. Saxton

The burden of chronic disease

Chronic diseases are *long-term conditions* that cannot be cured but can be controlled with medication and/or other therapies (DoH 2010). Examples include coronary heart disease (CHD), stroke, cancer, chronic respiratory diseases and diabetes, which together constitute the leading cause of mortality worldwide (60 per cent of all deaths) and are projected to increase by a further 17 per cent over the next 10 years (WHO 2010). In addition to the human cost however, chronic diseases place a heavy economic burden on healthcare systems. In England, there are currently 15.4 million people living with a chronic condition (DoH 2010), accounting for more than 50 per cent of all general practitioner appointments, 65 per cent of all outpatient appointments and over 70 per cent of all inpatient bed days (DoH 2010). The treatment and care of individuals with chronic disease accounts for 70 per cent of the total health and social care costs, and this is projected to rise dramatically over the next 12–15 years as the number of people aged over 65 years increases by an estimated 42 per cent (DoH 2010). In the USA, more than 109 million people report having at least one of the seven most common chronic conditions (CHD, hypertension, stroke, pulmonary conditions, cancer, diabetes, mental disorders), representing more than half the population, and a figure which is expected to increase by 42 per cent by 2023 (DeVol and Bedroussain 2007). The total impact of these diseases on the American economy is estimated to be $1.3 trillion annually ($1.1 trillion due to lost productivity and $277 billion spent annually on treatment). Table 1.1 shows 12 prevalent chronic disease conditions.

TABLE 1.1 Twelve prevalent chronic diseases

Chronic heart disease (CHD)
Stroke
COPD
Depression
Lung cancer
Diabetes
Arthritis
Colorectal cancer
Asthma
Kidney disease
Oral disease
Osteoporosis

Adapted from Carrier (2009).

The role of exercise in management of chronic disease

The rapidly expanding population of older people, coupled with factors such as health inequalities and poor health behaviours, means that the burden of chronic disease is an escalating problem that presents one of the major healthcare challenges of the twenty-first century. Hence, there has been a shift away from the traditional 'medical' model of care, with its emphasis on curative treatments and patients being regarded as passive recipients of care, to a model which is aimed at empowering patients with the skills and knowledge to manage their own condition (Carrier 2009). Evidence suggests that the majority of people with long-term conditions lead full and active lives (Corben and Rosen 2005) and over 90 per cent of people with LTCs say they are interested in being more active self-carers (DoH 2010). The need for effective self-care strategies is exemplified in the following quote taken from the UK Department of Health policy document *Supporting People with Long Term Conditions: an NHS and social care model to support local innovation and integration*:

> When you leave the clinic, you still have a long term condition. When the visiting nurse leaves your home, you still have a long term condition. In the middle of the night, you fight the pain alone. At the weekend, you manage without your home help. Living with a long term condition is a great deal more than medical or professional assistance.
>
> Harry Cayton, Director for Patients and the Public,
> Department of Health (DoH 2005)

Although chronic diseases such as CHD, stroke, cancer, and diabetes are among the most prevalent and costly conditions in modern society, they are also among the most preventable of all health problems (CDC 2010). Major risk factors for these conditions include physical inactivity, unhealthy diets and tobacco use and the World Health Organisation estimates that by eliminating these risk factors, at least 80 per cent of all cases of CHD, stroke and type 2 diabetes and 40 per cent of cancers would be prevented (WHO website). Regular physical activity is widely accepted as being beneficial for health and a substantial body of epidemiologic research has demonstrated inverse associations of varying strength between physical activity and the risk of several chronic diseases, including CHD, stroke, hypertension, type 2 diabetes mellitus, osteoporosis, obesity, anxiety and depression (Pate *et al.* 1995; Haskell *et al.* 2007; DoH 2004). Additionally, a growing body of research during the past twenty years has provided 'convincing' evidence of an inverse association between physical activity and risk of colon cancer (WCRF/AICR 2007). There is also evidence of a 'probable' inverse association between physical activity and risk of other cancers, including post-menopausal breast and endometrial cancer, and limited 'suggestive' evidence of a similar association between physical activity and lung, pancreatic and pre-menopausal breast cancer (WCRF/AICR 2007).

Aside from the important role it plays in the *primary prevention* of a range of chronic diseases, a physically active lifestyle can bring manifold health benefits to individuals who are carrying the burden of chronic disease. There is evidence that regular exercise is associated with physical and psychosocial health benefits in many chronic disease conditions (Pedersen and Saltin 2006) and hence, keeping fit and healthy is now promoted by government health departments as an essential element of self-care for boosting general wellbeing, improving mobility and easing of symptoms (NHS Choices 2010). A physically active lifestyle can have an important role in controlling or reducing the impact of a chronic disease, prolonging survival and enhancing overall health-related quality of life (*secondary* and *tertiary* prevention). In this respect, 'exercise rehabilitation' is increasingly being recognised amongst healthcare professionals as an effective adjuvant or adjunctive treatment for a growing number of chronic conditions. Table 1.2 shows some key research questions to consider when assessing the efficacy of exercise therapy as an adjuvant or adjunctive treatment for chronic disease.

TABLE 1.2 Some key research questions to address when assessing the efficacy of exercise therapy as an adjuvant or adjunctive treatment for chronic disease

---

Can exercise training counteract the adverse physiological and psychological sequelae of a chronic disease and its treatments? What is the role of exercise in chronic disease modification?

How does exercise interact with drug treatments for chronic disease? Can exercise counteract the side-effects of drug treatments?

How can exercise prescription be optimised to impact upon the broadest range of chronic disease specific health outcomes, e.g. frequency, intensity, duration and type of exercise, social setting, support structures, flexibility of provision, etc?

Why do some patients with a given chronic disease respond and/or adapt differently to exercise?

What are the contra-indications to exercise in different clinical groups?

Exercise terminology

'Exercise' and 'physical activity' are terms that are commonly used in the scientific literature. Caspersen *et al.* (1985) proposed definitions for *physical activity* and *exercise* to provide a framework in which studies could be interpreted and compared. *Physical activity* was defined as 'any bodily movement produced by skeletal muscles that results in energy expenditure'. *Exercise* was defined as a sub-category of physical activity which is 'planned, structured, repetitive and purposive' and which has the objective of improving or maintaining one or more components of physical fitness.

Winter and Fowler (2009) highlighted the limitations of these definitions, pointing out the shortfalls in relation to isometric exercise (static muscle actions) and argued that the two terms should be interchangeable, depending on circumstances and context. Nevertheless, *exercise* is more commonly used to refer to structured leisure time physical activities, such as swimming, jogging and recreational sports, rather than to common activities of daily living, e.g. walking and physical tasks in the home or work environment. The latter are more commonly categorised under the umbrella term of *physical activity*. For the purpose of this book, both *exercise* and *physical activity* are considered to mean any movement (or isometric exercise) of the skeletal muscles, in the context of recreational, occupational or activities of daily living, which increases energy expenditure.

Another term that is important in the context of exercise rehabilitation is *physical fitness*. *Physical fitness* generally refers to the characteristics of an individual that permit good performance of a given task in a specified physical, social and psychological environment (Bouchard *et al.* 1994). It is influenced by genetic factors but is sensitive to change in people of all ages and physical fitness levels who engage in regular exercise. *Physical fitness* can be sub-divided into smaller measureable components, e.g. aerobic power and endurance, muscular strength and endurance, speed, power, agility and flexibility. *Health-related fitness* is reserved for aspects of physical fitness and psychological wellbeing that can be improved by engaging in a physically active lifestyle. In a Scientific Consensus Statement (Bouchard *et al.* 1994), *health-related fitness* dimensions were categorised into morphological, muscular, motor, cardiorespiratory and metabolic. Whilst this model includes the main physical dimensions of health-related fitness, it fails to recognise psychosocial health benefits that can result from habitual exercise. Hence, a revised model, encompassing both physical (physiological) and psychosocial dimensions which can be influenced by exercise, potentially impacting upon health-related quality of life (QoL) and survival is presented in Figure 1.1.

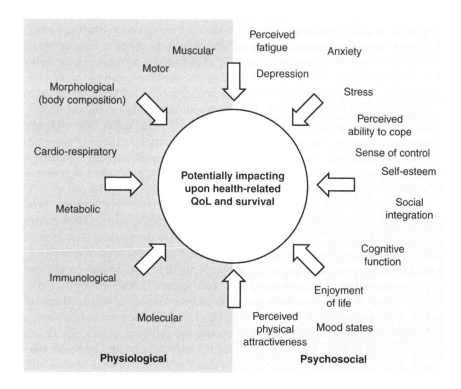

FIGURE 1.1 Physiological and psychosocial dimensions which can be influenced by exercise, potentially impacting upon health-related QoL and survival. Adapted from Saxton and Daley (2010).

Levels of evidence

A range of methodological approaches have been used to assess the impact of a physically active lifestyle on health outcomes which are relevant to people with chronic disease. These include observational studies (mainly case control and cohort studies), randomised controlled trials and non-randomised trials. *Observational studies* do not investigate cause and effect relationships but associations between outcomes and 'exposures' of interest (e.g. self-reported physical activity) and the data should be interpreted in this context. *Cohort studies* (prospective and retrospective) and *case-control* (or case comparison) studies are commonly used observational designs. In prospective cohort studies, physical activity status is assessed at some baseline time-point before participants are followed up (often at regular intervals) to see if they reach a pre-defined clinical endpoint (e.g. disease diagnosis, cardiovascular event, mortality). The frequency with which the outcome occurs is then compared between physically active and more sedentary participants to determine their relative chances of reaching the clinical end-point. Retrospective cohort studies use pre-existing data 'exposures' of interest and outcomes, and are quicker and cheaper to conduct. Limitations of cohort studies include failure to account for all potentially confounding variables in the analysis (although a greater number of potential confounders can be controlled for in larger cohort studies) and the time-scale needed to follow up large numbers of people over many years (prospective studies). In case-control studies, participants are selected on the basis of their disease status rather than exposure and the main outcome measure is the odds ratio of exposure (odds of exposure in cases divided by the odds of exposure in a matched or unmatched comparison group). Case-control studies are not as scientifically robust as cohort studies and are often nested within larger cohort studies.

Randomised controlled trials (RCTs) are considered to represent the 'gold standard' study design for establishing a cause and effect relationship between an intervention and an outcome. RCTs usually involve the random allocation of participants to an intervention group or a standard treatment control group (e.g. usual care, with or without placebo), although multiple intervention groups can also be compared with each other and the control group. This allows for the rigorous evaluation of a single variable (or complex intervention) in a defined patient group, as the assumption is that all confounding variables (known and unknown) are distributed randomly and equally between the different groups. RCTs are useful for investigating the effects of exercise interventions on key health outcomes in chronic disease populations and many examples of such studies will be discussed in the following chapters. Study outcomes often include physical (and functional) fitness, exercise adherence, perceptions of fatigue, indices of psychosocial wellbeing and health-related quality of life. A commonly used generic quality of life measure which has been validated for use in many clinical populations (e.g. Koloski *et al.* 2000; Ware *et al.* 1999) is the Medical Outcome Study Short Form-36 (SF-36; Ware and Sherbourne 1992). The SF-36 comprises eight health domains: physical functioning, role-physical, bodily pain, general health perceptions, vitality, social functioning, role-emotional and mental health. However, many other disease-specific health-related quality of life measures have been validated for use in different chronic disease populations and examples of these measures can be found in the following chapters.

Non-randomised intervention studies are also used to investigate the effects of structured exercise or non-structured physical activity on important health outcomes in chronic disease populations. Non-randomised parallel-arm trials (and single-group intervention studies) are more subject to bias, as confounding variables are unlikely to be equally distributed between groups and the participants volunteering for an intervention (or assigned to an intervention) may have certain characteristics which differ from the wider population (selection or allocation bias).

Dose-response issues

As for pharmacological treatments, it is important to establish whether dose-response relationships exist between the 'dose' of structured exercise or non-structured physical activity and health outcomes that are relevant for chronic disease populations. Measurable units of exercise are derived from knowledge of the frequency, intensity and duration of acute exercise bouts. Some combination of these factors can then be used to calculate total volume of exercise over a given period of time. Another important factor to consider is the type of exercise that is being undertaken. Purposeful structured exercise is often classified into aerobic activities that utilise large skeletal muscle groups in a rhythmic fashion (aimed at improving cardiopulmonary function and aerobic capacity) and resistance exercises (or strength training), in which skeletal muscles generate torque against an external resistance (e.g. free weights, body resistance, etc.).

In RCTs, the frequency, intensity and duration of supervised structured exercise can be precisely defined and the type(s) of exercise being undertaken easily recorded. For unsupervised exercise in the home or community setting (structured exercise or non-structured physical activity), exercise logs and objective free-living physical activity assessment tools (e.g. heart rate monitors, pedometers, accelerometers, etc.) are commonly used to quantify exercise dose. In many observational studies, self-report questionnaires or structured interviews are used to obtain information about the amount of structured exercise and non-structured physical activity that participants were engaged in at a set time point in their lives. Instruments include the Stanford Seven-Day Physical Activity Recall Interview (Sallis *et al.* 1985), the International Physical Activity Questionnaire (Craig *et al.* 2003) and the Godin Leisure Time Exercise Questionnaire (Godin *et al.* 1985). Questionnaire and interview techniques for assessing self-reported physical activity are susceptible to recall bias and hence, misclassification errors. Moreover, physical activity data tends to be assessed at a particular 'snap-shot' in time, with no indication of whether this is maintained in the follow-up period. However, these methods are highly pragmatic for large population studies and in some studies, the researchers have validated the questionnaires with objectively assessed physical activity data (e.g. accelerometry).

Multiples of the metabolic equivalent task (MET) is a commonly used method to quantify the intensity of physical activity. One MET is defined as the energy expended (or rate of oxygen consumed) by an average adult when sitting quietly (approximately 3.5 ml·kg^{-1}·min^{-1}). Thus, an individual who is performing an activity of 5 METs has an oxygen consumption which is five times higher than at rest. Using this method, exercise intensity is categorised in absolute terms as 'light' (< 3 METs), 'moderate' (3–6 METs) or 'vigorous' (> 6 METs). Compendium tables are available in the scientific literature (e.g. Ainsworth *et al.* 2000), which can be used to assign the MET level typically associated with a specific recreational, household or occupational task. When the intensity of self-reported physical activities (in METs) is then multiplied by the duration of specific physical activities, the total volume of physical activity in MET-hours·week^{-1} can be determined and used to assess associations between different levels of physical activity and other outcomes. When such a volume measurement is used to quantify exercise dose, it is useful to accompany it with additional information about the main types and intensities of exercise that the population under study were involved in.

Aims of the book

The role of exercise and other lifestyle interventions for promoting improvements in key health outcomes in chronic disease populations is increasingly being studied by research groups around the world. At the present time, we still have much to learn about the health impacts of regular exercise in different groups of patients undergoing different treatment regimens. Nevertheless, the weight of current evidence supports the assertion that a physically active lifestyle can have a positive impact on a wide range of physical and psychological outcomes in many chronic disease populations, with little evidence of adverse effects.

The key aim of this book is to present the most up-to-date synthesis of scientific evidence for exercise as a therapy in a range of chronic disease conditions. Fifteen active researchers or research groups in this field from around the world have each contributed a chapter to this book. The book includes both systematic reviews and narrative reviews, with each chapter designed to be standalone. The different chapters consider empirical evidence from a diversity of study designs, though an objective was to focus mainly on evidence from human RCTs. Although robust evidence-based recommendations for exercise are currently only possible for a few chronic diseases, where possible, suggestions for exercise prescription have been made on the basis of available evidence and experience of the research group. Future research will improve knowledge in relation to a number of key issues, including the impact of specific exercise modalities in different patient populations and during different phases of treatment, optimal dose of exercise for specific populations, the relative benefits of supervised and self-directed exercise programmes and how to optimise adherence to exercise rehabilitation.

I hope that this book will be of use to academics and health professionals, including clinical exercise physiologists, nutritionists, health promotion advisors, public health commissioners, health psychologists and exercise leaders. Some readers may choose to read this book in its entirety, whilst others may only read the chapters that are of most interest. I also hope that this book will provide impetus for further research in the field, so that ultimately, an increasing number of patients will understand the role of exercise in self-care and experience the full range of health benefits that exercise has to offer.

References

Ainsworth, B. E., Haskell, W. L., Whitt, M. C., Irwin, M. L., Swartz, A. M., Strath, S. J., O'Brien, W. L., Bassett, D. R. Jr, Schmitz, K. H., Emplaincourt, P. O., Jacobs, D. R. Jr and Leon, A. S. (2000) Compendium of physical activities: an update of activity codes and MET intensities. *Med Sci Sports Exerc*, 32 (9 Suppl), S498–504.

Bouchard, C., Shephard, R. J. and Stephens, T. (1994) *Physical Activity, Fitness, and Health Consensus Statement.* Champaign, IL: Human Kinetics Publishers.

Carrier, J. (2009) *Managing Long-Term Conditions and Chronic Illness in Primary Care: A Guide to Good Practice.* Oxford: Routledge.

Caspersen, C. J., Powell, K. E. and Christenson, G. M. (1985) Physical activity, exercise, and physical fitness: definitions and distinctions for health-related research. *Public Health Rep*, 100, 126–131.

Centers for Disease Control and Prevention (CDC) (2010) Available from http://www.dcd. gov. Accessed 15 May 2010.

Craig, C. L., Marshall, A. L., Sjöström, M., Bauman, A. E., Booth, M. L., Ainsworth, B. E., Pratt, M., Ekelund, U., Yngve, A., Sallis, J. F. and Oja, P. (2003) International physical activity questionnaire: 12-country reliability and validity. *Med Sci Sports Exerc*, 35, 1381–1395.

Corben, S. and Rosen R. (2005) *Self-management for Long-term Conditions.* London: King's Fund.

Department of Health (DoH) (2004) *Chief Medical Officer's Report. Evidence on the Impact of Physical Activity and Its Relationship to Health.* London: HSMO.

Department of Health (DoH) (2005) *Supporting People with Long-term Conditions. An NHS Social Care Model to Support Local Innovation and Integration.* London: Department of Health Publications.

Department of Health (DoH) (2010) *Improving the Health and Well-being of People with Long Term Conditions.* London: Department of Health Publications.

DeVol, R. and Bedroussian, A. (2007) *An Unhealthy America: The Economic Burden of Chronic Disease.* Santa Monica, CA: Milken Institute.

Godin, G. and Shephard, R. J. (1985) A simple method to assess exercise behavior in the community. *Can J Appl Sport Sci,* 10, 141–146.

Haskell, W. L., Lee, I. M., Pate, R. R., Powell, K. E., Blair, S. N., Franklin, B. A., Macera, C. A., Heath, G. W., Thompson, P. D. and Bauman, A. (2007) Physical activity and public health: updated recommendation for adults from the American College of Sports Medicine and the American Heart Association. *Med Sci Sports Exerc*, 39, 1423–1434.

Koloski, N. A., Talley, N. J. and Boyce, P. M. (2000) The impact of functional gastrointestinal disorders on quality of life. *Am J Gastroenterol,* (Jan) 95(1), 67–71.

NHS Choices (2010) *'Your Health, Your Way' NHS Guide to Long-term Conditions and Self Care.* Available from http://www.nhs.uk/planners/yourhealth/pages/yourhealth. aspx. Accessed 5 June 2010.

Pate, R. R., Pratt, M., Blair, S. N., Haskell, W. L., Macera, C. A., Bouchard, C., Buchner, D., Ettinger, W., Heath, G. W., King, A. C., Kriska, A., Leon, A. S., Marcus, B. H.,

Morris, J., Paffenbarger, R. S., Patrick, J., Pollock, M. L., Rippe, J. M., Sallis, J. and Wilmore, J. H. (1995) Physical activity and public health. A recommendation from the Centers for Disease Control and Prevention and the American College of Sports Medicine. *JAMA*, 273, 402–407.

Pedersen, B. K. and Saltin B. (2006) Evidence of prescribing exercise as a therapy in chronic disease. *Scand J Med Sci Sports*, 16 (Suppl 1), 3–63.

Sallis, J. F., Haskell, W. L., Wood, P. D., Fortmann, S. P., Rogers, T., Blair, S. N. and Paffenbarger, R. S. Jr. (1985) Physical activity assessment methodology in the Five-City Project. *Am J Epidemiol* (Jan), 121(1), 91–106.

Saxton, J. M. and Daley, A. (2010) *Exercise and Cancer Survivorship: Impact on Health Outcomes and Quality of Life.* New York: Springer.

Ware, J. E. Jr, Bayliss, M.S., Mannocchia, M. and Davis, G. L. (1999) Health-related quality of life in chronic hepatitis C: impact of disease and treatment response. The Interventional Therapy Group. *Hepatology* (Aug), 30(2), 550–555.

Ware, J. E. and Sherbourne, C. D. (1992) The MOS 36-item short-form health survey (SF-36). *Medical Care*, 30(6), 473–483.

Winter, E. M. and Fowler, N. (2009) Exercise defined and quantified according to the Systeme International d'Unites. *J Sports Sci*, 27, 447–460.

World Cancer Research Fund/American Institute for Cancer Research (WCRF/AICR) (2007) *Food, Nutrition, Physical Activity, and the Prevention of Cancer: A Global Perspective.* Washington DC: AICR.

World Health Organization (WHO) (2010) Available from http://www.who.int/en/. Accessed 15 May 2010.

2

CORONARY HEART DISEASE

Gavin Sandercock

Ageing and cardiovascular disease

The ageing cardiovascular system is unable to perform its various functions at the capacities once achieved during youth and young adulthood (Ferrari *et al.* 2003; Singh 2004). Yet despite this, the exercise capacity and cardiovascular functioning of master athletes shows that pronounced debilitating declines are not inevitable. In fact, many master athletes can 'out perform' younger individuals who do not engage in exercise training (Meredith *et al.* 1989; Tanaka and Seals *et al.* 2008) Hence, exercise training can forestall the declines in cardiovascular performance which play an integral role in impaired exercise capacity with increasing age (Kasch *et al.* 1993; Kasch *et al.* 1999; Tanaka and Seals 2008) and encouragingly, the elderly cardiovascular system retains plasticity and is able to respond positively to the demands of exercise training as it is in younger adulthood (Stratton *et al.* 1994; Singh 2004).

Preservation of cardiovascular function with ageing also depends on the health of the cardiovascular system. Unfortunately, post-mortem evidence suggests pathological processes within the cardiovascular system begin early in human life (Enos *et al.* 1953). Most significant of these, in terms of cardiovascular disease, is atherosclerosis, particularly when present in the coronary arteries (Berenson *et al.* 1998).

Atherosclerosis: risk factors, process, outcomes

A wide variety of pathological conditions are contained beneath the umbrella term of cardiovascular disease (CVD). These include any condition detrimental to normal functioning of either the heart or vasculature. For the purpose of this chapter, the term coronary heart disease (CHD) will be used to limit discussion to those diseases whose pathology mediates its effects, via acute and chronic ischae-mia, on the myocardium. Cardiac rehabilitation may be effective for many related conditions, including hypertension, the cardiovascular complications of type 2 diabetes, following valve replacement or repair surgery and heart failure but the evidence-base for efficacy is strongest for CHD.

The process by which atherosclerotic plaques develop in arteries is complex and the exact hypothesis is under constant scientific debate and review (Kent 1979; Wissler 1991; Libby *et al.* 2009). Very briefly, the lumen of coronary arteries nar-rows, initially due to the development of fatty streaks, then an atherosclerotic plaque comprising lipid or calcified matter. Minor occlusion of the lumen is usu-ally asymptomatic but the further development of a stable plaque creates angina pectoris due to myocardial ischaemia usually felt upon exertion. Parts of unstable plaques may detach and become thrombi. Passing down the ever-narrowing vas-cular tree these thrombi may partially or wholly (especially if further narrowing is evident at other regions) occlude the blood flow causing myocardial infarction or stroke. The severity of such episodes depends on the degree to which the vascular flow is occluded, the site of occlusion and the duration.

The economic cost of the CHD health burden is massive, and much of this health burden is directly attributable to ischaemic diseases due to atherosclerosis. Necrotic destruction of myocardial tissue due to obstruction of the coronary blood flow is termed myocardial infarction (MI). Improved emergency treatment of MI by thrombolysis and emergency revascularisation procedures and increased prev-alence of elective, preventive surgeries like coronary artery bypass grafting and angioplasty are increasingly effective. This means that many patients suffering from CHD are living longer. Although such treatments are effective in treating the disease's direct pathological consequences (atherosclerosis, thrombi) they do not return the patient to a full, active, high quality life. To do this and reduce the likelihood of more surgery and/or risk of a further MI, patients are offered cardiac rehabilitation.

Phases of cardiac rehabilitation

According to the World Health Organisation (WHO) Phase I is the education and encouragement given to the patient while in hospital. In the first instance, this is typically carried out by the emergency medical personnel if the patient is admitted for MI or the surgical care team for elective revascularisation patients. Following acute phase treatment, typically a specialist cardiac rehabilitation nurse or physi-otherapist will visit the patient pre-discharge to encourage mobilisation, provide reassurance and give information on the upcoming phases of cardiac rehabilita-tion the patient will be offered. Patients and carers are given educational advice and materials on: medications, diet, avoiding stress, emergency first aid and exer-cise guidance. In the UK, this advice is provided by specially trained facilitators who provide patients with the Heart Manual, a tool shown to reduce mortality and morbidity (Lewin *et al.* 1992). Phase II is the period at home between discharge from hospital and joining the supervised Phase III programme. During Phase II, either home visits or telephone contact may be used to reassure the patient and encourage further gradual mobilisation. This is usually carried out by a nurse specialist or Heart Manual Facilitator who encourages the patient to interact with the Heart Manual. Phase III comprises a supervised programme of graduated exercise together with monitoring of risk factors, education, stress management and relaxation training. This phase may be delivered via many staffing combinations (Brodie *et al.* 2006) but teams typically comprise a specialist cardiac rehabilitation nurse, who identifies patients and performs the risk assessments, a specialist cardiovascular physiotherapist or an exercise specialist who delivers the exercise programme. In North America, the cardiac rehabilitation team also commonly includes a dedicated cardiovascular clinician. For a detailed review of the components of cardiac rehabilitation, please refer to Bethell (2006). In the UK, guidance of delivering cardiac rehabilitation is provided by the NICE (2007) and SIGN (2002) but many other countries have their own guidance (Goble and Worcester 1999; NZGG 2002) including the AACVPR (Smith *et al.* 2006) in the USA (classification of cardiac rehabilitation phases is different in the USA).

Evidence for the effectiveness of cardiac rehabilitation

When assessing the efficacy of any medical intervention, the highest level of evidence must be sought. In the USA, the highest level of evidence for clinical efficacy (category 1) comes from randomised controlled trials (Smith *et al.* 2006). In the UK, this represents the second highest level of evidence (category 1b), as the combined evidence from numerous randomised controlled trials (via systematic review or meta-analysis) is assumed to represent the highest level of evidence (category 1a) (Harbour and Miller 2001; Atkins *et al.* 2004).

Several narrative reviews, systematic reviews and meta-analyses have considered the impact of cardiac rehabilitation on important health outcomes. These reviews and meta-analyses provide evidence for a positive effect on numerous outcome measures, including mortality, and this evidence is strong enough to support the recommendation of cardiac rehabilitation as a therapeutic intervention (Smith *et al.* 2006; NICE 2007). The following sections will consider this evidence in more detail.

Early reviews of cardiac rehabilitation trials suggested that post-myocardial infarction patients who were offered exercise therapy had a better prognosis than patients who did not (May *et al.* 1982). Statements like this, which seem obvious today, should be viewed in the context that until the 1970s, bed rest was still a recommended therapy for patients recovering from MI. Trials that attempted to mobilise patients or engage them in structured activities were in their infancy. For a more complete review of the history of cardiac rehabilitation, the reader is referred to Bethell (2006).

Systematic reviews are limited by individual trial outcomes and many early trials of cardiac rehabilitation suffered from poor methodology and small sample sizes. In such cases, it is preferable to pool the effect sizes from these heterogeneous trials (meta-analysis) and create a pooled effect size (ES) or pooled odds ratio (OR). This allows synthesis of the findings of many trials without comparing individuals within trials directly and yields greater statistical power than summarising findings from individual trials. Readers not familiar with the process and terminology of meta-analytical technique may find the information on the Cochrane Library website a useful starting point (www.thecochranelibrary.com).

Evidence for cardiac rehabilitation in reducing mortality

At first glance, the evidence for reductions in all cause mortality and cardiovascular mortality attributed to cardiac rehabilitation appear irrefutable. Four large-scale meta-analyses were performed on the data between 1988 and 2004, all showing statistically and clinically significant effects for cardiac rehabilitation on mortality.

Oldridge et al. (1988) analysed data from 2,202 controls and 2,145 patients randomly assigned to cardiac rehabilitation. Data were drawn from 10 trials (including the WHO multi-centre study trials) between 1972 and 1985. The odds ratio for all cause mortality was significantly reduced in the cardiac rehabilitation patients (OR = 0.76; 95% CI: 0.63–0.92) meaning that these patients were on average 24 per cent less likely to die within the two-year follow-up period. There was also a 25 per cent lower likelihood (OR = 0.75; 95% CI: 0.62–0.93) of cardiovascular death in patients receiving cardiac rehabilitation. The authors found no statistically significant difference in the rate of non-fatal re-infarction between the two groups (OR = 1.15; 95% CI: 0.93–1.42), although the odds ratio shows a trend towards a greater likelihood of this in cardiac rehabilitation patients.

Sub-group analysis for all cause mortality showed an added benefit of risk factor management combined with exercise in comparison to exercise therapy alone, and longer interventions (>36 months) were more effective than shorter ones (<12 weeks). The latter was also true for measures of cardiovascular mortality, where there was virtually no effect of <12 week cardiac rehabilitation (OR = 0.99; 95% CI: 0.78–1.26) but significant reductions for cardiac rehabilitation programmes lasting >12 weeks (OR = 0.65; 95% CI: 0.45–0.94).

One year later, O'Connor et al. (1989) analysed a similar data set but using slightly more stringent inclusion criteria. Like Oldridge et al. (1988), they found that cardiac rehabilitation produced significant reductions in all-cause (OR = 0.80; 95% CI: 0.66–0.96) and cardiovascular (OR = 0.78; 95% CI: 0.63–0.96) mortality. In addition, to the findings of the previous meta-analysis (Oldridge et al. 1988), O'Conner et al. (1989) also showed that there was a very large reduction in sudden death up to one year after randomisation (OR = 0.63; 95% CI: 0.41–0.97), which persisted (albeit non-significantly) at two and three years of follow-up. There was also a reduction in fatal re-infarctions (OR = 0.75; 95% CI: 0.59–0.95) for up to three years post-randomisation, but again, no difference in non-fatal re-infarction between the control and cardiac rehabilitation patients (OR = 1.09; 95% CI: 0.76–1.57). O'Connor *et al.* (1989) commented on the (non-significant) trend towards increased numbers of non-fatal re-infarctions observed in cardiac rehabilitation patients in their own meta-analysis and in that of Oldridge *et al.* (1988) and suggested that this could represent a real increase in non-fatal re-infarctions or an improved ability of post-cardiac rehabilitation patients to survive subsequent infarcts (as evidence by their lower fatal-re-infarction rates).

Considered together, these studies suggest a clinically important 20–25 per cent reduction in mortality due to cardiac rehabilitation programmes but the studies do have some inherent limitations. In both meta-analyses, women made up less than 3 per cent of the total population studied. In fact, only four of the 22 trials analysed by O'Connor *et al.* (1989) included any women at all. Also, participants over the age of 70 were generally excluded from the studies analysed and some of the larger studies (which excluded 55–65 year olds) investigated cohorts that would be considered young for cardiac rehabilitation patients by today's standards (Sanne 1973; Wilhelmsen *et al.* 1975). Additionally, the outcome measures considered in the trials did not permit the authors to postulate a mechanism by which cardiac rehabilitation might be effective in reducing mortality.

Jolliffe *et al.* (2001) analysed the effect of exercise-only cardiac rehabilitation on total mortality in 7,683 patients from 32 randomised controlled trials. This updated estimate of the effectiveness of exercise-only based cardiac rehabilitation produced evidence for an impressive 27 per cent reduction in all cause mortality (OR = 0.73; 95% CI: 0.54–0.98). Total cardiovascular disease mortality was also reduced to greater extent than in earlier meta-analyses, showing a 31 per cent decrease (OR = 0.69; 95% CI: 0.51–0.93) and this effect was even larger when deaths from coronary heart disease only were analysed, showing a 30 per cent reduction in cardiac deaths (OR = 0.70; 95% CI: 0.51–0.94).

Jolliffe *et al.* (2001) also systematically compared the effectiveness of exercise-only cardiac rehabilitation versus more comprehensive programmes (including education and/or psychosocial counselling) on clinical end points such as rehospitalisation and mortality. The authors also analysed how effective cardiac rehabilitation was at attenuating softer end points such as percutaneous transluminal coronary angioplasty (PTCA) or coronary artery bypass grafting (CABG) and, for the first time, outlined a potential mechanism for cardiac rehabilitation by summarising its effectiveness at risk factor modification. Interestingly, reductions were smaller for comprehensive cardiac rehabilitation compared with exercise-only cardiac rehabilitation. Exercise-only programmes reduced cardiac deaths by 31 per cent versus only 26 per cent in comprehensive programmes. Exercise-only programmes were also better at reducing cardiac deaths (35%) compared with comprehensive programmes (28%). Neither type of intervention produced a significant effect for sudden cardiac deaths or non-fatal re-infarctions.

Compared with analysis of hard end points such as mortality, analysis of 'soft' end points was limited by a lower number of studies being included, but neither exercise-based nor comprehensive cardiac rehabilitation showed a significant reduction in hospital admission rates for either PTCA or CABG. This finding may be explained, at least in part, by the reduction in certain risk factors which was observed, leading to a reduced need for revascularisation surgery.

Effects of cardiac rehabilitation on modifiable risk factors

The risk of atherosclerosis and CHD is altered by a number of risk factors that can be classified as either modifiable or non-modifiable (the latter being mainly heredity, age and sex). Modifiable risk factors are extremely well documented and a discussion is beyond the scope of this chapter. However, the importance (relative weighting) of the multiple modifiable risk factors is continually changing as new risk factors emerge (Hackam *et al.* 2003; Thomas *et al.* 2003; Cui *et al.* 2009; Libby *et al.* 2009). Considered next is the role that cardiac rehabilitation can have in improving some of the 'classic' risk factors, particularly those that are commonly used in risk stratification before (Eichler *et al.* 2007; Chen *et al.* 2009) and after MI (Cui *et al.* 2009).

Meta-analysis of comprehensive cardiac rehabilitation trials shows significant reductions in total cholesterol and low density lipoproteins (Jolliffe *et al.* 2001). Exercise-based interventions had no effect on any risk factor measures but the number of studies included was very small for both totals (Kentala 1972; Ballantyne *et al.* 1982; Wosornu *et al.* 1996) and LDL cholesterol (Ballantyne *et al.* 1982; Wosornu *et al.* 1996).

A more recent meta-analysis of exercise-only trials which contained data from many more studies (Taylor *et al.* 2004) showed that cardiac rehabilitation was effective in reducing triglycerides and total cholesterol but that it had no overall effect on LDL or HDL cholesterol levels. The potential impact that reductions in such risk factors may have on mortality is discussed in the next section.

How risk factor reduction influences outcome in cardiac rehabilitation

Taylor *et al.* (2006) calculated the reduction in mortality which could be attributed to risk factor reduction, further to their previous meta-analysis which showed cardiac rehabilitation could reduce total cholesterol and triglycerides (Taylor *et al.* 2004). These authors also demonstrated that cardiac rehabilitation significantly reduced systolic blood pressure. Smoking rates were also reduced although not significantly (OR = 0.82; 95% CI; 0.60–1.12). Taylor *et al.* (2006) calculated that 58.2 per cent of the reduction in mortality due to cardiac rehabilitation could be attributed to reductions in smoking (23.8%), cholesterol (19.7%) and blood pressure (14.7%).

Evidence for mortality and morbidity reduction are unequivocal and it is clear that risk factor modification plays a clear role in this success. Such trials provide information on long-term outcomes but have several shortcomings in that they tell us little about the patient in terms of their quality of life or functional capacity before, and particularly after, attending cardiac rehabilitation.

Jolliffe *et al.* (2001) also attempted to meta-analyse health-related quality of life (QoL) but the heterogeneity of tools (n=18 different instruments were identified) used to assess this construct did not facilitate statistical analysis. Bias in reporting and use of non-validated tools meant only four exercise-only cardiac rehabilitation trials were assessed; none of which showed clear changes in QoL. Seven comprehensive cardiac rehabilitation studies were reviewed but showed variable results. The largest effect was in the trial of the Heart Manual (Lewin *et al.* 1992) but it should be noted that this is given in phase II of cardiac rehabilitation whereas most interventions are based in phase III. Oldridge *et al.* (1991) reported significant improvements in QoL of patients recovering from MI over 12 months, but these improvements were no larger than those of the control group. Heterogeneity of methods and the small number of studies included in the analysis may have lead to a possible underestimation of the effectiveness of cardiac rehabilitation in improving QoL.

Given the particular weakness of evidence regarding improvements in quality of life it is difficult to determine from such data whether cardiac rehabilitation actually makes people 'feel better'. Clearly, one aim of cardiac rehabilitation should be to add life to years as well as years to life (Thompson 2009), allowing patients not only to survive, but also to lead fulfilling and, as much as possible, normal lives following CHD. The following section will examine the effect that exercise-based cardiac rehabilitation has on functional capacity. It should be borne in mind that functional capacity or fitness is an significant and independent prognosticator for mortality and morbidity (Williams 2001; Myers *et al.* 2002; Sui *et al.* 2007a; Sui *et al.* 2007b) (particularly that related to cardiovascular disease) may be thought of as a short-term, proxy measure for the potential long-term benefits of cardiac rehabilitation.

Does exercise-based cardiac rehabilitation increase patients' functional capacity?

Given the excellent evidence from randomised controlled trials for the effectiveness of cardiac rehabilitation, it is unsurprising that this type of trial became rarer after 2001. This is because it is unethical to withhold an effective treatment for research purposes. Much of the more recent evidence comes from cohort studies which, although they cannot demonstrate cause-and-effect relationships, often offer a more realistic view of how cardiac rehabilitation is carried out in clinical practice. In many of the older randomised trials, the training stimulus was large and may have exaggerated the effects of cardiac rehabilitation. For example one British trial (Bethell and Mullee 1990) used three one-hour exercise sessions per week at 75–85 per cent heart rate max, whereas a more recent UK survey suggested that the supervised training session frequency of between one and two times per week is more normal (Brodie *et al.* 2006). Other studies have included as many as five exercise sessions per week (Miller *et al.* 1984; Fletcher *et al.* 1994). Given Brodie *et al.*'s (2006) findings, and that most guidelines recommend two weekly supervised exercise sessions, it appears that the training stimulus which patients actually receive in cardiac rehabilitation may be far less than the average stimulus on which the evidence for reduced mortality has been calculated. The following review is not exhaustive but intends to demonstrate evidence for additional benefits of cardiac rehabilitation particularly when studied in a more naturalistic setting.

Despite recommendations to monitor cardiac rehabilitation patients' functional capacity, only 39 per cent of UK centres reported doing so both before and after rehabilitation (Brodie *et al.* 2006). A variety of exercise tests (step test, shuttle walking, cycle ergometry) were reported. Functional capacity testing pre- and post-rehabilitation appears to be more common in North America where it is also often carried out by maximal incremental treadmill testing. Still, the number of trials or retrospective analyses of changes in functional capacity remains relatively small. Balady *et al.* (1996) found baseline values of 8.6 ± 3.4 METs and 6.0 ± 2.6 METs for men and women respectively, who were entering a cardiac rehabilitation programme. Improvement in functional capacity varied by age and sex from 32 per cent in females >75 years to 50 per cent in females of 65–75 years. The authors concluded that all participants of all ages and both sexes could benefit from cardiac rehabilitation but particularly those with low (<5 METs) initial values.

Similarly, Lavie *et al.* (1993) increased estimated exercise capacity (METS) from 5.6 ± 1.6 to. 7.5 ± 2.3 in cardiac rehabilitation patients. These authors have also demonstrated the efficacy of cardiac rehabilitation in increasing exercise capacity and efficiency in obese patients (Lavie and Milani 1996; Lavie and Milani 1999).

More recently, one very large study (Ades *et al.* 2006) reported graded treadmill exercise test data on 2,896 patients entering cardiac rehabilitation and found that measured $\dot{V}O_2$ was low (around 40–60 per cent of age-predicted maximum). Factors which were associated with $\dot{V}O_2$ were: sex (men↑), age (older↓), treatment (PCI > MI > CABG), administration of β-blockers (↓), presence of hypertension (↓) and BMI (higher BMI↓). This study also demonstrated that standard (ACSM) prediction equations deriving METs from treadmill performance significantly overestimated the actual $\dot{V}O_2$ of cardiac rehabilitation patients. These authors also found increases in measured $\dot{V}O_2$ in 504 patients receiving 36 sessions of cardiac rehabilitation over a three-month period. But they also found this increase was modulated by factors including age and sex. Men's $\dot{V}O_2$ increased by 18 per cent compared with a 12 per cent increase in women of the same age.

US studies like those above have the luxury of drawing on pre- and post-cardiac rehabilitation graded exercise tests to assess changes in functional capacity. In many settings and in the UK particularly, alternative, cheaper and less time-consuming measures of functional capacity are used. One such measure is the 10m incremental shuttle-walking test. This has the advantage that it can be carried out without a cardiac technician or cardiologist, requires minimal equipment and does not include treadmill walking which may be unfamiliar to many patients. The test is safe, valid (Fowler and Singh 2005) and reliable over short (Jolly *et al.* 2008) and long (Pepera and Sandercock 2010) test–retest durations.

In centre-based cardiac rehabilitation programmes which have used this test as an estimate of functional capacity, there is good evidence that walking capacity is increased (Fowler and Singh 2005; Arnold *et al.* 2007; Sandercock *et al.* 2007). In general, patients can walk 350–400 metres at entry to cardiac rehabilitation and this capacity improves by an average of about 90 metres. Using standard MET equivalents for walking speed this is equal to about a 0.5 MET increase in capacity. As with treadmill exercise (Ades *et al.* 2006) however, shuttle-walking in cardiac rehabilitation patients has a higher VO_2 equivalent meaning that MET equivalents underestimate the true cost of this exercise in these patients groups (Woolf-May and Ferrett 2008). It appears, therefore, that hospital or centre-based cardiac rehabilitation is an effective therapy by which to increase the functional capacity of CHD patients.

Despite the wealth of evidence to support the efficacy of cardiac rehabilitation, recent UK data suggest that only 30 per cent of eligible patients attend cardiac rehabilitation; this is despite national targets of 85 per cent (NICE 2007). A number of clinical and psychosocial barriers to cardiac rehabilitation attendance (Cooper *et al.* 2002; Dunlay *et al.* 2009), adherence (Jackson *et al.* 2005) and drop-out (Yohannes *et al.* 2007) have been identified. Although a full review of these is beyond the scope of this chapter; one proposal to increase attendance is to offer home-based rehabilitation programmes as this may be preferable to certain patients less likely to attend centre-based programmes (Barber *et al.* 2001; Arthur *et al.* 2002; Arthur *et al.* 2006). Significant attention has been paid to the fact that home-based or unsupervised version of cardiac rehabilitation programmes may be more cost effective (Beswick *et al.* 2004; Salvetti *et al.* 2008; Jolly *et al.* 2009).

Trials of home- versus hospital-based cardiac rehabilitation have been meta-analysed (Jolly *et al.* 2006) and show some surprising results. The authors carried out two meta-analyses; one comparing home-based cardiac rehabilitation with usual care and one reporting home-based cardiac rehabilitation with hospital-based care. The latter analysis was encouraging showing significant differences for gains in functional capacity in home- versus centre-based rehabilitation. When compared with usual care, however, home-based rehabilitation did not significantly improve functional capacity, with only a 0.4 MET increase reported. In fact, home-based rehabilitation was only effective in reducing smoking at follow-up compared with usual care. The small number of studies included in this analysis may have influenced this result. More worrying is the increase in total mortality observed in the home-based group. Although not statistically significant, the odds ratios (1.39; 95% CI, 0.98–1.97) show a clear trend toward a higher mortality in patients receiving home-based cardiac rehabilitation. The inclusion of two large studies using mostly psychological interventions as home-based rehabilitation may, however, have biased this result.

Given the poor outcomes for mortality and the home-based rehabilitation's apparent inability it may seem futile to pursue such activity unless other benefits can be realised. In a cost-analysis of their multi-centre study, Jolly *et al.* (2009) found that the costs of home-based exercise were significantly higher than centre-based exercise. On a more positive note, higher adherence rates have been reported for home-based rehabilitation and it seems that behaviour change may be more long lasting in patients who receive their cardiac rehabilitation at home. One factor which is obvious from the literature is the selective nature of the samples in home-based cardiac rehabilitation studies. Typically, such studies use low risk patients (Jolly *et al.* 2006). Such patients usually have lower levels of classic risk factors and higher initial functional capacity than groups entering hospital-based programmes. Training responses (particularly changes in functional capacity) are subject to the law of initial values (Bouchard and Rankinen 2001), where smaller gains are observed in fitter patients and cardiac rehabilitation patients are no exception to this (Balady *et al.* 1996; Ades *et al.* 2006). More research is clearly needed to fully validate the use of home-based cardiac rehabilitation.

Exercise modality in cardiac rehabilitation: resistance versus aerobic exercise

The use of home-based exercise regimens obviously limits the choices and modalities of exercise available to practitioner and client. Much research has focused on the differences in training responses to resistance versus aerobic exercise. In their purest forms (for example continuous cycling for 30 minutes versus 3×8–10 repetitions at 65 per cent of a patient's one repetition maximum) the comparison of these two modalities is more or less academic because the majority of programmes use a combined approach to exercise whether through choice or necessity. Circuit training with both aerobic and resistive elements is the most commonly-used exercise modality (Brodie *et al.* 2006). When it is used, resistance exercise is often limited by equipment availability and safety concerns. This means that patients often perform exercises mainly at the high volume low end of the repetition continuum making the exercise a mixture of aerobic and resistive and not conducive to the continued development of strength.

Home and community versus hospital-based cardiac rehabilitation

Recent literature has focused on cost reduction and meeting the needs of patients. Undoubtedly, one reason for the slow uptake of exercise-based cardiac rehabilitation in light of evidence for its efficacy was safety concerns. Given that bed rest was still prescribed for those with damaged hearts into the late 1960s it is reassuring to know that there is good evidence for the safety of exercise-based cardiac rehabilitation as it is carried out today; this is undoubtedly due to the efficacy of risk stratification at entry to cardiac rehabilitation programmes.

Is exercise-based cardiac rehabilitation safe?

Safety of any intervention or health treatment is paramount and the overarching answer to the above question in terms of cardiac rehabilitation is yes. This is not coincidental but the result of carefully designed, evidence-based, exercise prescription coupled with careful risk stratification of all potential cardiac rehabilitation patients. Along with emotional triggers (Wilbert-Lampen *et al.* 2008), moderate and vigorous physical activity (PA) are two of the most common causes of sudden cardiac death (SCD) in the general population (Tofler and Muller 2006). It should always be remembered, however, that rates are low; estimates for exercise-induced myocardial infarction are 1 per 2500 (Mittleman *et al.* 1993). Estimates of SCD rates are even lower and predict only one such event is likely to occur for every half-million person-hours of exercise (Fletcher *et al.* 2001).

Nevertheless, the risk of adverse cardiac events is raised during exercise (Fletcher *et al.* 2001). This presents a paradox for health professionals in that it is known that long-term exercise training results in lower cardiovascular risk (Williams 2001) but that acute exposure to exercise may be an acute risk itself, particularly for those with cardiovascular disease (Cobb and Weaver 1986). A further paradox is that the acute risk associated with exercise is elevated significantly less in those who are regular exercisers (Siscovick *et al.* 1982; Mittleman *et al.* 1993). The practitioner is left, therefore, with a conundrum; do the chronic benefits of long-term exercise training outweigh the initial risks of (particularly initial) exercise sessions? In most cases, risk stratification protocols allow evidence-based decisions to be made. High risk individuals may need further treatment or investigation prior to starting an exercise-based programme of cardiac rehabilitation. In moderate risk individuals, a simple field test of cardiovascular function and/or functional capacity such the modified shuttle-walking test or 6 minute walking test may provide additional information. It should be noted that there is also a risk associated with performing such tests. Once initial peak work rate (usually reported as METs) has been established, exercise can be safely prescribed based on a submaximal percentage of this value. This exercise should be submaximal (50–75 per cent of maximum) and should adhere to simple procedures such as long warm-up (15–20 minutes) and cool-down (intervals). Such exercise is effective in increasing functional capacity, particularly in untrained or detrained individuals and a wealth of evidence from the cardiac rehabilitation literature suggests that it is also safe (Franklin *et al.* 1998; Pavy *et al.* 2006).

Conclusion

There is good scientific evidence that exercise-based programmes of cardiac rehabilitation significantly reduce mortality and morbidity from cardiovascular disease. Much of these reductions appear to be related to positive modification of cardiovascular disease risk factors. There is also fair evidence that exercise programmes can increase patients' functional capacity and quality of life. Despite such evidence, attendance at such programmes remains low and the focus of research has shifted from demonstrating the efficacy of cardiac rehabilitation, toward determining and overcoming barriers to attendance. Offering home-based programmes and those incorporating alternative exercise modalities may help to reduce these barriers but the efficacy and safety of such programmes should first be fully explored.

References

Ades, P.A., Savage, P. D., Brawner, C. A., Lyon, C. E., Ehrman, J. K., Bunn, J. Y. and Keteyian, S. J. (2006). Aerobic capacity in patients entering cardiac rehabilitation. *Circulation* 113(23): 2706–2712.

Arnold, H., Sewel, L. and Singh, S. (2007). A comparison of once versus twice per week cardiac rehabilitation. *British Journal of Cardiology* 14: 45–48.

Arthur, H. M., Patterson, C. and Stone, J. A. (2006). The role of complementary and alternative therapies in cardiac rehabilitation: a systematic evaluation. *Eur J Cardiovasc Prev Rehabil* 13(1): 3–9.

Arthur, H. M., Smith, K. M., Kodis, J. and McKelvie, R. (2002). A controlled trial of hospital versus home-based exercise in cardiac patients. *Med Sci Sports Exerc* 34(10): 1544–1550.

Atkins, D., Best, D., Briss, P. A., Eccles, M., Falck-Ytter, Y., Flottorp, S., Guyatt, G. H., Harbour, R. T., Haugh, M. C., Henry, D., Hill, S., Jaeschke, R., Leng, G., Liberati, A., Magrini, N., Mason, J., Middleton, P., Mrukowicz, J., O'Connell, D., Oxman, A. D., Phillips, B., Schunemann, H. J., Edejer, T. T., Varonen, H., Vist, G. E., Williams, J. W. Jr. and Zaza, S. (2004). Grading quality of evidence and strength of recommendations. *BMJ* 328(7454): 1490.

Balady, G. J., Jette, D., Scheer, J. and Downing, J. (1996). Changes in exercise capacity following cardiac rehabilitation in patients stratified according to age and gender. Results of the Massachusetts Association of Cardiovascular and Pulmonary Rehabilitation Multicenter Database. *J Cardiopulm Rehabil* 16(1): 38–46.

Ballantyne, F. C., Clark, R. S., Simpson, H. S. and Ballantyne, D. (1982). The effect of moderate physical exercise on the plasma lipoprotein subfractions of male survivors of myocardial infarction. *Circulation* 65(5): 913–918.

Barber, K., Stommel, M., Kroll, J, Holmes-Rovner, M. and McIntosh, B. (2001). Cardiac rehabilitation for community-based patients with myocardial infarction: factors predicting discharge recommendation and participation. *J Clin Epidemiol* 54(10): 1025–1030.

Berenson, G. S., Srinivasan, S. R., Bao, W., Newman, WP, 3rd, Tracy, R. E. and Wattigney, W. A. (1998). Association between multiple cardiovascular risk factors and atherosclerosis in children and young adults. The Bogalusa Heart Study. *N Engl J Med* 338(23): 1650–1656.

Beswick, A. D., Rees, K., Griebsch, I., Taylor, F. C., Burke, M., West, R. R., Victory, J., Brown, J., Taylor, R. S. and Ebrahim, S. (2004). Provision, uptake and cost of cardiac rehabilitation programmes: improving services to under-represented groups. *Health Technol Assess* 8(41): iii–iv, ix–x, 1–152.

Bethell, H. J. (2006). Exercise-based cardiac rehabilitation. *Medicine* 34(5): 195–196.

Bethell, H. J and Mullee, M. A. (1990). A controlled trial of community based coronary rehabilitation. *Br Heart J* 64(6): 370–375.

Bouchard, C. and Rankinen, T. (2001). Individual differences in response to regular physical activity. *Medicine and Science in Sports and Exercise* 33(6 Suppl): S446–451; discussion S452–443.

Brodie, D., Bethell, H. and Breen, S. (2006). Cardiac rehabilitation in England: a detailed national survey. *Eur J Cardiovasc Prev Rehabil* 13(1): 122–128.

Chen, L., Tonkin, A. M., Moon, L., Mitchell, P., Dobson, A., Giles, G., Hobbs, M., Phillips, P. J., Shaw, J. E., Simmons, D., Simons, L. A., Fitzgerald, A. P., De Backer, G. and De Bacquer, D. (2009). Recalibration and validation of the SCORE risk chart in the Australian population: the AusSCORE chart. *Eur J Cardiovasc Prev Rehabil* 16(5): 562–570.

Cobb, L. A and Weaver, W. D. (1986). Exercise: a risk for sudden death in patients with coronary heart disease. *J Am Coll Cardiol* 7(1): 215–219.

Cooper, A. F., Jackson, G., Weinman, J. and Horne, R. (2002). Factors associated with cardiac rehabilitation attendance: a systematic review of the literature. *Clin Rehabil* 16(5): 541–552.

Cui, J., Forbes, A., Kirby, A., Simes, J. and Tonkin, A. (2009). Laboratory and non-laboratory-based risk prediction models for secondary prevention of cardiovascular disease: the LIPID study. *Eur J Cardiovasc Prev Rehabil* 16(6): 660–668.

Dunlay, S. M., Witt, B. J., Allison, T. G., Hayes, S. N., Weston, S. A, Koepsell, E. and Roger, V. L. (2009). Barriers to participation in cardiac rehabilitation. *Am Heart J* 158(5): 852–859.

Eichler, K., Puhan, M. A., Steurer, J. and Bachmann, L. M. (2007). Prediction of first coronary events with the Framingham score: a systematic review. *Am Heart J* 153(5): 722–731.

Enos, W. F., Holmes, R. H. and Beyer, J. (1953). Coronary disease among United States soldiers killed in action in Korea; preliminary report. *J Am Med Assoc* 152(12): 1090–1093.

Ferrari, A. U., Radaelli, A. and Centola, M. (2003) Invited review: aging and the cardiovascular system. *J Appl Physiol* 95(6): 2591–2597.

Fletcher, B. J., Dunbar, S. B., Felner, J. M., Jensen, B. E., Almon, L., Cotsonis, G. and Fletcher, G. F. (1994). Exercise testing and training in physically disabled men with clinical evidence of coronary artery disease. *Am J Cardiol* 73(2): 170–174.

Fletcher, G. F., Balady, G. J., Amsterdam, E. A., Chaitman, B., Eckel, R., Fleg, J., Froelicher, V. F., Leon, A. S., Pina, I. L., Rodney, R., Simons-Morton, D. A., Williams, M. A. and Bazzarre, T. (2001). Exercise standards for testing and training: a statement for healthcare professionals from the American Heart Association. *Circulation* 104(14): 1694–1740.

Fowler, S. J. and Singh, S. (2005). Reproducibility and validity of the incremental shuttle walking test in patients following coronary artery bypass surgery. *Physiotherapy* 91: 22–27.

Franklin, B. A., Bonzheim, K., Gordon, S. and Timmis, G. C. (1998). Safety of medically supervised outpatient cardiac rehabilitation exercise therapy: a 16-year follow-up. *Chest* 114(3): 902–906.

Goble, A. and Worcester, M. (1999). *Best Practice Guidelines for Cardiac Rehabilitation and Secondary Prevention.* Victoria, National Heart Foundation of Australia.

Hackam, D. G. and Anand, S. S. (2003). Emerging risk factors for atherosclerotic vascular disease: a critical review of the evidence. *JAMA* 290(7): 932–940.

Harbour, R. and Miller, J. (2001). A new system for grading recommendations in evidence based guidelines. *BMJ* 323(7308): 334–336.

Jackson, L., Leclerc, J., Erskine, Y. and Linden, W. (2005). Getting the most out of cardiac rehabilitation: a review of referral and adherence predictors. *Heart* 91(1): 10–14.

Jolliffe, J. A., Rees, K., Taylor, R. S., Thompson, D., Oldridge, N. and Ebrahim, S. (2001). Exercise-based rehabilitation for coronary heart disease. *Cochrane Database Syst Rev* (1): CD001800.

Jolly, K., Lip, G. Y., Taylor, R. S., Raftery, J., Mant, J., Lane, D., Greenfield, S. and Stevens, A. (2009). The Birmingham Rehabilitation Uptake Maximisation study (BRUM): a randomised controlled trial comparing home-based with centre-based cardiac rehabilitation. *Heart* 95(1): 36–42.

Jolly, K., Taylor, R. S., Lip, G. Y. and Singh, S. (2008). Reproducibility and safety of the incremental shuttle walking test for cardiac rehabilitation. *Int J Cardiol* 125(1): 144–145.

Jolly, K., Taylor, R. S., Lip, G. Y. and Stevens, A. (2006). Home-based cardiac rehabilitation compared with centre-based rehabilitation and usual care: a systematic review and meta-analysis. *Int J Cardiol* 111(3): 343–351.

Kasch, F. W., Boyer, J. L., Schmidt, P. K., Wells, R. H., Wallace, J. P., Verity, L. S., Guy, H. and Schneider, D. (1999) Ageing of the cardiovascular system during 33 years of aerobic exercise. *Age Ageing* 28(6): 531–536.

Kasch, F. W., Boyer, J. L., Van Camp, S. P., Verity, L. S. and Wallace, J. P. (1993) Effect of exercise on cardiovascular ageing. *Age Ageing* 22(1): 5–10.

Kent, S. (1979). What causes atherosclerosis? *Geriatrics* 34(2): 85, 87, 89.

Kentala, E. (1972). Physical fitness and feasibility of physical rehabilitation after myocardial infarction in men of working age. *Ann Clin Res* 4: Suppl 9:1–84.

Lavie, C. J. and Milani, R. V. (1996). Effects of cardiac rehabilitation and exercise training in obese patients with coronary artery disease. *Chest* 109(1): 52–56.

Lavie, C. J. and Milani, R. V. (1999). Effects of cardiac rehabilitation and exercise training on peak aerobic capacity and work efficiency in obese patients with coronary artery disease. *Am J Cardiol* 83(10): 1477–1480, A1477.

Lavie, C. J., Milani, R. V. and Littman, A. B. (1993). Benefits of cardiac rehabilitation and exercise training in secondary coronary prevention in the elderly. *J Am Coll Cardiol* 22(3): 678–683.

Lewin, B., Robertson, I. H., Cay, E. L., Irving, J. B. and Campbell, M. (1992). Effects of self-help post-myocardial-infarction rehabilitation on psychological adjustment and use of health services. *Lancet* 339(8800): 1036–1040.

Libby, P., Ridker, P. M. and Hansson, G. K. (2009). Inflammation in atherosclerosis: from pathophysiology to practice. *J Am Coll Cardiol* 54(23): 2129–2138.

May, G. S., Eberlein, K. A., Furberg, C. D., Passamani, E. R. and DeMets, D. L. (1982). Secondary prevention after myocardial infarction: a review of long-term trials. *Prog Cardiovasc Dis* 24(4): 331–352.

Meredith, C. N., Frontera, W. R., Fisher, E. C., Hughes, V. A., Herland, J. C., Edwards, J. and Evans, W. J. (1989) Peripheral effects of endurance training in young and old subjects. *J Appl Physiol* 66(6): 2844–2849.

Miller, N. H., Haskell, W. L., Berra, K. and DeBusk, R. F. (1984). Home versus group exercise training for increasing functional capacity after myocardial infarction. *Circulation* 70(4): 645–649.

Mittleman, M. A., Maclure, M., Tofler, G. H., Sherwood, J. B., Goldberg, R. J. and Muller, J. E. (1993). Triggering of acute myocardial infarction by heavy physical exertion. Protection against triggering by regular exertion. Determinants of Myocardial Infarction Onset Study Investigators. *N Engl J Med* 329(23): 1677–1683.

Myers, J., Prakash, M., Froelicher, V., Do, D., Partington, S. and Atwood, J. E. (2002). Exercise capacity and mortality among men referred for exercise testing. *N Engl J Med* 346(11): 793–801.

NICE (2007). Secondary prevention in primary and secondary care for patient's following a myocardial infarction. Available at: http://guidance.nice.org.uk/CG48. [Accessed 10 May 2010].

NZGG (2002). *Best Practice Evidence-based Guideline: Cardiac Rehabilitation.* Auckland, New Zealand Guidelines Group.

O'Connor, G. T., Buring, J. E., Yusuf, S., Goldhaber, S. Z., Olmstead, E. M., Paffenbarger, R. S. Jr. and Hennekens, C. H. (1989). An overview of randomized trials of rehabilitation with exercise after myocardial infarction. *Circulation* 80(2): 234–244.

Oldridge, N. B., Guyatt, G. H., Fischer, M. E. and Rimm, A. A. (1988). Cardiac rehabilitation after myocardial infarction. Combined experience of randomized clinical trials. *JAMA* 260(7): 945–950.

Oldridge, N., Guyatt, G., Jones, N., Crowe, J., Singer, J., Feeny, D., McKelvie, R., Runions, J., Streiner, D. and Torrance, G. (1991). Effects on quality of life with comprehensive rehabilitation after acute myocardial infarction. *Am J Cardiol* 67: 1084–1089.

Pavy, B., Iliou, M. C., Meurin, P., Tabet, J. Y. and Corone, S. (2006). Safety of exercise training for cardiac patients: results of the French registry of complications during cardiac rehabilitation. *Arch Intern Med* 166(21): 2329–2334.

Pepera, G and Sandercock, GRH (2010). Long-term reliability of the incremental shuttle walking test in clinically stable cardiovascular disease patients. *Physiotherapy* 96(3): 222–227.

Salvetti, X. M., Oliveira, J. A., Servantes, D. M and Vincenzo de Paola, A. A. (2008). How much do the benefits cost? Effects of a home-based training programme on cardiovascular fitness, quality of life, programme cost and adherence for patients with coronary disease. *Clin Rehabil* 22(10–11): 987–996.

Sandercock, G. R., Grocott-Mason, R. and Brodie, D. A. (2007). Changes in short-term measures of heart rate variability after eight weeks of cardiac rehabilitation. *Clin Auton Res* 17(1): 39–45.

Sanne, H. (1973). Exercise tolerance and physical training of non-selected patients after myocardial infarction. *Acta Med Scand Suppl* 551: 1–124.

SIGN (2002). SIGN 57 Cardiac rehabilitation. A national clinical guideline. Edinburgh, Royal College of Physicians.

Singh, M. A. (2004) Exercise and aging. *Clin Geriatr Med* 20(2): 201–221.

Siscovick, D. S., Weiss, N. S., Hallstrom, A. P., Inui, T. S. and Peterson, D. R. (1982). Physical activity and primary cardiac arrest. *JAMA* 248(23): 3113–3117.

Smith, S.C. Jr., Allen, J., Blair, S. N., Bonow, R. O., Brass, L. M., Fonarow, G. C., Grundy, S. M., Hiratzka, L., Jones, D., Krumholz, H. M., Mosca, L., Pasternak, R. C., Pearson, T., Pfeffer, M. A. and Taubert, K. A. (2006). AHA/ACC guidelines for secondary prevention for patients with coronary and other atherosclerotic vascular disease: 2006 update: endorsed by the National Heart, Lung, and Blood Institute. *Circulation* 113(19): 2363–2372.

Stratton, J. R., Levy, W. C., Cerqueira, M. D., Schwartz, R. S. and Abrass, I. B. (1994). Cardiovascular responses to exercise. Effects of aging and exercise training in healthy men. *Circulation* 89(4): 1648–1655.

Sui, X., Laditka, J. N., Hardin, J. W. and Blair, S. N. (2007a). Estimated functional capacity predicts mortality in older adults. *J Am Geriatr Soc* 55(12): 1940–1947.

Sui, X., LaMonte, M. J. and Blair, S. N. (2007b). Cardiorespiratory fitness as a predictor of nonfatal cardiovascular events in asymptomatic women and men. *Am J Epidemiol* 165(12): 1413–1423.

Tanaka, H. and Seals, D. R. (2008). Endurance exercise performance in masters athletes: age-associated changes and underlying physiological mechanisms. *J Physiol* 586(1): 55–63.

Taylor, R. S., Brown, A., Ebrahim, S., Jolliffe, J., Noorani, H., Rees, K., Skidmore, B., Stone, J. A., Thompson, D. R. and Oldridge, N. (2004). Exercise-based rehabilitation for patients with coronary heart disease: systematic review and meta-analysis of randomized controlled trials. *Am J Med* 116(10): 682–692.

Taylor, R. S., Unal, B., Critchley, J. A. and Capewell, S. (2006). Mortality reductions in patients receiving exercise-based cardiac rehabilitation: how much can be attributed to cardiovascular risk factor improvements? *Eur J Cardiovasc Prev Rehabil* 13(3): 369–374.

Thomas, N. E., Baker, J. S. and Davies, B. (2003). Established and recently identified coronary heart disease risk factors in young people: the influence of physical activity and physical fitness. *Sports Med* 33(9): 633–650.

Thompson, D. (2009). Cardiac rehabilitation; adding years to life and life to years. *Journal of Reseach in Nursing* 14(3): 207–219.

Tofler, G. and Muller, J. (2006). Triggering of acute cardiovascular disease and potential preventive strategies. *Circulation* 114: 1863–1872.

Wilbert-Lampen, U., Leistner, D., Greven, S., Pohl, T., Sper, S., Volker, C., Guthlin, D., Plasse, A., Knez, A., Kuchenhoff, H. and Steinbeck, G. (2008). Cardiovascular events during World Cup soccer. *N Engl J Med* 358(5): 475–483.

Wilhelmsen, L., Sanne, H., Elmfeldt, D., Grimby, G., Tibblin, G. and Wedel, H. (1975). A controlled trial of physical training after myocardial infarction. Effects on risk factors, nonfatal reinfarction, and death. *Prev Med* 4(4): 491–508.

Williams, P. T. (2001). Physical fitness and activity as separate heart disease risk factors: a meta-analysis. *Med Sci Sports Exerc* 33(5): 754–761.

Wissler, R.W. (1991). Update on the pathogenesis of atherosclerosis. *Am J Med* 91(1B): 3S–9S.

Woolf-May, K. and Ferrett, D. (2008). Metabolic equivalents during the 10-m shuttle walking test for post- myocardial infarction patients. *Br J Sports Med* 42(1): 36–41; discussion 41.

Wosornu, D., Bedford, D. and Ballantyne, D. (1996). A comparison of the effects of strength and aerobic exercise training on exercise capacity and lipids after coronary artery bypass surgery. *Eur Heart J* 17(6): 854–863.

Yohannes, A. M., Yalfani, A., Doherty, P. and Bundy, C. (2007). Predictors of drop-out from an outpatient cardiac rehabilitation programme. *Clin Rehabil* 21(3): 222–229.

3

HYPERTENSION

V. A. Cornelissen and R. H. Fagard

Introduction

Hypertension is defined as a systolic blood pressure (BP) $\geq$ 140 mmHg or diastolic BP $\geq$ 90 mmHg or being on antihypertensive treatment. BP in excess of 140/90 mmHg is further categorized in terms of severity (Table 3.1) (Chobanian *et al.* 2003; Mancia *et al.* 2007). Although BP less than 140/90 mmHg was once considered normal, the Seventh Report of the Joint National Committee on Prevention, Detection, Evaluation and Treatment of High BP now includes the category of prehypertension, defined as the pressure range between 120/80 and 139/89 mmHg (Chobanian *et al.* 2003). Only pressures below 120/80 mmHg are considered optimal (Chobanian *et al.* 2003; Mancia *et al.* 2007). The morbidity and mortality associated with hypertension are substantial. Nearly one billion people in the world currently have hypertension, causing high BP to be one of the ten leading risk factors influencing the global burden of disease (WHO 2002; Kearney *et al.* 2005). It is estimated to lead to over seven million deaths each year, about 13 per cent of the total deaths worldwide (WHO 2002; Kearney *et al.* 2005).

TABLE 3.1 Definitions and classificiation of blood pressure levels

Category according to JNC VII**	Category according to guidelines ESH and ESC*	Systolic BP (mmHg)		Diastolic BP (mmHg)
Normal	Optimal	< 120	And	< 80
Prehypertension	Normal	120–129	And/or	80–84
	High Normal	130–139	And/or	85–89
Stage 1 hypertension	Grade 1 hypertension	140–159	And/or	90–99
Stage 2 hypertension	Grade 2 hypertension	160–179	And/or	100–109
	Grade 3 hypertension	$\geq$ 180	And/or	$\geq$ 110

Grades 1, 2 and 3 correspond to classification in mild, moderate and severe hypertension, respectively. Adapted from Chobanian *et al.*, 2003* and Mancia *et al.*, 2007**.

Average systolic BP increases approximately linearly with age, whereas diastolic BP plateaus in the sixth decade and decreases thereafter (Chobanian *et al.* 2003). Eventually, the lifetime risk of developing hypertension is approximately 90 per cent (Vasan *et al.* 2002). As a result, with the ageing of the population, the burden of hypertension is expected to increase significantly (Chobanian *et al.* 2003; Kearney *et al.* 2005). This growing epidemic of hypertension is thought to be predominantly due to lifestyle factors, including diminished physical activity and increased obesity, interacting with genetic susceptibility.

Data from observational studies in healthy individuals show a direct, strong, independent and continuous relation between BP and cardiovascular morbidity and mortality without any evidence of a threshold down to at least 115/75 mmHg (Lewington *et al.* 2002; Kannel *et al.* 2003). Therefore, adequate control of BP is of enormous public health importance. Irrespective of the level of BP, lowering of BP and prevention of hypertension is in the first instance preferable by lifestyle changes (Chobanian *et al.* 2003; Mancia *et al.* 2007). Given that epidemiological data suggest a strong relation between sedentary lifestyle and hypertension, all guidelines now recommend increased physical activity as a first line intervention for preventing high BP and treating patients with prehypertension or grade 1 or 2 hypertension (Chobanian *et al.* 2003; Pescatello *et al.* 2004a; Mancia *et al.* 2007). Unlike drug therapy, which may cause adverse effects and reduce the quality of life in a number of patients, a non-pharmacological therapy such as physical activity has no known harmful effects, may improve the sense of well-being of the patients and is often less expensive. Furthermore, it may interact favourably with other cardiovascular disease risk factors such as dyslipidemia and diabetes, which are often present in hypertensive individuals (Chobanian *et al.* 2003).

In this chapter, the impact of physical activity and fitness in relation to the prevention and management of high BP is evaluated from longitudinal observational data and from randomized controlled intervention studies in humans.

Physical activity, physical fitness and future hypertension: data from longitudinal observational studies

A considerable number of prospective cohort studies have investigated the role of physical activity and/or physical fitness in the prevention of hypertension. For the current overview, 20 studies were identified and these are summarized in Tables 3.2 and 3.3. At recruitment, the majority of participants were middle aged and were subsequently followed up for a mean duration of 1–25 years. Seven cohorts involved only men, two involved only women and eleven included both genders. Most participants were Caucasians living in the USA or Finland but studies in Japanese, Chinese or Korean individuals showed similar associations. Results in African–Americans (Pereira *et al.* 1999; Parker *et al.* 2007) were less consistent.

TABLE 3.2 Prospective cohort studies of physical activity and risk for developing hypertension

Author (country)	Participants	Follow-up	Physical activity assessments	Main findings
Paffenbarger et al. (1983) (USA)	14,998 male Harvard alumni	6–10 yrs	Daily number of city blocks walked, number of stairs climbed and type, frequency and duration of sports or recreational sports in hrs/week (none, light only, light and vigorous, vigorous only). Weekly EE in walking, stair climbing and sports (<500, 500–1999, ≥2000 kcal/wk)	Presence or absence of collegiate sports did not influence risk of hypertension, nor did stair climbing, walking or light sports. Absence of vigorous sports activity in postcollege years resulted in a 35% greater risk for hypertension
Folsom et al. (1985) (USA)	41,837 women, aged 55–69 yrs	2 yrs	Survey on LTPA (low, moderate, high)	High levels of LTPA were associated with significant reductions in risk of HTN [RR=0.70 (95% CI: 0.6–0.9)] compared to low levels of LTPA. However, in fully adjusted analyses (age, BMI, waist–hip ratio, smoking history) LTPA no longer contributed to HTN risk
Paffenbarger et al. (1991) (USA)	5,463 male University of Pennsylvania alumni, aged 39–55+	95,524 person years	Daily number of city block walked, number of stairs climbed and type, frequency and duration of sports or recreational sports in hrs/week (none, light only, light and vigorous, vigorous only) Weekly EE in walking, stair climbing and sports (<500, 500–1999, ≥2000 kcal/wk)	No association was observed with weekly distance walked or number of stairs climbed. Men who habitually engaged in vigorous sports play were at 19–29% less risk for HTN than those who reported no sports

Continued

TABLE 3.2 *continued*

Author (country)	Participants	Follow-up	Physical activity assessments	Main findings
Haapanen *et al.* (1997) (Finland)	731 men and 796 women, aged 35–63 yrs	10 yrs	Questionnaire including 23 questions regarding conditioning exercise, sports, physical recreation, different leisure time and household chores, and commuting to and from work. Weekly EE in LTPA. Men: low (0–1100), moderate (1101–1900), high (>1900) kcal/wk; women: low (0–900), moderate (901–1500), high (>1500) kcal/wk. Vigorous activity (≥6MET): ≥1time/wk or <1 time/wk	In men, high weekly EE (low relative to high category) and vigorous activity ≥ 1time/wk (reference) was associated with significant reduction in risk of HTN [age-adjusted RR=1.73 (1.13–2.65)] and [age-adjusted RR=1.56 (1.07–2.28)] respectively. These associations remained suggestively significant after adjustment for diabetes and BMI. These LTPA measures were not significantly associated with risk of HTN in women
Hayashi *et al.* (1999) (Japan)	6,017 men, aged 35–60 yrs	10 yrs	Questionnaire on LTPA, duration of walk to work, nature of occupation and level of activity involved. LTPA = regular physical exercise for at least 30 minutes enough to work up a sweat (0, 1, ≥2 times/wk). Commuting physical activity=duration of walk to work	Risk for HTN was reduced by 12% when the duration of the walk to work was increased by 10 minutes [RR=0.88 (0.79–0.98] and by 30% in men who engaged in regular physical activity at least once weekly [RR=0.70 (0.59–0.84)]
Pereira *et al.* (1999) (USA)	7,459 African-American and Caucasian men and women, aged 45–64 yrs	6 yrs	Baecke Physical Activity questionnaire LTPA: 4 questions on the frequency of television watching, walking, bicycling and walking/ bicycling to/from work or shopping and divided into quartiles. Sports index: average yearly freq and weekly duration of the respective sport or exercise. Work index: questions on individual main occupation	In Caucasian men a reduction in the odds of hypertension was observed with increasing quartile of LTPA and sports index. Baseline LTPA and sports index were not associated with future HTN in Caucasian women or in African–Americans. Work index was not related to future HTN in any group

Author (country)	Participants	Follow-up	Physical activity assessments	Main findings
Hernelahti et al. (2002) (Finland)	569 male former elite athletes and 319 male controls, aged ≤ 65 yrs	10 yrs	LTPA-index	Cumulative 10-year incidence of HTN was significantly lower in former endurance or mixed sports athletes whereas a history of being an athlete in power sports conferred no benefit. Odds ratio for HTN decreased by 12% per increasing quartile in LTPA- index
Hu et al. (2004) (Finland)	8,302 men and 9,139 women, aged 25–64 yrs	Mean: 11 yrs	Questionnaire on PA. Combination of CPA (walking or bicycling < 30 min or ≥ 30 min), OPA (light or moderate) and LTPA (low or moderate and high) merged to give 1) low, 2) moderate and 3) high PA category	RR of HTN associated with low, moderate and high PA were 1.0, 0.63 (0.5–0.8) and 0.59 (0.47–0.74) in men and 1.0, 0.82 (0.67–1.0) and 0.71(0.58–0.88) in women. These associations persisted in both overweight and none overweight subjects
Barengo et al. (2005) (Finland)	5,935 men and 6,227 women, aged 25–64 yrs	Mean: 11.3 yrs	Weekly LTPA: (low (inactive), moderate (moderate activity >4h/wk) high (vigorous activity > 3h/w) OPA: low/moderate/active CPA :motorized/walking or cycling >30 min/day walking or cycling >30 min/day	Multivariate adjusted risk for HTN, including occupational and commuting PA, was reduced with 24% in men with high LTPA (RR=0.79: 0.63–0.99) compared to low LTPA. Moderate LTPA did not show any statistically significant reduction of risk compared with low LTPA. No association could be detected for women. High OPA reduced the risk of HTN when men and women were combined (RR=0.83: 0.72–0.96). CPA was not associated with the risk of HTN
Nakanishi et al. (2005) (Japan)	2,548 male office workers, aged 35–59 yrs	7 yrs	Daily life EE estimated by a 1-day activity record during an ordinary weekday based on 20 selected daily life activities excluding regular PA: (<33.1, 33.1–36.7, 36.8–40.3, ≥40.4 kcal/wk)	RR for HTN across quartiles of daily life EE were 1.0, 0.84 (0.72–0.98), 0.75 (0.63–0.88) and 0.54 (0.45–0.64) (P<0.001 for trend). This association persisted in subjects divided according to BMI (< or ≥23.1.kg/m²).

Continued

TABLE 3.2 *continued*

Author (country)	Participants	Follow-up	Physical activity assessments	Main findings
Kim et al. (2006) (Korea)	2,802 men and 3,087 women, aged 40–69 yrs	2 yrs	Interview. Regular PA (≥2times/wk and ≥30 min each time): yes or no	Compared to those not exercising regularly, men [RR: 0.8 (0.6–1)] and women [RR: 0.6 (0.5–0.9)] exercising regularly had significantly lower odds of developing HTN
Gu et al. (2007) (China)	10,525 men and women, aged ≥ 40 yrs	Mean: 8.2 yrs	Work-related PA: low, moderate or high	Compared to the high category, men reporting low levels of work-related PA had a RR of HTN of 1.27 (1.1–1.47) and women had a RR of HTN of 1.22 (1.02–1.45)
Parker et al. (2007) (USA)	3,993 black and white men and women, aged 18–30 yrs	15 yrs	An interviewer-administered self-report of frequency of participation in each of 13 categories of sports and exercise, including 8 vigorous intensity activities and 5 moderate intensity activities, during the previous 12 months. An exercise score was computed and expressed in exercise units	Those who were more versus less physically active experienced a reduced risk [RR=0.83 (0.73–0.91)] for incident HTN (data shown for all combined)
Williams (2008) (USA)	29,139 men and 11,985 women	7.7 and 7.4 yrs	Average weekly running distance	Longer baseline distance predicted lower incident HTN

Author (country)	Participants	Follow-up	Physical activity assessments	Main findings
Chase et al. (2009) (USA)	16,601 men, aged 20–82 yrs,	Mean: 18.1 yrs	PA status was categorized into three mutually exclusive groups according to the type of PA reported during the three preceding months: sedentary = no to all activity questions; sport/fitness activity= no WJR but yes to participation in racquet sports, other strenuous sports, cycling, stair climbing, cross-country skiing, aerobic dancing or swimming; WJR= participating in a WJR-program in the last three months.	Men in WJR group had 13% lower [RR=0.87 (0.79–0.95)] and men in the sport category had 24% lower [(RR=0.76: 0.66–0.86)] HTN risk than sedentary men.

Values are multivariate adjusted risk unless otherwise stated.

CPA – commuting physical activity; EE – energy expenditure; HR – hazard ratio; RR – relative risk; LTPA – leisure time physical activity; OPA – occupational physical activity; PA – physical activity; HTN – hypertension; WJR – walking, jogging, running.

TABLE 3.3 Prospective cohort studies of physical fitness and risk for developing hypertension

Author (country)	Participants	Follow-up	Physical fitness assessment	Main findings
Blair et al. (1984) (USA)	4,820 men, 1,219 women, aged 20–65 yrs	1–12 yrs	Maximal treadmill test. High PF = subjects with excellent or superior fitness versus comparison group	Persons with low levels of PF had a RR of 1.52 for the development of HTN
Sawada et al. (1993) (Japan)	3,305 men, aged <50 yrs	5 yrs	Quintiles of estimated $\dot{V}O_{2max}$	Individuals in the least fit group had a 1.9 higher RR compared with the most fit group
Carnethon et al. (2003) (USA)	4,392 white and black men and women, aged 18–30 yrs	15 yrs	Duration of maximal treadmill test using Balke protocol. Low fitness= lowest quintile of sex specific duration; moderately fit = participants in the 20th to 60th percentile ; highly fit = participants above the 60th percentile of test	Individuals in the low fitness and moderate fitness category had a RR of 2.17 and 1.34 for the development of HTN compared to high fitness category. Further, each 1-min decrease in test duration was associated with a 19% higher 15-year risk of HTN
Barlow et al. (2005) (USA)	4,884 women, aged 20–79 yrs	Mean: 5 yrs	Duration of a maximal treadmill test using modified Balke protocol. Individuals were categorized into age-specific fitness categories: low fit = least-fit 20%, moderate fitness = next 40% and then high fitness	The odds ratios for HTN were 1, 0.61 and 0.35 in low, moderately and highly fit women. Each 1-MET increment in maximal exercise performance was associated with a 19% lower odds of incident hypertension. The inverse gradient of hypertension was seen across levels of fitness in women aged less than 55 years and those aged > 55 yrs
Mikkelsson et al. (2005) (Finland)	29 men and women, adolescents	25 yrs	Very slow versus very fast runner	Slow runners had a higher multivariate adjust risk of HTN (2.9; 1–8.3) compared to fast runners

Author (country)	Participants	Follow-up	Physical fitness Assessment	Main findings
Williams (2008) (USA)	29,139 men and 11,985 women	7.7 and 7.4 yrs	10 km performance	Compared to the least fit men, the fittest men had 62% lower risk for developing HTN
Chase et al. (2009) (USA)	16,601 men, aged 20–82 yrs	Mean 18.1yrs	Maximal treadmill test using modified Balke protocol. Individuals were categorized into thirds depending on age-specific distributions of treadmill time	An inverse gradient of incident hypertension event rates was observed across incremental thirds of PF. Men with middle and high PF had an 11% and 29% lower HTN risk than men with low PF

Values are multivariate adjusted risk unless otherwise stated.

Abbreviations: PF – physical fitness; RR – relative risk; HTN – hypertension.

Physical activity was assessed by questionnaires or sometimes an interview using a range of methodologies over time frames varying from one day to one year. The majority of authors assessed leisure-time physical activity and some also reported results for occupational physical activity and/or commuting physical activity. The most common physical activity variables measured were frequency, duration and estimated energy expenditure, and the dimensions of physical activity reported included light or low, moderate and vigorous or high, as well as physical activity accumulated in walking, jogging, running, cycling, stair climbing and a range of different sports.

In men, age-adjusted analysis showed that leisure time physical activity was, in general, inversely associated with hypertension risk, with participants recording the highest levels of physical activity having the lowest risk of hypertension compared with the least physically active. By contrast, none of the studies in women, except two (Hu *et al.* 2004; Kim *et al.* 2006), observed significant and independent relationships between the levels of leisure time physical activity and incident hypertension (Paffenbarger *et al.* 1991; Pereira *et al.* 1999; Haapanen *et al.* 1997; Barengo *et al.* 2005). If physical activity level was categorized, most studies reported a dose-response relation between the amount of physical activity and reduction in hypertension risk. With regard to the mode of exercise, Hernelathi *et al.* (2002) reported that the cumulative 10-year risk for developing hypertension was significantly lower in former athletes of endurance and mixed sports whereas a history of being a power athlete conferred no benefit.

Fewer studies have investigated the effect of commuting physical activity and physical activity at work on the risk of hypertension. Hayashi *et al.* (1999) found that multivariable adjusted risk for hypertension was significantly reduced by 12 per cent when the duration of the walk to work was increased by 10 minutes. By contrast, commuting physical activity was not associated with the risk of hypertension in Finnish men and women (Hayashi *et al.* 1999). Further, whereas the work index was not independently predictive for future hypertension in either black or white men and women (Pereira *et al.* 1999), Barengo *et al.* (2005) reported significant associations between high levels of occupational physical activity and reduced risk of hypertension when men and women were combined, and low levels of work-related physical activity resulted in a 22 to 27 per cent higher risk of developing hypertension when compared with the high category in Chinese individuals (Gu *et al.* 2007).

Although estimation of physical activity by questionnaire or interview is useful, and often the best available tool, it must be acknowledged that self-reported measures of physical activity are only modestly correlated with objective measures obtained using criterium methods (Aadahl *et al.* 2007). One approach to more objectively assess recent physical activity is to measure cardiorespiratory fitness or aerobic power. As shown in Table 3.3, all studies report a dose-response relation between increasing levels of physical fitness and the risk for developing hypertension. Further, higher physical fitness reduced the odds for hypertension, independent of physical activity, and is therefore an important risk factor separate from physical activity (Williams 2008; Chase *et al.* 2009).

Overweight, obesity and weight gain have been shown to be important and independent risk factors for the development of hypertension. It has therefore been hypothesized that increasing physical activity might reduce BP through decreased body weight. Adjustment for body mass index (BMI) did result in an attenuation of the association between physical activity and hypertension risk in most cases, but in the majority of studies the association remained statistically significant. Furthermore, high levels of physical activity were associated with a lower risk of hypertension across different BMI-categories (Nakanishi *et al.* 2005; Gu *et al.* 2007). Therefore, the reduced risk of hypertension in physically active and fit individuals cannot be explained by a decrease in BMI alone.

At last, a few investigators have examined prospectively the influence of changes in physical fitness on changes in BP. Sawada and colleagues (1993) showed that subjects whose maximal oxygen uptake ($\dot{V}O_{2max}$) improved > 15 per cent over a 5-year follow-up period showed a smaller increase in systolic and diastolic BP than other groups who showed no change or a deterioration of aerobic fitness. Similarly, Sedgwick *et al.* (1993) reported that women who improved their aerobic fitness by > 5 per cent over a four-year period experienced an improvement in SBP (by 4 mmHg) in comparison to women who showed a lower fitness gain. Such an association could however not be demonstrated in men. Finally, Williams (2008) reported that reduction of vigorous physical activity over a 7.4 year period of follow-up increased the odds of developing hypertension. Moreover, it was shown that the odds of developing hypertension depended on the follow-up running distance without relation to baseline activity which implies that success in motivating the population to become more active will not yield its expected anti-hypertensive effect if the activity is not sustained.

In summary, the current evidence suggests that higher levels of physical activity, especially leisure time physical activity, are associated with a reduced incidence of hypertension, but the results are not always consistent, especially in women and African–Americans and with regard to occupational and commuting activities, for which more data are needed. Without exception, higher levels of physical fitness are inversely and in a dose-dependent manner associated with the incidence of hypertension, independent of physical activity. Finally, increasing levels of physical fitness seem to be associated with reductions in BP over time.

Exercise in the prevention, treatment and management of hypertension: data from randomised controlled trials

A difficulty in the interpretation of the epidemiological data is distinguishing cause and effect: that is to ascribe differences in BP or in the incidence of hypertension to differences in levels of physical activity or fitness because of confounding factors that cannot be accounted for. These include self-selection, interindividual differences and limitations of statistical adjustment for confounders that have or have not been taken into consideration. Furthermore, questions on the role of different characteristics of physical activity in the prevention and treatment of hypertension are difficult to answer on the basis of epidemiological data: i.e. the health effects of varying exercise intensity, duration and/or total volume remains largely unsolved (Pescatello *et al.* 2004a). Therefore, randomized controlled trials are of paramount importance, since they can evaluate the effectiveness of interventions while controlling for each of the individual confounders. However, the evidence provided by a single study is often insufficient to arrive at definite and generalizable conclusions and the findings of single studies remain often imprecise estimates of the hypothetical true effect (Fagard *et al.* 1996). This is mostly due to an insufficient number of participants, variable characteristics of participants and the way the exercise study is done. Therefore, meta-analysis is probably the best method to systematically review previous work. Meta-analyses provide more precise estimates of the effects of interventions than individual trials and make it possible to assess the generalizability of the conclusions to a more varied range of individuals or treatment protocols (Fagard *et al.* 1996).

A number of meta-analyses investigating the effect of dynamic aerobic endurance training (Kelley *et al.* 2001; Kelley and Kelley 2001; Fagard 2001; Whelton *et al.* 2002; Cornelissen and Fagard 2005a) or resistance training (Kelley 1997; Kelley and Kelley 2000; Cornelissen and Fagard 2005b) on BP have been performed over the last several decades. The current overview is based on two meta-analyses (Cornelissen and Fagard 2005a; Cornelissen and Fagard 2005b) which have been performed recently by our laboratory, but in general the results concur with previous meta-analyses. Common inclusion criteria of the two meta-analyses were 1) inclusion of a randomized non-exercise control group or phase, 2) aerobic exercise training or resistance exercise as the only intervention, 3) exercise intervention for a minimum of 4 weeks, 4) inclusion of participants who were sedentary normotensive and or hypertensive adults with no other concomitant disease, 5) published in a peer-reviewed journal up to December 2003. Weighted meta-regression analysis was applied to assess whether variations in results were related to variations in study groups or training characteristics.

Dynamic aerobic endurance training

A total of 72 randomized controlled trials met the inclusion criteria involving 105 exercise training groups and 3,936 participants. The average age of the study groups ranged from 21 to 83 years (median 47) and 57 per cent of the participants were men. The duration of exercise training ranged from 4 to 52 weeks (median 16). The frequency of exercise ranged from one to seven days per week (median 3) and exercise intensity was between 30 and 87.5 per cent of the heart rate reserve (HRR; median 65 per cent). Each exercise session lasted from 15 to 63 minutes (median 40 minutes) after exclusion of warm-up and cool-down activities and involved mainly walking, jogging, running or cycling. The overall changes of resting heart rate and $\dot{V}O_{2peak}$ averaged -4.8 beats per minute (95% CI: -5.7 to -3.9) and $+4$ ml.min^{-1}.kg^{-1} ($+3.5$ to $+4.5$) respectively, demonstrating the overall efficacy of the exercise training programmes. The average change of BP in response to aerobic endurance training, after adjustment for control observations, ranged from –20 to +9 mmHg for systolic BP and from –11 to +11.3 mmHg for diastolic BP. The overall net change of systolic BP/diastolic BP averaged –3.0 (–4.0 to –2.0) /–2.4 (–3.1 to –1.7) mmHg ($P<0.001$), that is after adjustment for control observations and after weighting for the number of exercise trained participants, which could be analyzed in each study group. BP reduction is even more important in patients with hypertension. When we analyzed the effects of exercise training according to the recent Seventh Report of the Joint National Committee on Prevention, Detection, Evaluation and Treatment of high BP classification[2] the net effect was greatest in the hypertensives compared to the normotensives (Table 3.4).

Do age, gender or ethnicity affect the BP response to aerobic endurance training? By applying univariate regression analyses, weighting for the number of subjects in each trained group, the exercise training-induced changes in systolic and diastolic BP did not seem to depend on age (Cornelissen and Fagard 2005a). Further, meta-analytic research by Kelley and collegues (Kelley *et al.* 2001) reported no significant differences between the resting exercise training-induced BP response of normotensive or hypertensive men and women. With regard to ethnicity, a meta-analysis by Whelton *et al.* (2002) reported that black participants had significantly greater reduction in systolic BP [–10.96 mmHg (–21.0 to –0.89) vs –3.44 mmHg (–5.3 to –1.6)] and Asian participants had significantly greater reduction in diastolic BP [–6.6 mmHg (–8.4 to –4.7) vs –2.6 mmHg (–3.8 to –1.4)] compared with white participants. These results were however based on four studies in blacks and six studies in Asians, so further research is needed to study how and why ethnic differences in the BP response to endurance training exist, if they exist at all.

TABLE 3.4 Baseline BP for the exercise groups and weighted net changes in response to dynamic aerobic exercise training

Variable	Sub-group	Baseline	Net Change	P-value within groups	P among groups
Systolic BP (mmHg)	Normotension	114.3	–2.4 (–4.2 to –0.6)	<0.01	
	Prehypertension	127.2	–1.7 (–3.1 to –0.29)	<0.05	<0.001
	Hypertension	145.4	–6.9 (–9.1 to –4.6)	<0.001	
Diastolic BP (mmHg)	Normotension	73	–1.6 (–2.4 to –0.74)	<0.001	
	Prehypertension	80.3	–1.7(–2.6 to –0.75)	<0.001	<0.001
	Hypertension	92.3	–4.9(–6.5 to –3.3)	<0.001	

Values are given as weighted mean (95 per cent Confidence Limits). Net mean changes were calculated as the difference between the mean changes in the training group and mean changes in the control group in case of a parallel group design, and as the differences measured at the end of the training period and at the end of the sedentary period in case of a cross-over design. Adapted from Cornelissen and Fagard (2005a).

A limitation of this meta-analysis is the small number of trials using blinded (n=10) or automated BP (ABP) measurements (n=9). ABP is less subjective to observer bias and white-coat effect than casual determinations and reflects more accurately the BP a person maintains during activities of daily living (Aihara *et al.* 1998). Reproducibility of home BP has been reported to be even better than that of ABP, since ABP may be influenced by physical and mental activity on any given day (Musso *et al.* 1997). Among randomized controlled trials, only nine trials, involving 11 study groups, performed ABP monitoring. Nine groups reported average daytime BP from early morning to late evening and two reported average 24-hour BP. Because earlier analyses found that nighttime BP is either not affected or much less influenced by exercise training (Fagard 2000), the analysis was based on daytime BP from nine studies and on 24-hour BP in the two studies that did not report day ABP (Cornelissen and Fagard 2005a). Baseline ABP averaged 134.8/85.6 mmHg and the exercise-induced weighted net reduction of –3.3/–3.5 mmHg in BP was significant, thereby adding further support to the BP-lowering effect of aerobic exercise training. Likewise, the only study that reported home BP found that aerobic exercise decreased BP by an average of 5 mmHg for systolic BP and 4 mmHg for diastolic BP (Ohkubo *et al.* 2001).

Resistance, strength, weight and isometric training

In the past, resistance exercise training was contra-indicated for individuals with hypertension as it was thought to cause a chronic elevation of resting BP by inducing vascular hypertrophy and increasing vascular resistance due to large acute increases in BP elicited by this type of exercise. Nowadays, both the American Heart Association (Williams *et al.* 2007) and the American College of Sports Medicine (Pescatello *et al.* 2004a) each support moderate intensity resistance exercise as a complement to aerobic exercise programmes in the prevention and management of hypertension. Justification for resistance exercise as an adjunct to aerobic exercise for controlling BP stems from several studies which were summarized in three meta-analyses (Kelley 1997; Kelley and Kelley 2000; Cornelissen and Fagard 2005b).

Contrary to the large amount of evidence on the benefits of dynamic aerobic exercise training on BP, research on the effect of resistance exercise is less compelling. Only nine randomized controlled trials could be identified in our most recent meta-analysis involving 12 study groups and 341 participants (Cornelissen and Fagard 2005b). The average age of the study groups ranged from 20 to 72 years (median 69 years) and 61 per cent of the participants were men. Study durations varied from 6 to 26 weeks (median 14 weeks). The frequency of exercise training was two or three weekly sessions in two and ten study groups, respectively, and intensity ranged from 30 to 90 per cent of the one repetition maximum (1RM) strength for each exercise (mean 61 per cent). The duration of each session is difficult to assess from the reported data. The number of different exercises performed ranged from 1 to 14 (mean 10) and involved the use of arms, trunk and legs in the majority of them. The number of sets for each type of exercise ranged from 1 to 4 (mean 2) and the number of repetitions per set ranged from 1 to 25. Three trials reported using a circuit training protocol and one trial involved only static hand-grip exercises. At baseline, BP averaged 131 (123 to 138.8) / 81.1 (74.5 to 87.7) mmHg. In agreement with previous narrative reviews (Hurley and Roth 2000; Schwartz and Hirth 1995) and two older meta-analysis (Kelley 1997; Kelley and Kelley 2000) we reported that the resistance training programmes resulted in an overall weighted net change in resting systolic BP of –3.2 (–7.1 to +0.7) mmHg (P=0.10) and in diastolic BP of –3.5 (–6.1 to –0.9) mmHg (P<0.01), which was approximately of the same magnitude as seen after aerobic endurance training. The lack of data on the effects of resistance training on ABP warrants further investigation because this may be more indicative of future CVD morbidity and mortality (Fagard et al. 2005a). Furthermore, in contrast to aerobic exercise training, a non-significant trend of smaller reductions in BP in the hypertensive as compared to the normotensive groups was observed after resistance training (Cornelissen and Fagard 2005b). However, caution is warranted when interpreting these results as only 3 of the 12 study groups involved hypertensive subjects. Therefore, more trials are needed in hypertensive participants.

Additional benefits of exercise training for the (pre)-hypertensive patient

Nowadays, guidelines emphasize that BP control and the diagnosis of hypertension should be related to quantification of total cardiovascular risk (Chobanian et al. 2003; Mancia et al. 2007). This is based on the fact that only a small fraction of the hypertensive population has an elevation of BP alone, with the great majority exhibiting additional cardiovascular risk factors and there is a relationship between the severity of the BP elevation and that of alterations in glucose and lipid metabolism (Meigs et al. 1997; Stamler et al. 1986). Therefore, it is important to know to what extent one particular BP lowering tool, such as physical activity, also concomitantly influences other important cardiovascular risk factors and improves long-term prognosis.

Whereas BP increases with increasing age, aerobic power and muscle mass are significantly reduced by normal ageing. Independently of BP status, a significant enhancement of VO_{2max} was reported after aerobic exercise training (Cornelissen and Fagard 2005a) and, to a lesser extent, also after dynamic resistance training (Cornelissen and Fagard 2005b). On top of this, dynamic resistance training increased muscular strength in the studies included in the meta-analysis (Cornelissen and Fagard 2005b). These improvements are important since aerobic power is a strong and independent predictor of cardiovascular mortality and morbidity in normotensive and hypertensive individuals (Kokkinos et al. 2009a; Kokkinos et al. 2009b); and muscular strength has been shown to be inversely associated with all-cause mortality independent of aerobic power (FitzGerald et al. 2004).

In addition, aerobic exercise training resulted in various other cardioprotective benefits: i.e. improved body composition with significant reductions of body weight (–1.2 kg), waist circumference (–2.8 cm) and percentage body fat (–1.4 per cent), as well as favourable effects on lipid profile (HDL +0.032 mmol/l, triglycerides –0.11 mmol/l) and insulin resistance (HOMA –0.31) (Cornelissen and Fagard 2005a). More recent studies have also reported positive effects on non-traditional risk factors associated with hypertension, such as diminished amounts of circulating clotting and inflammatory factors (Edwards *et al.* 2007). Furthermore, skeletal muscle is the primary metabolic site for glucose and triglyceride disposal and is an important determinant of resting metabolic rate (Braith and Stewart 2006). As a consequence, resistance exercise and subsequent increases in skeletal muscle mass have been shown to increase basal metabolism, reduce total body fat mass and visceral adipose tissue (Hurley and Roth 2000; Braith and Stewart 2006; Haskell *et al.* 2007). Resistance exercise may also effectively modify cardiovascular risk factors such as lipoprotein lipid profiles and glucose metabolism, though to a lesser extent than aerobic exercise training (Braith and Stewart 2006). However, by preventing the decline in muscle mass and function, resistance training more importantly contributes to the maintenance of functional abilities and prevents osteoporosis, sarcopenia and accompanying falls, fractures and disabilities which increase with increasing age and are common in elderly hypertensive patients (Ohkubo *et al.* 2001; Braith and Stewart 2006; Haskell *et al.* 2007).

Finally, cross-sectional studies demonstrate positive associations between physical activity (Fossum *et al.* 2007) or physical fitness (Bize *et al.* 2007) and health-related quality of life. It is generally accepted that in people who have a level of fitness that compromises their daily physical functioning, both aerobic and resistance training may contribute to an improved health-related quality of life (Izawa *et al.* 2004). Recently a positive dose-response relationship between the amount of exercise performed and improvements in physical and mental quality of life measures was also observed in healthy sedentary postmenopausal women with elevated systolic BP (Martin *et al.* 2009) For a more comprehensive overview of the acute and chronic effects of aerobic and resistance exercise in multiple organ systems the reader is referred to expanded resources (Williams *et al.* 2007; Haskell *et al.* 2007; Thompson *et al.* 2001; Thompson *et al.* 2003).

In summary, on a population average, the reduction in systolic and diastolic BP for those who undertake regular aerobic or resistance exercise is approximately 3 to 4 mmHg. These reductions are of major clinical significance because it has been estimated that a 2 mmHg reduction of SBP results in a 6 per cent reduction in stroke mortality and a 4 per cent reduction in mortality attributable to coronary heart disease; the percentage reductions amount to 14 per cent and 9 per cent, respectively, for a 5 mmHg decrease in BP (Chobanian *et al.* 2003). Furthermore, both dynamic aerobic exercise training and dynamic resistance training have additional benefits for cardiovascular risk factors and other health-related parameters on top of BP reductions. These findings are compatible with the evidence from epidemiological prospective follow-up studies that physical activity and fitness are inversely related to the incidence of cardiovascular and all-cause disease and mortality (Thompson *et al.* 2003).

Exercise characteristics and the blood pressure response

To effectively prescribe exercise for hypertension management, the optimal exercise dose or frequency, intensity, time and type of exercise (FITT) for evoking anti-hypertensive effects needs to be quantified. We will discuss each of these individual components in relation to its current known effect on BP.

Frequency

In univariate weighted regression analysis, weekly training frequency did not contribute significantly to explain the inter-study variance of the BP response to aerobic exercise training, i.e. training frequencies between 3 and 7 days per week lowered BP in our meta-analysis (Cornelissen *et al.* 2005a). However, Tully *et al.* (2007) observed a slightly larger, although not significant, BP reduction in participants randomised to the 5-day walking group compared to those randomized to the 3-day walking group. Similarly, Jennings *et al.* (1986) in normotensives and Nelson *et al.* (1986) in hypertensives found that the fall in BP was significantly greater on a seven-times-per-week schedule than when the participants exercised thrice weekly. In all resistance training studies, except two, participants were exercising thrice weekly, which makes it difficult to investigate the effect of training frequency and, therefore, more studies are warranted (Cornelissen and Fagard 2005b).

Importantly, during the last two decades, several investigators have shown that a single bout of exercise may result in immediate BP reductions that persist for a major portion of the day (Pescatello and Kulikowich 2001; MacDonald 2002). This acute affect, which has been shown after both acute aerobic and acute resistance exercise training, may add significant benefits for patients with hypertension by lowering their BP into normotensive ranges for certain periods of the day. Furthermore, it might contribute to the BP reductions resulting from exercise training (Pescatello and Kulikowich 2001). This underlines the importance of recommending daily aerobic exercise, especially in the hypertensives. With regard to resistance exercise, it has been shown that 75 per cent of the musculoskeletal improvement that occurs with a three-days-per-week resistance programme can also be attained with a two-days-per-week regimen, but more research is warranted regarding changes in BP (Williams *et al.* 2007; Braith and Stewart 2006).

Intensity

Current guidelines recommend aerobic exercise training at moderate intensity (Chobanian *et al.* 2003; Mancia *et al.* 2007; Pescatello *et al.* 2004a;

Haskell *et al.* 2007). However, the majority of patients with hypertension are older, sedentary and often overweight individuals who are limited in the level of physical activity that they can undertake. Our meta-analysis revealed no significant relation between exercise intensity and BP decrease (Cornelissen and Fagard 2005a) but this should be confirmed by randomized controlled trials. For that reason, we recently performed a study to investigate whether exercising at lower intensity (33 per cent of HRR) has an effect on BP and whether the effect is comparable to an identical exercise training programme at higher intensity (66 per cent of HRR) in older sedentary subjects (Cornelissen *et al.* 2009). The rationale was that if effective, physical activity might be more easily recommended and implemented in daily life. Both exercise programmes equally reduced systolic BP at rest, during submaximal exercise and during recovery following exercise by an average of 4.5–6 mmHg; whereas diastolic BP was significantly reduced after exercise training at higher intensity only. In addition, Pescatello *et al.* (2004b) showed similar results after acute bouts of aerobic exercise, i.e. low intensity (40 per cent $\dot{V}O_{2max}$) was as effective as moderate intensity (60 per cent $\dot{V}O_{2max}$) in eliciting post-exercise hypotension. Therefore, BP lowering seems to occur at a low-intensity threshold. A meta-analysis examining the effect of walking intervention programmes on BP confirmed that low-intensity exercises such as walking can effectively lower both systolic and diastole BP (Murphy *et al.* 2007). Therefore, recommendations to increase the amount of walking that people undertake in their daily routines could be an easy way to promote physical activity and contribute to the prevention and control of high BP in the general population. In this regard, unsupervised home-based/community low intensity programmes (Kolbe-Alexander *et al.* 2006) and worksite-based walking programmes (Murphy *et al.* 2006) have shown to effectively lower BP by –4 to –9 mmHg in middle-aged to older Caucasian and African American individuals with mild to moderate hypertension (Staffileno *et al.* 2007; Sohn *et al.* 2007).

BP reductions did not differ significantly with intensity (> 55 per cent of 1RM or > 55 per cent of 1RM) in dynamic resistance exercise studies (Cornelissen and Fagard 2005b). Also no significant difference could be observed after static leg exercise, thrice weekly for eight weeks at low (10 per cent of 1RM) or high (20 per cent of 1RM) intensity (Wiles *et al.* 2010). Likewise, an acute dynamic resistance exercise session at 40 per cent or 80 per cent of 1RM resulted in similar acute reductions of systolic BP (Rezk *et al.* 2006). Earlier, Simao *et al.* (2005) had suggested that intensity has no effect on the magnitude of the hypotensive response after resistance exercise. However, high intensity isometric exercise such as heavy weightlifting should be avoided (Pescatello *et al.* 2004a; Mancia *et al.* 2007).

Time of session

The magnitude of reduction in BP after aerobic exercise training did not appear to be correlated with the duration of exercise sessions, which ranged from 15 and 63 minutes per session (Cornelissen and Fagard 2005b). Dalleck and colleagues

(2009) reported similar BP reductions in postmenopausal women randomized to either 30 or 45 minutes of moderate exercise (five days a week for 12 weeks), adding further support to the current recommendations of '30 minutes' of exercise on most days of the week. Given that a lack of time is a frequently cited barrier to physical activity, a recommendation that allows individuals to perform short bouts of activity throughout the day rather than having to put aside a continuous time slot seems attractive. Chronic intervention studies comparing continuous (e.g. 40 minutes) versus intermittent exercise (e.g. 4×10 minutes) found similar decreases in BP, with no differences between the two patterns of exercise (Murphy et al. 2009). Furthermore, roughly similar BP reductions were observed following an acute session of 10, 15, 30 and 45 minutes of aerobic exercise at 70 per cent of $\dot{V}O_{2peak}$ (MacDonald 2002). Therefore, a short bout of exercise that is repeated several times throughout the day could be an important non-pharmacological tool for the prevention of hypertension, but more notably a vital component in the daily control of BP in the hypertensive patient.

Type of exercise

Most of the previous aerobic exercise training studies used walking, jogging, cycling or a combination of these, and no difference in BP reduction has been observed between these different modalities (Cornelissen and Fagard 2005a). Therefore, any activity that uses large muscle groups, can be maintained continuously, and is rhythmical and aerobic in nature is recommended as the primary modality for those with hypertension (Pescatello et al. 2004a). Although swimming is also frequently recommended as a form of exercise to improve health, little data are available on its BP lowering effects. When comparing the effect of walking and swimming training on resting BP in older normotensive and pre-hypertensive individuals, a significant main effect of swimming compared with walking was observed, i.e. increasing systolic BP by 4.4 mmHg more than walking after six months and a trend to increased diastolic BP, which was maintained at 12 months (Cox et al. 2006). Therefore, it was suggested that any recommendation for older sedentary novice swimmers to take up swimming should be made with caution and that they should have regular BP monitoring (Cox et al. 2006). Nevertheless, the clinical significance of these findings needs to be evaluated further, especially in other populations, such as those diagnosed with hypertension.

With regard to resistance exercise, all but one study used dynamic exercises and therefore involving movements of the arms, legs and/or trunk (Cornelissen and Fagard 2005b). This is likely to introduce an aerobic component to the work-out as suggested by the significant increase in $\dot{V}O_{2max}$ (Cornelissen and Fagard 2005b). Furthermore, there were no differences in the BP reduction between conventional resistance training programmes or circuit protocols (Cornelissen and Fagard 2005b). Recently, the effect of pure static training has also been addressed in an additional small number of randomized controlled trials (McGowan et al. 2007; Wiles et al. 2010). These studies, using almost invariably a training intensity of 30 per cent of the maximal voluntary contraction force and involving only hand-grip exercises, reported statistically significant reductions in resting BP for both normotensive individuals and older hypertensives (McGowan *et al.* 2007). Finally, promising results in terms of BP reductions where shown following alternative disciplines such as tai chi (Yeh *et al.* 2008) or Qigong (Rogers *et al.* 2009).

Exercise recommendations

The exact frequency, intensity, time and type of exercise required to optimally lower BP remains to be elucidated. However, the recommendations in Table 3.5 are predicted to result in a control and/or lowering of BP for both the prevention and management of hypertension (Pescatello *et al.* 2004a). Ideally, exercise prescription aimed at prevention or management of hypertension requires aerobic exercise, supplemented by resistance exercise on most, or preferably all, days of the week. Exercise should be performed at moderate intensity for a minimum of 30 minutes of continuous or accumulated physical activity per day. Given that a single bout of low-intensity exercise can cause acute reductions in BP that last many hours, augmenting or contributing to the reductions in BP resulting from chronic exercise training, daily exercise should be emphasized in the hypertensive patient. Furthermore, just as one BP drug and one dose are not suitable for all patients, one exercise prescription is unlikely to fit all individuals. Therefore, the above described prescription requires individualization, especially in terms of intensity and duration.

TABLE 3.5 Minimum exercise prescription recommendations in the prevention and management of hypertension

Mode	Intensity	Duration	Frequecy
Aerobic (endurance) Walking Cycling Jogging Running	Moderate: 40–60% of HRR or 12–13 RPE or	30 min	5 days/week
	Vigorous: 60–84% of HRR or 14–16 RPE AND	20 min	3 days/week
Resistance (strength) Progressive weight training using major muscles Body weight exercise Theraband exercise	8–12 repetitions resulting in substantial fatigue	One set of 8–10 exercise (multiple sets if time allows)	2 or more non-consecutive days/ week

HRR = heart rate reserve; RPE = Borg rating of perceived exertion (6–20 point scale). Combinations of moderate and vigorous intensity aerobic activity can be performed to meet the weekly recommendations (e.g. 2 × 30 min moderate sessions and 2×20 min vigorous sessions). Adapted from Sharman and Stowasser (2009).

Since the largest public health benefits appear to result from going from no exercise to some exercise, and given that BP reductions occur at a low intensity threshold, sedentary people should be encouraged to build up gradually from a low intensity to the recommended dose of physical activity. Having achieved at least 30 minutes on most and preferably all days of the week, progression to moderate intensity should be considered if possible. That is, due to the dose-response relationship between physical activity and cardiovascular health in general, levels of exercise performed beyond the minimum recommendations are expected to provide greater health benefits (Haskell *et al.* 2007). Finally, since after the cessation of chronic exercise training, BP values rapidly return to pre-exercise training levels (Manfredini *et al.* 2009), individuals should continuously seek, with help from their clinicians and health care providers, enjoyable exercise programmes that will encourage lifelong habitual physical activity.

Safety considerations

Evaluation

Any pre-activity evaluation should involve a medical review, physical examination, assessment of cardiovascular disease risk and, in the case of hypertension, screening tests for secondary causes, target organ damage and cardiovascular disease complications according to current guidelines (Chobanian *et al.* 2003; Mancia *et al.* 2007; Pescatello *et al.* 2004a). The further extent of the pre-exercise training evaluation depends on the intensity of the anticipated exercise and on the patient's symptoms, overall cardiovascular risk (Chobanian *et al.* 2003; Mancia *et al.* 2007) and presence of other comorbidities (Pescatello *et al.* 2004a; Fagard *et al.* 2005b; Fagard and Cornelissen 2007). In patients with hypertension about to engage in hard or very hard exercise (intensity ≥ 60 per cent of $\dot{V}O_{2max}$), a medically supervised peak or symptom limited exercise test with electrocardiography (ECG) and BP monitoring is warranted. In men or women with low or moderate added risk, but without any overt signs and symptoms of CV disease, who engage in light-to-moderate dynamic physical activity, there is generally no need for further testing beyond the routine evaluation. Asymptomatic individuals with high or very high added risk may benefit from exercise testing before engaging in moderate intensity (40–60 per cent of maximum) exercise but not for light or very light activity (< 40 per cent of maximum) (Fagard *et al.* 2005b; Fagard and Cornelissen 2007). Patients with exertional dyspnoea, chest discomfort or palpitations need further examination, which includes exercise testing, echocardiography, Holter monitoring, or combinations thereof (Fagard *et al.* 2005b). In case of a comorbid clinical condition, the recommendations for the specific condition should be observed (Peliccia *et al.* 2005). Finally, systematic follow-up should be provided and all exercising patients should be advised on exercise-related warning signs and symptoms, such as chest pain or discomfort, abnormal dyspnoea, dizziness, or malaise, which would necessitate consulting a qualified physician (Pescatello *et al.* 2004a; Fagard *et al.* 2005b; Fagard and Cornelissen 2007).

Exercise and anti-hypertensive medication

Exercising hypertensive patients should be treated according to current guidelines (Chobanian *et al.* 2003; Mancia *et al.* 2007). In general BP lowering medications do not preclude participation in exercise programmes. However, beta blockers reduce $\dot{V}O_{2max}$ and exercise heart rate (Pescatello *et al.* 2004a). It may therefore, be more appropriate to use ratings of perceived exertion rather than target heart rates to gauge the intensity of prescribed exercise. Furthermore, beta blockers and diuretics may impair thermoregulation during exercise in hot and/or humid environments. As a precaution, people taking these agents should be advised to limit the amount and intensity of exercise in hot weather as well as to ensure appropriate hydration and clothing (Pescatello *et al.* 2004a).

Future research opportunities

Although there is sufficient evidence that both dynamic aerobic exercise training and, to some extent, resistance exercise are beneficial in the prevention and management of hypertension, additional investigations are warranted, regarding the unanswered questions identified in this chapter. Furthermore, despite the well-known health benefits of exercise, there remains a broad range of evidence to underscore concerns that the majority of adults in Western societies are still not active enough, and that long-term compliance to physical activity is poor (Haskell *et al.* 2007). Large gaps in knowledge exist on the most effective means to promote a physically active lifestyle. Similarly, further knowledge on factors influencing the maintenance of a physically active lifestyle is required. Additional physiological and basic research is necessary to provide a scientific rationale to underpin the importance of physical activity in hypertension management (Pescatello *et al.* 2004a). Such research should focus on the mechanisms by which different exercise programmes reduce BP and how this interacts with other traditional and non-traditional risk factors as well as how genetic polymorphism may influence the BP response to exercise training.

The optimal and minimal amounts of exercise needed to obtain BP reductions still need to be clarified (Pescatello *et al.* 2004a). Trials aimed at addressing these questions should take into account the interaction with ethnicity, age, gender, various medical conditions and other important cardiovascular risk factors as well as genetic variation between participants. More research is needed to determine if even shorter bouts of low or high intensity accumulated exercise throughout the day confer a health benefit, and whether an accumulated approach to physical activity can increase adherence among sedentary hypertensive elderly populations and those at increased risk of developing hypertension. Regarding the type of exercise, there is very limited data on optimal dose of dynamic (aerobic or resistance) exercise or isometric resistance exercise for hypertension management and more research is clearly warranted.

Finally, since home and ABP monitoring are more predictive than 'snap-shot' BP monitoring by healthcare professionals for predicting morbidity and mortality (Fagard *et al.* 2005a), future exercise trials should incorporate these measurement procedures, particularly in resistance training studies where it has not, to our knowledge, previously been investigated.

Summary and conclusions

In this chapter we have shown that there is clear evidence from prospective cohort studies and randomized controlled intervention trials that physical activity plays an important role in the prevention, treatment and management of hypertension. Both dynamic aerobic exercise training and to some extent resistance exercise are effective non-pharmacological interventions that provide multiple additional benefits beyond BP reduction. Although additional and larger randomized controlled trials are needed to allow a more precise definition of the optimal exercise training characteristics for lowering BP in different populations, based on the current evidence, the following exercise prescription is recommended for the general population (Pescatello *et al.* 2004a):

- frequency: most, preferably all days of the week
- intensity: moderate intensity
- time: at least 30 minutes of continuous or accumulated physical activity per day
- type: primarily exercise exercise supplemented by resistance exercise.

Furthermore, individuals who wish to further improve their personal fitness, reduce their risk of chronic diseases and disabilities and/or prevent unhealthy weight gain might benefit from exceeding the minimum recommended amounts of physical activity (Haskell *et al.* 2007).

References

Aadahl, M., Kjaer, M., Kristensen, J.H., Mollerup, B. and Jorgensen, T. (2007). Self-reported physical activity compared with maximal oxygen uptake in adults. *Eur J Cardiovasc Prev Rehabil*, 14: 422–428.

Aihara, A., Imai, Y., Sekino, M., Kato, J., Ito, S., Ohkubo, T., Tsuji, I., Satoh, H., Hisamichi, S. and Nagai, K. (1998). Discrepancy between screening blood pressure and ambulatory blood pressure: a community-based study in Ohasama. *Hypertens Res*, 21: 127–136.

Barengo, N.C., Hu, G., Kastarinen, M., Lakka, T.A., Pekkarinen, H., Nissinen, A. and Tuomilehto, J. (2005) Low physical activity as a predictor for antihypertensive drug treatment in 25–64 year old populations in eastern and south western Finland. *J Hypertens*, 23: 293–299.

Barlow, C.E., LaMonte, M.J., Fitzgerald, S.J., Kampert, J.B., Perrin, J.L. and Blair, S.N. (2005). Cardiorespiratory fitness is an independent predictor of hypertension incidence among initially normotensive healthy women. *Am J Epidemiol*, 163: 142–150.

Bize, R., Johnson, J.A. and Plotnikoff, R.C. (2007). Physical activity level and health-related quality of life in the general adult population: a systematic review. *Prev Med*, 45: 401–15.

Blair, S.N., Goodyear, N.N., Gibbons, L.W. and Cooper, K.H. (1984). Physical fitness and incidence of hypertension in healthy normotensive men and women. *JAMA*, 252: 487–490.

Braith, R.W. and Stewart, K.J. (2006) Resistance exercise training: its role in the prevention of cardiovascular disease. *Circulation*, 113: 2642–2650.

Carnethon, M.R., Gidding, S.S., Nehgme, R., Sidney, S., Jacobs, D.R. and Liu, K. (2003). Cardiorespiratory fitness in young adulthood and the development of cardiovascular disease risk factors. *JAMA*, 290: 3092–3100.

Chase, N.L., Lee, D.C. and Blair, S.N. (2009). The association of cardiorespiratory fitness and physical activity with incidence of hypertension in men. *Am J Hypertens*, 22: 417–424.

Chobanian, A.V., Bakris, G.L., Black, H.R., Cushman, W.C., Green, L.A., Izzo, J.L., Jones, D.W., Materson, B.J., Oparil, S., Wright, J.T. and Roccella, E.J., National High Blood Pressure Education Program Coordination Committee. (2003) Seventh report of the Joint National Committee on Prevention, Detection, Evaluation and Treatment of High Blood Pressure. *Hypertension*, 42: 1206–1252.

Cornelissen, V.A. and Fagard, R.H. (2005a). Effects of dynamic aerobic endurance training on blood pressure, blood pressure-regulating mechanisms and cardiovascular risk factors. *Hypertension*, 46: 667–675.

Cornelissen, V.A. and Fagard, R.H. (2005b). Effect of resistance training on resting blood pressure: a meta-analysis of randomized controlled trials. *J Hypertens*, 23: 251–259.

Cornelissen, V.A., Arnout, J., Holvoet, P. and Fagard, R.H. (2009). Influence of exercise at lower and higher intensity on blood pressure and cardiovascular risk factors at older age. *J Hypertens*, 27: 753–62.

Cox, K.L., Burke, V., Beilin, L.J., Grove, J.R., Blanksby, B.A. and Puddey, I.B. (2006). Blood pressure rise with swimming versus walking in older women: the sedentary women exercise adherence trial 2 (SWEAT 2). *J Hypertens*, 24: 307–314.

Dalleck, L.C., Allen, B.A., Hanson, B.A., Borresen, E.C., Erickson, B.S. and De Lap, S.L. (2009). Dose-response relationship between moderate intensity exercise duration and coronary heart disease risk factors in postmenopausal women. *J Womens Health*, 18: 105–113.

Edwards, K.M., Ziegler, M.G. and Mills, P.J. (2007). The potential anti-inflammatory benefits of improving physical fitness in hypertension. *J Hypertens*, 25: 1533–1542.

Fagard, R.H., Staessen, J.A. and Thijs, L. (1996). Advantages and disadvantages of the meta-analysis approach. *J Hypertens*, 14: S9-S13.

Fagard, R.H. (2000) Physical activity, fitness and blood pressure. In Birkenhäger WH, Reid JL, Bulpitt CJ, (eds) *Handbook of Hypertension* vol. 20. Epidemiology of hypertension. Amsterdam; Elsevier: pp.191–211.

Fagard, R.H. (2001). Exercise characteristics and the blood pressure response to dynamic physical training', *Med Sci Sports Exerc*, 33:S484–492.

Fagard, R.H., Van Den Broeke, C. and De Cort, P. (2005a). Prognostic significance of blood pressure measured in the office, at home and during ambulatory monitoring in older patients in general practice. *J Hum Hypertens*, 19: 801–7.

Fagard, R.H., Björnstad, H.H., Borjesson, M., Carré, F., Deligiannis, A. and Vanhees, L. (2005b). ESC study group of sports cardiology recommendations for participation in leisure-time physical activity and competitive sports for patients with hypertension. *Eur J Cardiovasc Prev Rehabil*, 12: 326–331.

Fagard, R.H. and Cornelissen, V.A. (2007). Effect of exercise on blood pressure control in hypertensive patients. *Eur J Cardiovasc Prev Rehabil*, 14: 12–7.

FitzGerald, S.J., Barlow, C.E., Kampert, J.B., Morrow,J.R., Jackson, A.W. and Blair, S.N. (2004). Muscular fitness and all-cause mortality: prospective observations. *J Phys Act Health*, 1:7–18.

Folsom, A.R., Caspersen, C.J., Taylor, H.L., Jacobs, D.R., Luepker, R.V., Gomez-Marin, O., Gillum, R.F. and Blackburn, H. (1985). Leisure time physical activity and its relationship to coronary risk factors in a population based sample. The Minnesota Heart Survey. *Am J Epidemiol*, 121:570–579.

Fossum, E., Gleim, G.W., Kjeldsen, S.E., Kizer, J.R., Julius, S., Devereux, R.B., Brady, W.E., Hille, D.A., Lyle, P.A. and Dahlof, B. (2007). The effect of baseline physical activity on cardiovascular outcomes and new-onset diabetes in patients treated for hypertension and left ventricular hypertrophy: the LIFE study. *J Intern Med*, 262: 439–448.

Gu, D., Wildman, R.P., Wu, X., Reynolds, K., Huang, J., Chen, C.S. and He, J. (2007). Incidence and predictors of hypertension over 8 years among chinese men and women. *J Hypertens*, 25: 517–523.

Haapanen, N., Miilunpàalo, S., Vuori, I., Oja, P. and Pasanen, M. (1997). Association of leisure time physical activity with the risk of coronary heart disease, hypertension and diabetes in middle-aged men and women. *Int J Epidemiol*, 26: 739–747.

Haskell, W.L., Lee, I.M., Pate, R.R., Powell, K.E., Blair, S.N., Franklin, B.A., Macera, C.A., Heath, G.W., Thompson, P.D., Bauman, A. – American College of Sports Medicine – American Heart Association. (2007). Physical activity and public health: updated recommendation for adults from the American College of Sports Medicine and the American Heart Association. *Circulation*, 116: 1081–93.

Hayashi, T., Tsumura, K., Suematso, C., Okada, K., Fujii, S. and Endo, G. (1999). Walking to work and the risk for hypertension in men: the Osaka Health Survey. *Ann Intern Med*, 13: 21–26.

Hernelathi, M., Kujala, M., Kaprio, J. and Sarna, S. (2002). Long-term vigorous training in young adulthood and later physical activity as predictors of hypertension in middle-aged and older men. *Int J Sports Med*, 23: 178–182.

Hu, G. Barengo, N.C., Tuomilehto, J., Lakka, T.A., Nissinene, A. and Jousilahti, P. (2004). Relationship of physical activity and body mass index to the risk of hypertension: a prospective study in Finland. *Hypertension*, 43: 25–30.

Hurley, B.F. and Roth, S.M. (2000). Strength training in the elderly: effects on risk factors for age-related diseases. *Sports Med* 30: 249–268.

Izawa, K.P., Yamada, S., Oka, K., Watanabe, S., Omiya, K., Iijima, S., Hirano, Y., Kobayashi, T., Kasahara, Y., Samejima, H. and Osada, N. (2004). Long-term exercise maintenance, physical activity, and health-related quality of life after cardiac rehabilitation. *Am J Phys Med Rehabil*, 83: 884–92.

Jennings, G., Nelson, L., Nestel, P., Esler, M., Korner, P., Burton, D. and Bazelmans, J. (1986). The effects of changes in physical activity on major cardiovascular risk factors, hemodynamics, sympathetic function, and glucose utilization in man: a controlled study of four levels of activity. *Circulation*, 73: 30–40.

Kannel, W.B., Vasan, R.S. and Levy, D. (2003). Is the relation of systolic blood pressure to risk of cardiovascular disease continuous and graded, or are there critical values. *Hypertension*, 42: 453–456.

Kearney, P.M., Whelton, M., Reynolds, K., Muntner, P., Whelton, P.K. and He, J. (2005). Global burden of hypertension: analysis of worldwide data. *Lancet*, 365: 217–223.

Kelley, G. (1997). Dynamic resistance exercise and resting blood pressure in adults: a meta-analysis. *J Appl Physiol*, 82: 1559–1565.

Kelley, G.A. and Kelley, K.S. (2000). Progressive resistance exercise and resting blood pressure: a meta-analysis of randomized controlled trials. *Hypertension*, 35: 838–843.

Kelley, G.A., Kelley, K.A. and Tran, Z.V. (2001) Aerobic exercise and resting blood pressure: a meta-analytic review of randomized controlled trials. *Prev Cardiol*, 4: 73–86.

Kelley, G.A. and Kelley, K.S. (2001). Aerobic exercise and resting blood pressure in older adults: a meta-analytic review of randomized controlled trials. *J Gerontol A Biol Sci Med Sci*, 56: M298-M303.

Kim, J., Kim, E., Yi, H., Joo, S., Shin, K., Kim, J., Kimm, K. and Shin, C. (2006). Short-term incidence rate of hypertension in Korea middle-aged adults. *J Hypertens,* 24: 2177–2182.

Kokkinos, P., Manolis, A., Pittaras, A., Doumas, M., Giannelou, A., Panagiotakos, D.B., Faselis, C., Narayan, P., Singh, S. and Myers, J. (2009a). Exercise capacity and mortality in hypertensive men with and without additional risk factors. *Hypertension*, 53: 494–499.

Kokkinos, P., Myers, J., Doumas, M., Faselis, C., Manolis, A., Pittaras, A., Kokkonos, J.P. and Fletcher, R.D. (2009b). Exercise capacity and all-cause mortality in prehypertensives men. *Am J Hypertens*, 22: 735–741.

Kolbe-Alexander, T.L., Lambert, E.V. and Charlton, K.E. (2006). Effectiveness of a community based low intensity exercise program for older adults. *J Nutr Health Aging*, 10: 21–29.

Lewington, S., Clarke, R., Qizilbash, N., Peto, R. and Collins, R. (2002). Age-specific relevance of usual blood pressure to vascular mortality: a meta-analysis of individual data for one million adults in 61 prospective studies, Prospective Studies Collaboration. *Lancet*, 360: 1903–1913.

MacDonald J.R. (2002). Potential causes, mechanisms, and implications of post exercise hypotension. *J Hum Hypertens*, 16: 225–36.

Mancia, G., De Backer, G., Dominiczak, A., Cifkova, R., Fagard, R., Germano, G., Grassi, G., Heagerty, A.M., Kjeldsen, S.E., Laurent, S., Narkiewicz, K., Ruilope, L., Rynkiewicz, A,. Schmieder, R.E., Boudier, H.A. and Zanchetti, A. (2007). Guidelines for the Management of Arterial Hypertension – The Task Force for the Management of Arterial Hypertension of the European Society of Hypertension (ESH) and of the European Society of Cardiology (ESC). *J Hypertens*, 25: 1105–1187.

Manfredini, F., Malagoni, A.M., Mandini, S., Boari, B., Felisatti, M., Zamboni, P., Manfredini, R. (2009).Sport therapy for hypertension: why, how and how much. *Angiology*, 60: 207–16.

Martin, C.K., Church, T.S., Thompson, A.M., Earnest, C.P. and Blair, S.N. (2009). Exercise dose and quality of life – a randomized controlled trial. *Arch Intern Med*, 169: 269–278.

McGowan, C.L., Visocchi, A., Faulkner, M., Verduyn, R., Rakobowchuk, M., Levy, A.S., McCartney, N. and MacDonald, M.J. (2007). Isometric handgrip training improves local flow-mediated dilation in medicated hypertensives. *Eur J Appl Physiol*, 99: 227–234.

Meigs, J.B., D'Agostino, R.B. Sr, Wilson, P.W., Cupples, L.A., Nathan, D.M. and Singer, D.E. (1997). Risk variable clustering in the insulin resistance syndrome -The Framingham Offspring Study. *Diabetes*, 46: 1594–1600.

Mikkelsson, L., Kaprio, J., Kautiainen, H., Nupponen, H., Tikkanen, M.J. and Kujala, U.M. (2005). Endurance running ability at adolescence as a predictor of blood pressure levels and hypertension in men: a 25-year follow-up study. *Int J Sports Med*, 26: 448–452.

Murphy, M.H., Blair, S.N. and Murtagh, E.M. (2009). Accumulated versus continuous exercise for health benefit – a review of empirical studies. *Sports Med*, 39: 29–43.

Murphy, M.H., Murtagh, E.M., Boreham, C.A., Hare, L.G. and Nevill, A.M. (2006). The effect of a worksite based walking programme on cardiovascular risk in previously sedentary civil servants. *BMC Public Health*, 22: 136.

Murphy, M.H., Nevill, A.M., Murtagh, E.M. and Holder, R.L. (2007). The effect of walking on fitness, fatness and resting blood pressure: a meta-analysis of randomized, controlled trials. *Prev Med*, 44: 377–385.

Musso, N.R., Vergassola, C., Barone, C. and Lotti, G. (1997). Ambulatory blood pressure monitoring: how reproducible is it?. *Am J Hypertens*, 10: 936–939.

Nakanishi, N. and Suzuki, K., (2005). Daily life activity and the risk of developing hypertension in middle-aged Japanese men. *Arch Intern Med*, 165: 214–220.

Nelson, L., Esler, M.D., Jennings, G.L. and Korner, P.I. (1986). Effect of changing levels of physical activity on blood pressure and haemodynamics in essential hypertension. *Lancet*, 2:473–476.

Ohkubo, T., Hozawa, A., Nagatomi, R., Fujita, K., Sauvaget, C., Watanabe, Y., Anzai, Y., Tamagawa, A., Tsuji, I., Imai, Y., Ohmori, H. and Hisamichi, S. (2001). Effect of exercise training on home blood pressure values in older adults: a randomized controlled trial. *J Hypertens*, 19: 1045–1052.

Paffenbarger, R.S. Jr, Wing, A.L., Hyde, R.T. and Jung, D.L. (1983). Physical activity and incidence of hypertension in college alumni. *Am J Epidemiol*, 117: 245–257.

Paffenbarger, R.S. Jr, Jung, D.L., Leung, R.W. and Hyde, R.T. (1991). Physical activity and hypertension: an epidemiological view. *Ann Med*, 23: 319–327.

Parker, E.D., Schmitz, K.H., Jacobs, D.R., Dengel, D.R. and Schreiner, P.J. (2007). Physical activity in young adults and incident hypertension over 15 years of follow-up: the CARDIA study. *Am J Public Health*, 97: 703–709.

Peliccia, A., Fagard, R., Bjornstad, H.H., Anastassakis, A., Arbustini, E., Assanelli, D., Biffi, A., Borjesson, M., Carrè, F., Corrado, D., Delise, P., Dorwarth, U., Hirth, A., Heidbuchel, H., Hoffmann, E., Mellwig, K.P., Panhuyzen-Goedkoop, N., Pisani, A., Solberg, E.E., van-Buuren, F. and Vanhees, L. (2005). Recommendations for competitive sports participation in athletes with cardiovascular disease – A consensus document from the Study Group of Sports Cardiology of the Working group of Cardiac Rehabilitation and exercise Physiology and the Working Group of Myocardial and Pericardial Diseases of the European Society of Cardiology. *Eur Heart J*, 26: 1422–1445.

Pereira, M.A., Folsom, A.R., Mc Govern, P.G., Carpenter, M., Arnett, D.K., Liao, D., Szklo, M. and Hutchinson, R.G. (1999). Physical activity and incident hypertension in black and white adults: the atherosclerosis risk in communities study. *Prev Med*, 28: 304–312.

Pescatello, L.S. and Kulikowich, J.M. (2001). The aftereffects of dynamic exercise on ambulatory blood pressure. *Med Sci Sports Exerc*, 33: 1855–61.

Pescatello, L.S., Franklin, B.A., Fagard, R., Farquhar, W.B., Kelley, G.A. and Ray, C.A. (2004a). Exercise and hypertension: position stand of the American College of Sports Medicine. *Med Sci Sports Exerc*, 36: 533–553.

Pescatello, L.S., Guidry, M.A., Blanchard, B.E., Kerr, A., Taylor, A.L., Johnson , A.N., Maresh, C.M., Rodriguez, N. and Thompson, P;D. (2004b). Exercise intensity alters postexercise hypotension. *J Hypertens*, 22: 1881–1888.

Rezk, C.C., Marrache, R.C., Tinucci, T., Mion, D.Jr, and Forjaz, C.L. (2006). Post-resistance exercise hypotension, hemodynamics, and heart rate variability: influence of exercise intensity. *Eur J Appl Physiol*, 98: 105–12.

Rogers, C.E., Larkey, L.K. and Keller, C. (2009). A review of clinical trials of tai chi and qigong in older adults. *West J Nurs Res*, 31: 245–279.

Sawada, S., Tanaka, H., Funakoshi, M., Shindo, M., Kono, S. and Ishiko, T. (1993). Five-year prospective study on blood pressure and maximal oxygen uptake. *Clin Exp Pharmacol Physiol*, 20:483–487.

Schwartz, R.S. and Hirth, V.A. (1995). The effects of endurance and resistance training on blood pressure. *Int J Obesity*, 19: S52–S57.

Sedgwick, A.W., Thomas, D.W. and Davies, M. (1993). Relationships between change in aerobic fitness and changes in blood pressure and plasma lipids in men and women: the 'Adelaide 1000' 4-year follow-up. *J Clin Epidemiol*, 46: 141–151.

Sharman, J.E. and Stowasser, M. (2009). Australian association for exercise and sports science position statement on exercise and hypertension. *J Sci Med Sport*, 12: 252–257.

Simao, R., Fleck, S.J., Polito, M., Monteiro, W. and Farinatti, P. (2005). Effects of resistance training intensity, volume and session format on the postexercise hypotensive response. *J Strength Cond Res*, 19: 853–858.

Sohn, A.J., Hasnain, M. and Sinacore, J.M. (2007). Impact of exercise (walking) on blood pressure levels in African American adults with newly diagnosed hypertension. *Ethn Dis*, 17: 503–507.

Staffileno, B.A., Minnick, A., Coke, L.A. and Hollenberg, S.M. (2007). Blood pressure responses to lifestyle physical activity among young, hypertension-prone African-American women. *J Cardiovasc Nurs*, 22: 107–17.

Stamler, J., Wentworth, D. and Neaton, J.D. (1986). Is relationship between serum cholesterol and risk of premature death from coronary heart disease continuous and graded? Findings in 356,222 primary screenees of the Multiple Risk Factor Intervention Trial (MRFIT). *JAMA*, 256: 256–282.

Thompson, P.D., Crouse, S.F., Goodpaster, B., Kelley, D., Moyna, N., Pescatello, L. (2001). The acute versus the chronic response to exercise. *Med Sci Sports Exerc*, 33: S438–45.

Thompson, P.D., Buchner, D., Pina, I.L., Balady, G.J., Williams, M.A., Berra, K., Blair, S.N., Costa, F., Franklin, B., Fletcher, G.F., Gordon, N.F., Pate, R.R., Rodriguez, B.L., Yancey, A.K., Wenger, N.K., American Heart Association Council on Clinical Cardiology Subcommittee on Exercise, Rehabilitation, and Prevention, American Heart Association Council on Nutrition, Physical Activity, and Metabolism Subcommittee on Physical Activity. (2003). Exercise and physical activity in the prevention and treatment of atherosclerotic cardiovascular disease: a statement from the council on clinical cardiology: subcommittee on exercise, rehabilitation and prevention and the council on nutrition, physical activity, and metabolism (subcommittee on physical activity). *Circulation*, 107: 3109–3116.

Tully, M.A., Cupples, M.E., Hart, N.D., McEneny, J., McGlade, K.J., Chan, W.S. and Young, I.S. (2007). Randomised controlled trial of home-based walking programmes at and below current recommended levels of exercise in sedentary adults. *J Epidemiol Community Health*, 61: 778–83.

Vasan, R.S., Beiser, A., Seshadri, S., Larson, M.G., Kannel, W.B., D'Agostino, R.B. and Levy, D. (2002). Residual lifetime risk for developing hypertension in middle-aged women and men: the Framingham Heart Study. *JAMA*, 287: 1003–1010.

Whelton, S.P., Chin, A., Xin, X. and He, J. (2002). Effect of aerobic exercise on blood pressure: a meta-analysis of randomized controlled trials. *Ann Intern Med*, 136: 493–503.

Wiles, J.D., Coleman, D.A. and Swaine, I.L. (2010). The effects of performing isometric training at two exercise intensities in healthy young males. *Eur J Appl Physiol*, 108: 419–28.

Williams, M.A., Haskell, W.L., Ades, P.A., Amsterdam, E.A., Bittner, V., Franklin, B.A., Gulanick, M., Laing, S.T. and Stewart, K.J., American Heart Association Council on Clinical Cardiology, American Heart Association Council on Nutrition, Physical Activity, and Metabolism. (2007). Resistance exercise in individuals with and without cardiovascular disease: 2007 update: a scientific statement from the American Heart Association Council on Clinical Cardiology and Council on Nutrition, Physical Activity, and Metabolism. *Circulation*, 116: 572–84.

Williams, P.T. (2008). A cohort study of incident hypertension in relation to changes in vigorous physical activity in men and women. *J Hypertens*, 26: 1085–1093.

World Health Organization (WHO) (2002) *World health report: Quantifying selected major risks to health – other diet-related risk factors and physical inactivity.* http://who.int/whr/2002/chapter4/en/index4.html. Accessed 1 August 2009.

Yeh, G.H., Wang, C., Wayne, P.M. and Phillips, R.S. (2008).The effect of tai chi exercise on blood pressure: a systematic review. *Prev Cardiol*, 11: 82–89.

4

STROKE

Frederick M. Ivey, Alice S. Ryan, Charlene E. Hafer-Macko and Richard F. Macko

Introduction

Stroke-related disability causes profound physiological and activity behavior changes, resulting in peak fitness levels that are approximately half those in age-matched sedentary controls (Ivey *et al.* 2005; Ivey and Macko 2009). Peak fitness levels in disabled stroke survivors indicate functional aerobic impairment (Ivey *et al.* 2005; Potempa *et al.* 1995; Chu *et al.* 2004; Rimmer *et al.* 2009) and may compromise the capacity of stroke patients to meet the elevated energy demands of hemiparetic gait (Corcoran *et al.* 1970; Fisher and Gullickson 1978; Olney *et al.* 1986). Diminished physiological fitness reserve limits basic activities-of-daily-living (ADL) capacity after stroke, contributing to activity intolerance and subjective fatigue (Michael *et al.* 2002; 2006). These changes severely impact function and cardiometabolic health in this population (Ivey *et al.* 2006a; 2009).

A variety of different exercise training modalities including treadmill walking (Macko *et al.* 2005b), cycling (Potempa *et al.* 1995), home-based (Duncan *et al.* 1998) and aquatic exercise (Chu *et al.* 2004) have been safely used to improve cardiovascular fitness after stroke. Recent studies also suggest that structured physical activity programmes, particularly those employing task-oriented exercises that simulate elements of basic mobility function, can improve walking and balance even years after stroke (Ivey *et al.* 2009; Macko *et al.* 2005a; 2005b). Locomotor-based exercise regimens have been shown to increase both fitness and improve gait patterning to reduce the energy costs of hemiparetic gait (Macko *et al.* 1997a; Macko *et al.* 2001; Ivey *et al.* 2009). Since evidence-based studies show that such physiologic and functional benefits are attainable irrespective of time elapsed since the index disabling stroke (Ivey *et al.* 2009), structured exercise constitutes a potential health strategy to improve mobility function, basic ADL capacity and cardiometabolic health over the longer-term for stroke survivors (Ivey *et al.* 2008).

Stroke often produces residual deficits in muscular strength that persistently impair function (Patten *et al.* 2004). Research is now examining the effects of strength training on important health outcomes after stroke (Patten *et al.* 2004; Pak and Patten 2008). While initially encouraging, based on the strength and function gains observed in stroke survivors (Pak and Patten 2008), more work is needed to better understand the full range of adaptations possible with this type of intervention. It is likely that skeletal muscle changes on the paretic side underlie some of the aforementioned adverse changes in fitness, function and general health (Hafer-Macko *et al.* 2008). For this reason, we devote a section of this chapter to advances in our understanding of the body composition and tissue-level abnormalities that result after stroke. There is reason to believe, extrapolating from research in non-neurological populations (McGuigan *et al.* 2001; Martel *et al.* 2005; Kryger and Andersen 2007), that strength training may potentially improve hemiparetic skeletal muscle quantity and quality for ageing individuals with chronic disability post-stroke.

A final section provides some exercise recommendations for stroke survivors based on best available evidence. Current health care recommendations endorse exercise as an adjunct to pharmacological treatment for optimal risk factor management after stroke (Gordon *et al.* 2004). While further research is needed to optimize exercise design, new evidence regarding dose-intensity and health benefits of exercise after stroke is presented. General guidelines for implementing exercise programmes after stroke should take into account the multiple facets of stroke disability. Goals should be oriented towards a multiple-physiological systems approach, intended to improve musculoskeletal fitness, sensorimotor function, and cardiovascular-metabolic health (Ivey *et al.* 2009). Further, exercise therapy interventions should be evaluated on the basis of their potential for preventing or reducing stroke-related abnormalities in body composition, skeletal muscle and bone health. There are also unique safety and feasibility issues to consider when implementing exercise programmes after stroke. Recommendations are provided for initial medical evaluation to optimize safety and address the barriers to exercise participation after stroke. Finally, we outline some new directions regarding how models of exercise for stroke survivors may evolve in the near future, and the potential effects on cognitive function, motor learning and cerebrovascular health.

Physiological impairments after stroke

Cardiopulmonary impairment after stroke

Conventional sub-acute stroke rehabilitation focuses primarily on optimizing basic ADL skills and functional independence, and preventing complications that impact upon recovery during the critical sub-acute period (USDHHS 1995). It is unlikely that the most commonly applied forms of stroke rehabilitation provide an adequate exercise stimulus to reverse the profound cardiopulmonary deconditioning associated with stroke. Cardiac monitoring during typical sub-acute stroke physical therapy in a major academic hospital in Canada revealed that an aerobic intensity of 40 per cent of the measured heart rate reserve (HRR) was reached in less than 3 minutes per session (MacKay-Lyons and Makrides 2002a). HRR is calculated with the Karvonen formula (HRR = maximum heart rate – resting heart rate; target heart rate = (HRR × training per cent) + resting heart rate). Maximum heart rate can be estimated from the formula 220 – age of the patient.

While the practice of stroke rehabilitation varies tremendously across different health care systems and countries, one large study in the United States (mid-west region) reported that only 9 ± 5 (mean $\pm$ SD) outpatient physical therapy visits are attended by the average stroke patient. Further, this study showed that therapy had usually concluded between 30 and 180 days post stroke (Duncan *et al.* 2003). This pattern exemplifies a global impression that conventional physical therapy during the sub-acute recovery phase provides an inadequate cardiopulmonary stimulus to address the level of cardiometabolic deconditioning encountered, and this probably contributes to extended disability and worsened recurrent stroke profiles.

TABLE 4.1 Peak aerobic fitness after stroke

Study	Subjects	Testing device	Mean $\dot{V}O_{2\,peak}$ (ml/kg/min)
Potempa *et al.* (1995)	42 chronic stroke, 43–72 y	Cycle ergometer	15.9
Fujitani *et al.* (1999)	2–49 months post-stroke (n=30), 53.6 y	Cycle ergometer	17.7
Rimmer *et al.* (2000)	35 chronic stroke, 53 ± 8 y	Cycle ergometer	13.3
Mackay-Lyons *et al.* (2002b)	29 sub-acute, 65 ± 14 yr	Treadmill 15% BWS	14.4
Duncan *et al.* (2003)	92 sub-acute, 69 ± 10 yr	Cycle ergometer	11.5
Kelly *et al.* (2003)	17 sub-acute, 61 ± 16 y	Semi-recumbent cycle	15.0
Chu *et al.* (2004)	12 chronic, 62 ± 9 y	Cycle ergometer	17.2
Ivey *et al.* (2005)	131 chronic, 64 ± 7 yr	Treadmill full BWS	13.6
Rimmer *et al.* (2009)	55 chronic, 60 ± 10 y	Cycle ergometer	13.0

BWS = Body Weight Support.

Studies that have measured cardiopulmonary fitness levels after stroke show a consistent and dramatic reduction in this parameter (Table 4.1). Older individuals (60–70 years) are expected to have peak oxygen levels ranging between 25 and 30 ml.kg^{-1}.min^{-1} depending on a number of factors (Bruce *et al*. 1973; ACSM 2006). Thus, the mean peak oxygen consumption level in stroke patients is roughly half that of apparently healthy age-matched individuals.

$\dot{V}O_{2peak}$ levels in this range compromise functional status as they are below the oxygen consumption requirements for some basic ADLs. The human body at rest consumes roughly 3.5 ml.kg^{-1}.min^{-1} of oxygen or 1 metabolic equivalent task (MET) (Jette *et al*. 1990). The MET calculations associated with various forms of activity (Ainsworth *et al*. 2000) reveal that light instrumental activities of daily living (IADLs) generally require approximately up to 3 METs of oxygen consumption, equating to 10.5 ml.kg^{-1}.min^{-1}, whereas more strenuous ADLs require approximately 5 METS or 17.5 ml.kg^{-1}.min^{-1}(Ainsworth *et al*. 2000). The impact of low cardiopulmonary fitness on function after stroke is best illustrated when peak fitness values are considered in the context of the range of energy expenditure necessary to perform daily activities (Figure 4.1) (Ivey *et al*. 2005). While peak values for age-matched healthy individuals far exceed the approximated ADL range, the exhaustion value falls in the middle of the zone for most stroke patients. Thus, many stroke patients must exercise to exhaustive levels to achieve the middle of the established ADL range, making mid to upper level ADLs either impossible or unsustainable.

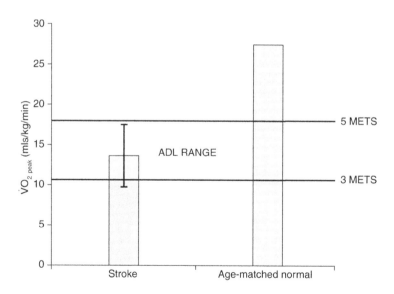

FIGURE 4.1 Peak aerobic fitness levels of chronic stroke patients (n=131) relative to the energy requirements for activities of daily living. Reproduced with permission from Topics in Stroke Rehabilitation (Ivey *et al*. 2005).

Skeletal muscle targets for exercise therapies after stroke

The underlying biological mechanisms for post-stroke deconditioning and adaptation to exercise therapy have not been systematically investigated. The disability of stroke is widely attributed to brain injury alone, and the diminished fitness attributed to reduced 'central' neural drive. However, there are a number of changes in skeletal muscle and surrounding tissues that propagate disability and contribute to low fitness levels, including skeletal muscle atrophy, muscle fiber type changes and tissue inflammation (Hafer-Macko et al. 2008). Hence, these could be primary mechanistic targets around which to focus the design of rehabilitation therapies after stroke.

Skeletal muscle atrophy

The quantity and quality of metabolically active tissue partially accounts for the amount of oxygen a person can utilize. Ryan et al. (2000) reported a strong relationship between total body muscle mass by Dual Energy X-ray Absorbtiometry (DXA) and peak $\dot{V}O_2$ after stroke. In this study, $\dot{V}O_2$ was also strongly associated with the lean muscle mass of both thighs, with lean mass predicting over 40 per cent of the variance in peak aerobic fitness (Ryan et al. 2000). These results suggest that muscle atrophy is a significant contributor to the poor physical performance in this population, regardless of the time elapsed since the disabling stroke event.

Bilateral mid-thigh computer tomography (CT) scans can be used to illustrate the severe atrophy caused by chronic hemiparesis (Figure 4.2) (Ryan et al. 2002). There is extreme gross muscular atrophy in the paretic leg mid-thigh CT scans, showing 20 per cent lower muscle area compared to the non-paretic thigh. In addition, intramuscular area fat is 25 per cent greater in the paretic thigh compared to the non-paretic thigh (Ryan et al. 2002). Elevated intramuscular fat is linked to insulin resistance and its complications (Frontera et al. 1997). These body composition abnormalities may impact upon whole body metabolic health and function.

| Paretic | Non-paretic | Paretic | Non-paretic |

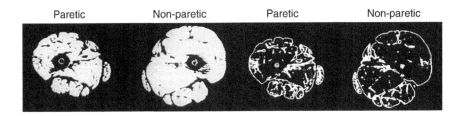

FIGURE 4.2 Bilateral CT Scan illustrating muscle atrophy (left) and elevated intramuscular area fat (right) on the paretic side. Reproduced with permission from Topics in Stroke Rehabilitation (Ivey et al. 2005).

To date, treadmill (TM) aerobic exercise models have been unsuccessful for restoring paretic limb muscle tissue in stroke survivors. For this reason, studies are now underway to assess the extent to which skeletal muscle atrophy can be modified with strength training after stroke.

Unilateral muscle fiber-type changes

Cellular changes in skeletal muscle contribute to poor fitness and worsening CVD risk after stroke. Prior studies of hemiparetic muscle reveal variable findings related to altered fiber type proportions, loss of type I muscle fibers, fiber atrophy and reduced oxidative capacity (Chokroverty *et al.* 1976; Landin *et al.* 1977; Scelsi *et al.* 1984; Frontera *et al.* 1997; Hachisuka *et al.* 1997; Jakobsson *et al.* 1991). A slow-to-fast fiber type conversion has been reported (Frontera *et al.* 1997; Landin *et al.* 1977; De Deyne *et al.* 2004). Skeletal muscles are composed of fibers that express different myosin heavy chain (MHC) isoforms. Slow (Type I) MHC isoform fibers have higher oxidative function, are more fatigue resistant and are more sensitive to insulin-mediated glucose uptake. Fast (Type II) MHC fibers are recruited for more powerful movements; they fatigue rapidly and are less sensitive to the action of insulin (Daugaard and Richter 2001). Routine ATPase staining of paretic leg muscle biopsies show elevated proportions of fast type II fibers in the paretic leg of stroke survivors (Figure 4.3) (Ivey *et al.* 2005).

Paretic   Non-paretic

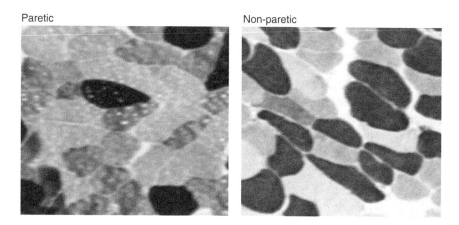

FIGURE 4.3 Fiber-type shift on paretic side. Reproduced with permission from Topics in Stroke Rehabilitation (Ivey *et al.* 2005).

Similar findings are reported in the hemiparetic upper extremity (Landin *et al.* 1977). Further, densitometric analysis of MHC gel electrophoresis shows significantly elevated proportion of fast MHC isoforms in the paretic versus non-paretic vastus lateralis muscle (DeDeyne *et al.* 2004). These findings contrast with the relatively equal proportions of slow and fast MHC fibers found in vastus lateralis of individuals without stroke (Landin *et al.* 1977). Interestingly, a shift to fast MHC composition in the paretic muscle is also seen in animals and humans after spinal cord injury (Huey *et al.* 2001). This suggests that neurological alterations may be partially responsible for the shift of muscle phenotype. A switch to fast MHC can occur with muscle unloading or disuse, suggesting that the relative inactivity after stroke could also be facilitating these changes. The shift to fast MHC after stroke contrasts to the changes seen in normal ageing, where fast MHC fibers are preferentially lost through denervation and slow MHC fiber density increases (Kandarian and Stevenson 2002). Hence, the predominance of fast MHC in the hemiparetic leg is an abnormal muscle molecular phenotype that would be expected to result in a more fatigable, insulin resistant muscle.

Inflammatory pathway activation in hemiparetic skeletal muscle

Inflammation may be central to much of the skeletal muscle and metabolic changes observed after stroke. The inflammatory molecule tumor necrosis factor-alpha (TNF-alpha) blocks insulin signaling and mediates muscle atrophy (de Alvaro *et al.* 2004; Greiwe *et al.* 2001; Hunter *et al.* 2002; Saghizadeh *et al.* 1996). Bilateral biopsies from vastus lateralis muscle of chronic stroke patients reveal a nearly threefold increased tumor necrosis factor-alpha mRNA expression in hemiparetic leg muscle, compared to age-matched non-stroke controls (Hafer-Macko *et al.* 2005). In addition, there is a significant 1.6-fold increased TNF-alpha mRNA expression in the non-paretic leg muscle of stroke patients compared to controls (Hafer-Macko *et al.* 2005), evidence of a bilateral or systemic process conferring more widespread inflammatory effects. Immunohistochemical studies further show that TNF-alpha localizes to the inter-fascicular space, as well as the muscle fascicle, suggesting that increased inflammatory cytokine production may arise from both muscle and surrounding adipocytes (Ivey *et al.* 2005).

Systemic metabolic abnormalities after stroke

Aside from the functional impact of reduced aerobic capacity and skeletal muscle function, there are also systemic metabolic abnormalities to consider. Kernan *et al.* (2003) reported a high prevalence of insulin resistance during the sub-acute stroke recovery period. Subsequent findings in chronic stroke patients reveal an extremely high prevalence of abnormal glucose metabolism (Ivey *et al.* 2006b). Specifically, out of over 200 chronically disabled stroke survivor volunteers studied, 35 per cent screened had documented diabetes by

medical history and another 45 per cent had fasting and/or post-load hyperglycemia. These findings suggest that the rate of abnormal glucose metabolism may
be as high as 80 per cent in chronic stroke patients (Ivey *et al.* 2006b). This is
clinically relevant, given that impaired and diabetic glucose tolerance prospectively predict a 2–3-fold increased risk for recurrent cerebrovascular events
(Vermeer *et al.* 2006). Other findings suggest that de-conditioned stroke survivors
suffer extraordinary high rates of other metabolic risk factors such as hyperlipidemia (Kopunek *et al.* 2007).

Impact of exercise therapy on key health outcomes

Although a comprehensive review of the stroke literature exceeds the scope of
this chapter, details related to some of the more widely cited studies are provided in the following sections. Our summary of stroke-exercise research focuses
on programmes involving the lower extremities or whole body, consistent with
the mission of improving mobility function, fitness and metabolic health, and
countering the secondary body composition abnormalities that occur as a consequence of stroke and physical inactivity. Upper extremity therapeutic research
is referenced in several other review articles (Lum *et al.* 2009; Alon *et al.* 2009;
Timmermans *et al.* 2009). Many of the exercise studies cited in this chapter include elements of aerobic exercise that incorporate larger muscle groups
to provide a cardiovascular exercise stimulus for improving metabolic health.
These exercise modalities are consistent with consensus statements for exercise recommendations in high cardiovascular disease risk populations, and are
similar to recommendations for normal, healthy individuals (ACSM 2009). We
also include recent advances in the application of resistance training to stroke
survivors, providing evidence of strength gains and paretic leg performance
capacity (Patten *et al.* 2004; Pak and Patten 2008), without deleterious increases
in spasticity (Teixeira-Salmela *et al.* 1999). Finally, reference is made to commu-
nity-feasible and home-based exercise models, which may afford opportunities
to better disseminate health and function, by promoting exercise programmes to
larger numbers of stroke survivors.

Exercise and peak aerobic capacity after stroke

Several exercise modalities have been shown to be successful for increasing
cardiovascular fitness in stroke survivors. A synthesis of these studies suggests
that approaches to exercise training necessarily vary as a function of neurological deficit severity, baseline fitness levels and the time phase of recovery after
stroke (Ivey *et al.* 2006a; 2009). Moreover, differing elements of exercise training prescriptions and their progression (e.g. aerobic intensity, training velocity,
repetition) may further determine the nature and magnitude of change in exercise-
mediated outcomes. Table 4.2 summarizes some of the more widely cited exercise
intervention studies, which have measured the impact on peak aerobic capacity.

TABLE 4.2 Exercise intervention studies and their impact on peak aerobic fitness

Study	Design/ population	Intervention	$\Delta \dot{V}O_{2peak}$
Potempa et al. (1995)	Randomized/ chronic stroke	10 weeks cycle training 3×/wk vs. passive range of motion	Treatment: +13%** Control: +1 %
Rimmer et al. (2000)	Randomized/ chronic stroke	12 weeks on a variety of aerobic (30 min.) and strength equipment (20 min.) 3×/wk vs. delayed entry controls	Treatment: +8%** Control: –10%
Macko et al. (2001)	Non-controlled/ chronic stroke	6 months treadmill exercise 3×/wk	Treatment: +10%*
Duncan et al. (2003)	Randomized/ subacute stroke	12 week in-home therapist supervised program emphasizing strength, balance, endurance (cycle) vs. usual care	Treatment: +9%** Control: +1%
Chu et al. (2004)	Randomized/ chronic stroke	8 weeks water based aerobics up to 80% HRR vs. upper extremity functional exercise	Treatment: +23%** Control: +3%
Macko et al. (2005)	Randomized/ chronic stroke	6 month progressive treadmill training 3×/wk. vs. attention controls (stretching)	Treatment: +17%** Control: +3%
Pang et al. (2005)	Randomized/ chronic stroke	Community-based UE vs. LE exercise 3×/wk 19 weeks	Treatment (LE): +11%**
Michael et al. (2009)	Non-controlled/ chronic stroke	Gymnasium-based progressive adaptive physical activity exercise class	Treatment: +15%*
Rimmer et al. (2009)	Randomized/ chronic stroke	12 weeks of moderate intensity cycle training 3×/wk	Treatment: +5.6% Control: –2.8%
Tang et al. (2009)	Controlled/ subacute stroke	Semi recumbent bicycle training + rehab – 3×/wk vs. inpatient rehabilitation only very early after stroke	Treatment: +13%* Control: +8%

**significant between groups across time. *significant within group.

LE = Lower Extremity; UE = Upper Extremity; HRR = Heart Rate Reserve.

There is limited evidence that exercise training can improve peripheral vascular function in stroke patients. Billinger et al. (2009) showed that single-leg flexion-extension exercise increases femoral artery blood flow and produces Doppler ultrasound evidence of vascular remodeling, implying that exercise training may be effective for helping to reverse the known deficits in blood flow and vasomotor reactivity (Ivey et al. 2004) that may contribute to physiological dysfunction in the hemiparetic leg (Hafer-Macko et al. 2008). Further studies are needed to determine the extent to which various types of exercise impact upon blood flow parameters and the associated mechanisms.

Peak aerobic fitness gains of as little as 1 MET (3.5 ml/kg/min) prospectively predict 17–29 per cent lower non-fatal and 28–51 per cent fatal cardiac events in men with various risk profiles (Laukanen *et al.* 2004). Hence, the importance of some observed gains after stroke cannot be overstated from the standpoint of clinical relevance. It is clear that a variety of exercise interventions can improve this important parameter after stoke and it is likely that intensity variations, which are often not systematically reported, strongly influence gains. Most recently, our group has applied a carefully controlled higher intensity treadmill stimulus to chronically disabled stroke survivors and surprisingly observed improvements in $\dot{V}O_{2peak}$ that were more than 2-fold greater than prior reports. (Ivey, Macko *et al.* unpublished data).

Cardiovascular risk factor modification after stroke

Beyond the goals of improving aerobic fitness after stroke, tertiary stroke prevention and cardiovascular disease risk factor modification should be a major objective of exercise prescription in this population (Gordon *et al.* 2004). In non-stroke populations at high risk of cardiovascular disease, exercise has been shown to improve a number of physiological factors linked to stroke and cardiac event risk, including insulin sensitivity (Holloszy 2005), hemostatic and inflammatory markers (Womack *et al.* 2003; Hjelstuen *et al.* 2006) and indices of vascular endothelial dependent vasomotor reactivity in coronary and peripheral arteries (Green *et al.* 2004). Other health benefits include improved lipid profiles (Buyukyazi 2005) and improved autonomic tone, which is linked to lower cardiac mortality (Rosenwinkel *et al.* 2001). Exercise is established as an adjunct to best medical care in the management of obesity, dyslipidemia, diabetes and hypertension, strongly supporting a role for exercise to address cardiovascular comorbidities in stroke survivors (Gordon *et al.* 2004). Recent evidence from our laboratory shows that moderate intensity treadmill exercise therapy improves the insulin (Figure 4.4) and glucose response to oral glucose load in stroke survivors (Ivey *et al.* 2007), suggesting improvements in insulin sensitivity across a 6-month intervention period. Results showed that stroke survivors with impaired glucose tolerance (IGT) and hyperinsulinemia have the most to gain metabolically from a treadmill exercise programme (Ivey *et al.* 2007).

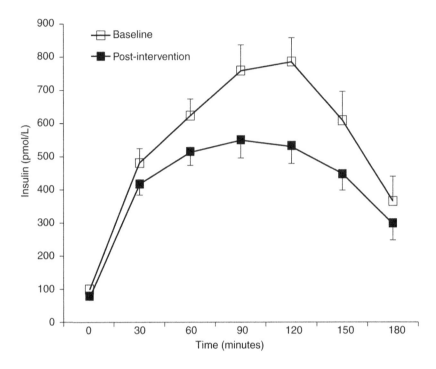

FIGURE 4.4 Change in 3-hour insulin area across 6-months of moderate intensity treadmill exercise rehabilitation. Significant changes were observed for total area as well as the 60, 90, 120 and 150 minute time-points *p<0.01. Reproduced with permission from Stroke (Ivey *et al.* 2007).

The requisite and optimal dosage of aerobic exercise training for improving cardiopulmonary fitness and cardiovascular risk profile after stroke is not fully established. A preliminary report by Rimmer *et al.* (2009) suggested that 12 weeks of moderate intensity aerobic exercise is more effective than low-intensity or conventional therapeutic exercise regimens for improving blood pressure and lowering total cholesterol in stroke patients. Further studies are needed to determine whether exercise training is effective for improving long-term cardiovascular health outcomes. It is also important to determine the threshold dose-intensity for these types of adaptations after stroke.

Functional capacity after stroke

A recent meta-analysis suggests that the overground gait training, which forms a major part of physical therapy services for stroke survivors, does not conclusively demonstrate evidence of improved gait function (States *et al.* 2009). This is significant in that approximately 75 per cent of stroke survivors are left with residual deficits that persistently impair function (Jorgensen *et al.* 1995; Paolucci *et al.* 2001). In particular, hemiparetic and other sensorimotor deficits that impair gait and balance limit basic ADL mobility function and promote a sedentary lifestyle that leads to profound physical deconditioning. Until recently, the temporal window for recovery of motor function was widely considered to be only about 3 to 6 months, with little hope for significant improvement thereafter (Jorgensen *et al.* 1995). Seminal studies in rehabilitation of the paretic upper extremity now inform us that task-repetitive training can improve arm motor function in chronic stroke, and that these gains are linked to brain plasticity (Luft *et al.* 2004). Similarly, a model has begun to emerge that motor learning associated with brain plasticity can be mediated by structured physical activity of the lower extremity (to improve mobility function) even years post-stroke (Luft *et al.* 2008; Forrester *et al.* 2008; Pattersen *et al.* 2008). These advances have prompted a paradigm shift in stroke rehabilitation. In the United States, the most recent National Institute of Health, National Institute for Neurological Disorders and Stroke Progress Review Group provided consensus that task-oriented training has emerged as the dominant evidence-based approach to motor restoration after stroke (NINDS 2006). While a thorough discussion of task-oriented training is beyond the scope of this text, key elements such as motor skill training and behavioral demands that facilitate brain plasticity can be implemented in exercise models to improve both cardiovascular health and functional motor outcomes (Winstein and Wolf 2009). Table 4.3 presents several examples of exercise intervention studies that have produced significant improvements in motor outcomes having relevance to basic ADL function in sub-acute and chronic stroke patients (Ivey *et al.* 2006a; 2009).

TABLE 4.3 Exercise intervention studies and their impact on selected functional and physical performance outcomes

Study	Design/ population	Intervention	Δ function
Hesse et al. (1994)	Non-controlled/ subacute and chronic stroke	5 weeks 5×/wk off partial weight support treadmill walking	Rivermead Mobility Treatment: +110% Gait velocity: Treatment: +250%
Potempa et al. (1995)	Randomized/ chronic stroke	10 weeks cycle training 3×/wk vs. passive range of motion	Fugl-Meyer Index Treatment: No change Control: No change
Duncan et al. (1998)	Randomized/ subacute stroke	12 weeks home based. Theraband, walking or bike for 20 minutes vs. usual care	10-min gait velocity Treatment: +37.3 % Control: +12.3% 6-min walk Treatment: +28% Control: +17%
Teixeira-Salmela et al. (1999)	Non-controlled/ chronic stroke	10 weeks aerobic + strength training 3×/ wk	30-min gait speed (m/s) Treatment: +21.2%*
Rimmer et al. (2000)	Randomized/ chronic stroke	12 weeks on a variety of aerobic (30 min.) and strength equipment (20 min.) 3×/wk vs. delayed entry controls	Exercise time Treatment: +29% Control: +15%
Katz-Leurer et al. (2003)	Randomized/ acute stroke	8 weeks cycle ergometer 2×/wk at 60% HRR vs. usual care	Post-intervention walk distance Treatment: 143 m Control: 108 m Stair climbing Treatment: 26 Control: 18
Eng et al. (2003)	Non-controlled/ chronic stroke	8 weeks community-based 3×/wk aerobic stepping, stretching, functional LE strengthening (chair rise)	12-min walk Treatment: +9.5% 10-min walk speed Treatment: +14.4% (self-selected) +9.3% (fastest)
Duncan et al. (2003)	Randomized/ subacute stroke	12 week in-home therapist supervised programme, emphasising strength, balance, endurance vs. usual care	10-min gait velocity Treatment: +25.7% Control: +18 % 6-min walk distance Treatment: +26% Control: +15%

Study	Design/population	Intervention	Δ function
Chu et al. (2004)	Randomized/chronic stroke	8 weeks water based aerobics up to 80% HRR vs. upper extremity functional exercise	Self selected gait speed (m/s) Treatment: +16.1% Control: +2.9%
Eich et al. (2004)	Randomized/subacute stroke	6 weeks 5×/wk harness secured and minimally supported treadmill walking (30 min) plus physiotherapy (30 min) vs. physiotherapy alone (60 min)	10-min walk Treatment: +78% Control: +36% 6-min walk Treatment: +84% Control: +51%
Macko et al. (2005b)	Randomized/chronic stroke	6 month progressive treadmill training vs. attention controls (stretching)	6-min walk Treatment: +30% Control: +11% WIQ Distance Treatment: +56% Control: +12%
Pang et al. (2005)	Randomized/chronic stroke	Community-based UE vs. LE exercise 3×/wk for 19 weeks	6-min walk Treatment (LE): +19.7%
Pang et al. (2006)	Randomized/chronic stroke	Community-based UE vs. LE exercise 3×/wk for 19 weeks	Wolf Motor Function LE: 0% UE: +7% Fugl-Meyer Assessment LE: +2% UE: +12% Dynamometry (grip strength) LE: +2% UE: 17%

Continued

TABLE 4.3 *continued*

Study	Design/ population	Intervention	Δ *function*
Macko *et al.* (2008)	Non-controlled/ chronic stroke	Group exercise in hospital gymnasium (Italy)	6-minute walk Treatment: +23% Berg Balance Score Treatment +32% Short Physical Performance Battery Treatment: +59%
Stuart *et al.* (2009)	Controlled/ chronic stroke	Community-based adaptive physical activity class vs. natural history controls for 6 months	Berg Balance Score Treatment: +5 pts Control: −1.5 6-minute walk Treatment: +14% Control: −9%
Michael *et al.* (2009)	Non-controlled/ chronic stroke	Low-intensity group exercise in hospital gymnasium 3×/wk for 6 months	Berg Balance: Treatment: +36% Dynamic Gait Index: Treatment: +39% 6-minute walk Treatment: +11%

LE = Lower Extremity; UE = Upper Extremity.

The impact of specific exercise modalities after stroke

The remaining sections of the chapter consider the impact of specific exercise modalities, including cycle ergometry, water-based exercise, strength training, treadmill training, partial body weight support treadmill training, multi-modal therapy, as well as home and community-based interventions, on important health outcomes in stroke patients. Much work remains before the exercise format for producing optimal gains in fitness and function to delay disability and cardiovascular morbidity/mortality after stroke can be established.

Cycle ergometry and single limb flexion-extension exercise

A seminal study conducted by Potempa *et al.* (1995) compared 10 weeks of adapted cycle ergometer exercise with a control intervention consisting of passive range of motion exercise in chronic stroke patients. Results showed a significant between group difference in $\dot{V}O_{2peak}$ change over time, with the cycle ergometer group achieving 13 per cent gains compared to no change for controls. Though Fugl-Meyer sensorimotor scores were positively correlated with gains in peak $\dot{V}O_2$, neither of the treatment groups showed significant differences in functional outcome scores. This study showed that aerobic exercise using cycle ergometry is feasible and improves fitness in chronic hemiparetic stroke, but provided no clear evidence that cycle exercise could improve neuromuscular function or functional mobility. However, Tang *et al.* (2009) recently investigated the benefits of adding 30 minutes of cycle ergometry to conventional early stroke rehabilitation. Importantly, they found a trend toward improved $\dot{V}O_{2peak}$, peak power output and 6-minute walk distance, suggesting that early initiation of cycle exercise may enhance cardiovascular and functional mobility outcomes. Another 2009 study reported that moderate intensity cycle training is effective for achieving reductions in blood pressure and hyperlipidemia after stroke (Rimmer *et al.* 2009). Larger studies are needed to develop a clear picture of how cycle ergometry impacts upon important health outcomes in stroke survivors in both the subacute and chronic phases of recovery.

Water-based exercise

Chu *et al.* (2004) conducted a water-based exercise study lasting 12 weeks. Those in the experimental group exercised for one hour, three days per week in a swimming pool. The patients were progressed to 30 minutes of water aerobics at 80 per cent HRR, with the remainder of time consisting of stretching and warm-up/cool down. Although this study had a very small sample size (7 treatment and 5 controls) the intervention produced the greatest relative gains in peak aerobic capacity shown to date (23 per cent), perhaps arguing for strong consideration of this form of intervention for stroke survivors. Importantly, this type of intervention has recently been shown to produce benefits for balance and function after stroke (Noh *et al.* 2008). Specifically, postural balance and knee flexor strength were improved in stroke participants following aquatic therapy (Noh *et al.* 2008).

Strength training

There are now eight randomized controlled trials examining the effects of progressive lower extremity strength training alone or in combination with other therapies after stroke (Teixeira-Salmela *et al.* 1999; Kim *et al.* 2001; Sullivan *et al.* 2007; Ouellette *et al.* 2004; Flansbjer *et al.* 2008; Lee *et al.* 2008; Sims *et al.* 2009; Bale and Strand 2008). Of these, only four looked at the effects of strength training exclusively (Kim *et al.* 2001; Ouellette *et al.* 2004; Flansbjer *et al.* 2008; Bale and Strand 2008), with the remaining four studies being hybrid interventions. Teixeira-Salmela *et al.* (1999) reported the effects of lower extremity strength training in combination with aerobic exercise and showed improvements in strength, gait speed and stair climbing compared to controls, without concomitant increases in spasticity after the combined programme. Similarly, a recently conducted randomized trial by Sullivan *et al.* (2007) combined strength training with treadmill training, showing significant increases in walking speed and 6-minute walk distance. Kim *et al.* (2001) attempted to isolate the effects of progressive isokinetic strength training on strength and function after stroke. After a 6-week programme, the strength training group had superior strength gains compared to controls, although walking function improved in both groups (Kim *et al.* 2001). In a 12-week randomized trial comparing high-intensity lower extremity strength training to a stretching control group, Oulette *et al.* (2004) showed greater gains in strength, self-reported function, and disability in strength trainers compared to controls. Randomized trials of the past two years have confirmed the beneficial effects of strength training on strength, stair climbing power, and balance after stroke (Flansbjer *et al.* 2008; Lee *et al.* 2008; Bale and Strand 2008). One more recent strength training trial also supports the use of strength training for combating post-stroke depression (Sims *et al.* 2009). Finally, several important reviews on this topic detail results of all controlled and non-controlled strength-training trials performed in the stroke population to date (Patten *et al.* 2004; Pak and Patten 2008; Lexell *et al.* 2008). No studies have considered the metabolic impact of strength training after stroke. Similarly, there have not been any attempts to investigate tissue-level adaptations on the hemiparetic side with strength training. More work in these novel areas is necessary before a complete picture of this therapy's potential can be established.

Treadmill-based training approaches

Based on pioneering studies of hind limb stepping recovery in despinalized cats, variants of treadmill-based training have emerged to promote locomotor learning after stroke (Barbeau and Rossignol 1987; Richards *et al.* 1993). A biomechanical basis for this approach is supported by findings that treadmill walking improves reflexive gait patterning in hemiparetic patients (Hesse *et al.* 1999; Silver *et al.* 2000). The facilitation of gait patterning with treadmill is well characterized for both body weight-supported (BWS) (Hesse *et al.* 1994) and self-supported full weight-bearing treadmill exercise conditions (Macko *et al.* 2005a). Treadmill walking produces a 50 per cent improvement in inter-limb stance to swing symmetry ratios, 30 per cent improvement in impulse symmetry, and improved timing of quadriceps activation compared to over-ground walking in hemiparetic stroke patients (Harris-Love *et al.* 2001). Treadmill-based training also provides task-repetition that animal and human studies suggest is requisite to mediate motor learning and neuroplasticity (Dobkin *et al.* 2007; Schmidt and Lee 1999). Randomized studies show benefits of treadmill training translate into improved over-ground walking, and can be extended to more severely impaired subjects using BWS strategies (Hesse *et al.* 1994). Treadmill-based training can also be combined with progressive aerobic exercise to improve both fitness and ambulatory function (Macko *et al.* 2005b), as discussed in the following sections.

Partial body-weight support (BWS) treadmill training

Partial BWS treadmill exercise has received much investigation, particularly as a means to provide a physiological gait training stimulus to more impaired subjects across earlier phases of stroke recovery (Hesse *et al.* 1999; 2008; McCain *et al.* 2008). This approach utilizes a suspensory harness to progress patients from 30–40 per cent BWS to full weight-bearing treadmill walking, typically with 1–2 therapists facilitating stepping and truncal stability across 4–6 weeks. Early studies by Hesse *et al.* (1995; 1994; 1999) provide evidence that BWS treadmill exercise may restore gait in severely affected non-ambulatory patients. Subsequent randomized studies confirm that BWS treadmill exercise training is better tolerated and more effective than full weight-bearing treadmill to improve gait and balance function in more severely hemiplegic patients, specifically the subset with lower gait velocities (<0.2 m/s), poorer balance (Berg Scores <15 points) (Visintin *et al.* 1998; Barbeau and Visintin 2003), and of more advanced age. The latter finding may be explained by the significantly lower oxygen demands of BWS treadmill exercise; a finding which raises the question of whether BWS treadmill exercise, using current protocols, provides an adequate aerobic exercise intensity for evoking metabolic health benefits (Danielsson and Sunnerhagen 2000).

Despite some positive findings, a Cochrane Review concluded that there were no significant effects from BWS treadmill exercise, except greater walking speed in those already ambulatory (Mosely *et al.* 2004). Whether BWS treadmill exercise or other treadmill-based training strategies are more effective than conventional therapy to durably improve function or fitness after stroke remains unclear (Nilsson *et al.* 2001). However, few studies have systematically investigated the specific training parameters or conditions of BWS treadmill exercise in relation to key health outcomes. One promising avenue is that BWS treadmill exercise at higher velocities may be more efficacious to improve walking velocity during the sub-acute stroke period (Sullivan *et al.* 2002). These findings have spurred important clinical trials investigating the relative benefits of BWS treadmill exercise across the sub-acute versus chronic stroke phases.

Full body-weight support treadmill exercise

Although partial body-weight support treadmill exercise might be an effective means of initiating exercise training, particularly for those with greater gait impairments (Barbeau and Visintin 2003), this form of exercise rehabilitation has not traditionally utilized aerobic progression formulas (Danielsson and Sunnerhagen 2000). Thus, based on studies of exercise rehabilitation in the frail elderly, we have studied the profile of fitness and mobility function gains across six months of progressive full body-weight support treadmill aerobic exercise training in stroke survivors with chronic hemiparesis (Macko *et al.* 1997a; 2001; 2005a; 2005b). This is a much longer therapeutic duration than is typical for most stroke rehabilitation programmes. Our results show that the time profile of cardiovascular fitness gains with regular treadmill exercise training are progressive and nearly equal across the initial three months and third to sixth month of training (Figure 4.5) (Macko *et al.* 2005b). There is no evidence of plateau, suggesting that training even beyond six months may produce further benefits in peak fitness levels. In addition, full body-weight support treadmill exercise also improves 6-minute walk performance and self-reported indices of functional mobility across six months, with greater gains in 6-minute walk occurring within the initial three months of training (Macko *et al.* 2005b).

Prospective studies show a plateau in mobility recovery within three months after stroke in 95 per cent of hemiparetic patients receiving conventional rehabilitation care (Jorgensen *et al.* 1995). Our findings in a randomized study show that treadmill exercise improves both fitness and mobility function long after conventional rehabilitation care has ended, and that the duration of exercise therapy to optimize these outcomes is at least six months. These results support a rationale for long-term exercise rehabilitation after stroke, consistent with public health recommendations for sustained regular exercise to improve fitness and cardiovascular health for all Americans (Gordon *et al.* 2004). Although studies conducted beyond six months are lacking, we hypothesize that additional gains over a longer intervention period are possible after stroke.

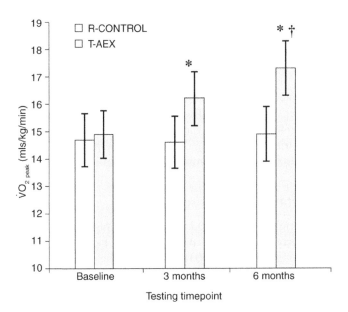

FIGURE 4.5 Progression of improvement in $\dot{V}O_{2peak}$ across six months with progressive, full BWS treadmill exercise in chronic hemiparetic stroke patients. Reproduced with permission from Stroke (Macko *et al.* 2005).

Robotics-assisted treadmill rehabilitation is a rapidly evolving area with recent technological advances now enabling mobility-based exercise training (Hornby *et al.* 2008; Krebs *et al.* 2008). Several studies report that robotic devices that precisely guide the lower extremity through a consistent kinematic pattern are less effective than therapist assistance for durably improving consistency of hemiparetic leg movements, gait velocity and cadence (Lewek *et al.* 2009; Hidler *et al.* 2009). Hence, intra-limb variability and the need for volitional motor learning with therapist assisted training appears to have enhanced gait outcomes. Other studies show that the robotics assisted locomotion condition requires significantly less energy consumption than treadmill-based hemiparetic ambulation (Hidler *et al.* 2008), which may alter the aerobic conditioning impact. Further studies are needed to optimize programmable robotics applications to help customize motor learning and enhance access to exercise training by even more disabled stroke survivors.

Multi-modal exercise

A trial involving primarily African–American stroke survivors utilized a multi-modal intervention (Rimmer *et al.* 2000). A delayed-entry controlled design was used to provide training to all 35 participants. Outcome testing included measures of peak $\dot{V}O_2$, strength, flexibility and body composition. The 3×/week training protocol consisted of the following components: cardiovascular endurance (30 minutes), muscle strength and endurance (20 minutes) and flexibility (10 minutes). Results showed significant time by group interactions for the following measures during cycle ergometer fitness testing: $\dot{V}O_{2peak}$, time to exhaustion and maximal workload. This was among the first randomized exercise studies in stroke to show significant between group effects for muscular strength and endurance as well as improvements in body composition (body weight, BMI, total skinfolds) (Rimmer *et al.* 2000). Other multi-modal exercise therapies have also been successful after stroke (Cheng *et al.* 2001; Marigold *et al.* 2005; Vearrier *et al.* 2005), particularly in the context of falls prevention.

Community-translation of exercise studies for stroke survivors

There are a number of psychosocial, economic, as well as practical geographic issues that affect longitudinal participation of exercise rehabilitation in stroke survivors (Rimmer *et al.* 2008; Resnick *et al.* 2008; Shaughnessy and Resnick 2009). Principal among them are limited access to facilities, transportation, and the cost and labor intensity of maintaining stroke therapies in the setting of limited resources for health care support (Rimmer *et al.* 2008). While both home and rehabilitation centre-based programmes have been studied, there is a relative paucity of data regarding how to safely and effectively translate structured exercise programmes for stroke survivors to the community level. Implementation of community-based exercise programmes for disabled stroke survivors is also complicated by the heterogeneity in deficit profiles that may influence the nature of the training regimens and the safety of their conduct. However, group exercise research programmes targeted toward individuals with mild to moderate gait deficit severity have recently emerged as a first step in community translation. Such group programmes increase geographical access, and may in the future provide a more cost-effective and socially reinforced model to sustain structured physical activity across the continuum of stroke care.

Duncan *et al.* (1998) was the first of the randomized studies to utilize a home-based intervention model. The programme consisted of 36 sessions of 90-minute duration over 12–14 weeks. Participants in the usual care group had services as prescribed by their physicians. All sessions for the exercise group were supervised by a physical or occupational therapist at home. Components of the programme were range of motion and flexibility, strength, balance, upper extremity functional use and endurance training (riding a stationary bike for 30 minutes). Although both the intervention and usual care groups improved in balance, upper- and lower-extremity motor control, upper-extremity function and gait velocity, gains for the intervention group exceeded those in the usual care group in balance, endurance, peak aerobic capacity and mobility. The study was important in demonstrating the practical utility of home-based interventions compared to the more frequently applied hospital-based intervention programmes for improving fitness and function after stroke. However, it should be noted that there was still a high level of supervision despite the study being home-based. Additional studies are required to further substantiate the benefits of home-based exercise therapy as well as to clarify the recommendations and guidelines for this type of intervention. A study by Pang *et al.* (2005; 2006) in Canada was among the first to examine effects of community-based group exercise on mobility and bone health for individuals with chronic stroke. Individuals with chronic stroke (>1 yr) that could walk 10 metres independently (with or without assistive device) were randomized to 19 weeks of three one-hour sessions per week of arm exercise or a fitness and mobility exercise treatment group that included brisk walking, sit-to-stand exercises, stepping onto low platforms, walking an obstacle course, and partial squats and toe rises to improve strength. The fitness and mobility group significantly increased $\dot{V}O_{2peak}$ by 9 per cent, 6-minute walk distance by 20 per cent, and improved paretic leg strength, but not Berg Balance Scores. This exercise programme prevented the declines in femoral neck bone mineral density that occurred in the Arm Group, and increased distal tibial trabecular bone mineral content on the paretic side. Hence, this study shows that a lower intensity community-based exercise class produces modest gains in fitness, walking velocity, leg strength and helps preserve bone health for older individuals with milder chronic deficits post-stroke (Pang *et al.* 2005; 2006).

In the Empoli region of Tuscany, Italy, an ongoing adaptive physical activity (APA) exercise programme for management of older individuals with chronic stroke has been developed and sponsored by the local Public Health Authorities in conjunction with Italian and United States National Institutes of Health

(Macko *et al.* 2008; Stuart *et al.* 2009). This programme is based on models of task-oriented exercise and has gymnasium-based group exercises, leveraging social support to facilitate exercise compliance, and a homework component to help translate these gains into ADL function. Training includes a walking warm-up, seated stretching exercises (including reach across the midline to enhance truncal control), sit-to stand, weight shifting and partial squats at a ballet bar for strength and balance. Sessions conclude with a walking 'obstacle course' for mobility and all exercises are progressed. A hospital-based two-month duration pilot study of APA showed improved Berg Balance Scores, 6-minute walk distance and Barthel Index Scores in 20 older subjects with chronic deficits (Macko *et al.* 2008). A subsequent community-based clinical trial including 93 individuals with mild-moderately impaired gait deficits showed improved 6-minute walks, Berg Balance and Short Physical Performance Battery Scores compared to controls (Stuart *et al.* 2009). Notably, APA also reduced the insulin response to oral glucose challenge, suggesting that lower aerobic intensity activity may be sufficient to reduce insulin resistance after stroke (unpublished Stuart, Macko *et al.*). A more progressive version of the APA class is reported to robustly improve Berg Balance and Dynamic Gait Index Scores sufficiently to reduce fall risk category (Michael *et al.* 2009). Furthermore, this more intense version of APA improved VO_{2peak} by 15 per cent; a similar gain in cardiopulmonary fitness to that reported with modified cycle ergometry or treadmill walking (Michael *et al.* 2009). While further research is needed to establish whether community-based programmes reduce falls and help prevent diabetes and recurrent stroke, these studies suggest that community-based group exercise studies are sustainable and effective to improve balance and mobility function. If careful attention is placed on progression and compliance, these community group exercise programmes may be suitable for rectifying reduced levels of fitness and hyperinsulinemia after stroke.

Goals of exercise therapy after stroke

Exercise programmes should be considered as an adjunct to best medical care for risk factor modification and to optimize fitness and motor function for all stroke survivors that are medically eligible and have adequate baseline neuromotor function to participate. The goals are to improve functional mobility, aerobic capacity and body composition, as well as to prevent and reverse IGT, diabetes and other vascular event risk factors. There is now consensus that task-oriented rehabilitation can improve motor function by leveraging principles of motor learning, even years after stroke (NINDS 2006). Though basic questions remain regarding how to optimize exercise training programmes, the gains in fitness, sensorimotor function and the systemic adaptations in insulin sensitivity and glucose tolerance attainable have much potential to improve key health outcomes and quality of life for stroke survivors (Gordon *et al.* 2004).

Exercise programmes for stroke patients should be initiated at the earliest feasible time-point. As most stroke survivors and their families have little knowledge about the importance of exercise after stroke, education needs to be provided early to outline its role in stroke risk factor modification and for increasing fitness levels. Likewise, most stroke survivors and many health care providers outside the field of rehabilitation care are unaware that gait and balance can be improved by task-oriented training, even years after the initial stroke event (Macko *et al.* 2005b; Wolf *et al.* 2006). Physical inactivity is an independent risk factor for stroke (Hooker *et al.* 2008; Liang *et al.* 2009; Stroud *et al.* 2009) and 'disuse' leads to deconditioning (Ivey *et al.* 2005), which worsens disability and stroke risk. These are understated health concerns that need reinforcement. Patients and their families should also be informed that consensus statements strongly recommend regular exercise as an adjunct to best medical treatment for management of insulin resistance (Gordon *et al.* 2004), which is highly prevalent after stroke (Kernan *et al.* 2003; Ivey *et al.* 2006b).

Medical eligibility and timing of exercise initiation

Stroke patients have a high prevalence of medical and cardiovascular comorbid conditions that can influence their exercise capacity and safety (Kopunek *et al.* 2007). Evaluation for eligibility in an exercise programme should begin with a medical history, physical and cardiopulmonary examination. Exclusions for exercise post-stroke are consistent with American College of Sports Medicine (ACSM) criteria for high cardiovascular disease (CVD) risk subjects (ACSM 2006). In brief, exclusion criteria employed for exercise research studies have generally included symptomatic heart failure, unstable angina, symptomatic peripheral arterial occlusive disease, chronic pain syndromes, dementia or severe aphasia (operationally defined as incapacity to follow 2-point commands) (Macko *et al.* 2005a) and other medical conditions that preclude participation in low intensity aerobic exercise, consistent with ACSM guidelines (ACSM 2006). These research criteria do not reflect the full scope of the stroke population that could potentially benefit from exercise. Some medical conditions that are exclusions for specific research reasons may be quite amenable to supervised exercise, with proper medical oversight. Regardless, using these criterion along with entry exercise stress tests, our safety data including >16,000 treadmill exercise training and >400 peak exercise tests in chronic hemiparetic stroke patients reveals no study-related serious adverse events. Composite analyses from our treadmill-based exercise studies reveals only occasional minor musculoskeletal complaints at a rate not different from controls performing supervised stretching exercises (Macko *et al.* 2005b).

Clinical research has not yet determined precisely when it is best to start exercise programmes for stroke survivors, or which exercise training modality(s) or dose-intensity are optimal across the different phases of stroke recovery. Initiating exercise during the early stroke recovery period is complicated by greater deficit profiles (Jorgensen 1995; Hesse *et al.* 1999; Barbeau and Visintin 2003), high prevalence of cardiac comorbid conditions (Roth 1993, 1994), and medical problems such as autonomic deconditioning and pain syndromes that are common post stroke (USDHHS 1995). Such factors may limit patients' activity tolerance, forcing clinicians to weigh the benefit and feasibility of adding additional structured activity to intensive early inpatient rehabilitation regimens. Despite these limitations, physical inactivity can produce rapid declines in cardiopulmonary fitness and muscle mass that worsen functional aerobic impairment, which is already present in the early stroke period, supporting a rationale for early initiation of exercise intervention (MacKay-Lyons and Makrides 2002b).

A starting point during sub-acute stroke recovery period is to assess the profile of exercise during rehabilitation and free-living physical activity. Although most conventional rehabilitation does not provide an adequate exercise intensity stimulus to reverse deconditioning after stroke (Hjeltnes 1982; MacKay-Lyons and Makrides 2002b), practice patterns differ considerably, as can the cardiopulmonary response and tolerability to exertion during rehabilitation in different stroke patients (Roth 1994). One practical approach is to assess the exercise intensity of usual physical therapy, focusing on upright and transitional movements that produce the greatest exertion (MacKay-Lyons and Makrides 2002b). Heart rate monitoring and Ratings of Perceived Exertion (RPE) scales can be used to better estimate exercise intensity and subjective exercise tolerance. Therapists can consider adding a component of low intensity exercise, contingent on the cardiopulmonary safety profile and rehabilitation needs for each patient. While the longitudinal health benefits of initiating specific exercise modalities early post-stroke are not yet established, protocols that engage large muscle groups are considered optimal for cardiovascular conditioning (Macko *et al.* 2005a), and task-oriented training that may enhance mobility recovery seems most efficacious for improving function (NINDS 2006). Some individuals may be too impaired to perform modified cycle ergometry or full weight bearing treadmill exercise. Randomized studies suggest that BWS treadmill exercise is better tolerated by individuals with more severe gait and balance deficits (Barbeau and Visintin 2003), can provide an aerobic stimulus if properly applied and, hence, warrants consideration during early stroke recovery.

By the chronic phase of stroke, most patients have achieved some degree of ambulatory function and may not require BWS exercise or more dependent exercise modalities for rehabilitation. Structured exercise programmes can be implemented using specific progression formulas, including the use of cardiopulmonary exercise testing where available to enhance the safety and prescription accuracy of aerobic training, as outlined below.

Exercise testing

Studies show that approximately 75 per cent of stroke survivors have some form of concurrent cardiovascular disease; perhaps half with coronary artery disease (Roth 1993; 1994). Albeit uncommon, exertion-related myocardial events or cardiopulmonary intolerance such as electrocardiography (ECG) abnormalities and blood pressure drops are possible during exercise in some individuals with pre-existing cardiac conditions (Macko *et al.* 2005a). Hence, consideration should be given to cardiopulmonary assessment, including exercise testing. In the USA, clinicians often relegate stroke patients with gait deficits to pharmacologic cardiac stress tests with radionuclide imaging that offer high sensitivity and specificity for detecting reversible myocardial ischemia, and do not require physical effort or impart fall risk to the patient. These tests are costly, provide limited information on which to design an aerobic exercise prescription and do not reveal the neuromotor capacity or cardiopulmonary tolerability of patients to undertake any specific exercise regimen. With proper safeguards, cardiopulmonary exercise stress testing is well tolerated by many stroke survivors with mild-moderate hemiparetic gait deficits, reveals previously undiagnosed or asymptomatic coronary artery disease in 20–40 per cent of stroke survivors and provides useful information to customize design and optimize safety (Macko *et al.* 2005a; Ivey and Macko 2009). Treadmill exercise testing protocols validated in our laboratory for gait impaired stroke patients are outlined in Table 4.4.

Symptom-limited maximal effort or submaximal effort exercise testing is recommended where available to best define cardiopulmonary safety and the tolerability of stroke patients to physical exertion before starting formal exercise. In addition, exercise testing with open circuit spirometry can provide a reliable and valid means for quantifying fitness gains for both treadmill and bicycle testing modalities in hemiparetic stroke patients (Potempa *et al.* 1995; Macko *et al.* 2005b; Rimmer *et al.* 2009l). Protocols for exercise testing with open circuit spirometry are validated for both treadmill and modified cycle ergometry (Potempa *et al.* 1995; Dobrovolny *et al.* 2003).

There are currently no empiric data to guide the decision between choices of submaximal versus symptom-limited peak effort exercise testing in stroke patients. Peak effort rather than the maximal exercise test is used here because most stroke patients do not achieve the full criterion for $\dot{V}O_{2max}$ (Macko *et al.* 1997b). Peak exercise heart rates are the most accurate and have proven useful for managing exercise progression. For high cardiac risk stroke patients, conservative guidelines extrapolated from the cardiac population suggest that exercise should be conducted at least 10 beats per minute below the exercise intensity that produces systolic blood pressures >250 mm Hg, diastolic blood pressure >115 mmHg, ST segment depression >1 mm or other significant ECG abnormalities or clinical cardiopulmonary intolerance (ACSM 2006).

TABLE 4.4 Exercise testing protocols adjusted according to gait deficit severity

1 Start at 0.1 mph and increase gradually to velocity determined from zero incline TM test.
2 Fastest comfortable walking velocity maintained at no incline for initial 2 minutes, then:
   • Milder gait deficits: advance to 4% incline for next 2 minutes, then increase incline 2% every minute thereafter (velocity constant) to peak volitional exertion.
   • Moderate-to-severe deficits: advance to 2% incline for next 2 minutes, then increase incline by 2% every 2 minutes thereafter, with velocity held constant.

Peak effort exercise testing may not be available or the preferred option for some patients, depending on their deficit profiles, latency since stroke and medical history. While few studies have systematically investigated submaximal effort exercise protocols to design aerobic prescriptions for stroke survivors, precedence in the field of cardiac rehabilitation supports this approach. American Heart Association consensus statements conclude that submaximal effort exercise testing with predetermined endpoints of 70 per cent of age-predicted maximum HRR is consistent with best practice in post-myocardial infarction patients (Gordon *et al.* 2004). A period of ECG telemetry monitoring is recommended for those patients deemed at high cardiac risk that cannot undergo any formal exercise testing (ACSM 2006). Recent studies provide initial evidence that even low intensity exercise classes produce modest gains in fitness and walking function, and may reduce insulin resistance for chronic hemiparetic stroke patients (Pang *et al.* 2005; Stuart *et al.* 2009; Michael *et al.* 2009). While some of these programmes have simply required physician clearance for participation, their long-term benefits to modify cardiovascular risks, prevent diabetes or reduce recurrent stroke and vascular cognitive impairment has not yet been tested.

Guidelines for exercise therapy progression

The target training parameters used in chronic stroke patients from our laboratory (Macko *et al.* 2005b) consist of three 40–45 minute sessions per week of treadmill walking at 60 per cent to 70 per cent of HRR. Creating a zone of 60–70 per cent simply requires performing the calculation twice to come up with an upper and lower limit for the desired range. Training is initiated conservatively at 40 per cent of HRR for durations of 10–15 minutes and advanced as tolerated. Discontinuous training epochs consisting of 3–5 minutes treadmill walking with similar duration interval rests are used in those highly deconditioned or more severely disabled patients incapable of continuous exercise. Total exercise duration is then advanced as tolerated toward the target. Handrail support is used, and 5-minute treadmill warm-up and cool-down periods at approximately 30 per cent of HRR are phased into each workout as participants develop the necessary endurance for longer bouts of training (Macko *et al.* 2005b). Regression analyses of clinical factors related to training safety reveal that arm hemiplegia (inability to grasp treadmill handrail for support) and presence of major sensory deficit is associated with increased risk of falls during treadmill training (Macko *et al.* 2005a). While such events are uncommon and low impact, we use suspensory safety harnesses in a non-weight-bearing fashion (e.g. Biodex Medical, Shirley, NY) to eliminate the risk of fall injury in our patients. Heart rate is monitored continuously by two-lead ECG (Polar Electro, Woodbury, NY), and blood pressure recordings are taken before, at the mid-point, and at the conclusion of each exercise session to ensure safety and to document the intensity of the exercise session (Macko *et al.* 2005a; 2005b).

Progression of training workload is determined bi-weekly by monitoring each patient's gait, heart rate response and patient-reported level of fatigue at the end of the session. If no gait instability, exaggerated heart rate response (HRR >80 per cent) or extreme fatigue is noted (Borg Perceived Exertion used as adjunct to rate tolerability), an increase in training speed by 0.1-mph increments is prioritized to reach the target training intensity. Increase in treadmill grade (1 per cent increments) is utilized secondarily to achieve target aerobic intensity for those individuals who do not tolerate further treadmill velocity progression to meet this goal. Exercise duration is typically advanced approximately 5 minutes every two weeks, as tolerated, to arrive at a total 45 minutes of exercise by the third month. For those completing intermittent bouts of exercise, only duration is altered in order to progress to one continuous bout of 15 minutes (Macko *et al.* 2005a).

Summary and future directions

In summary, exercise therapy programmes have been shown to improve fitness, function, body composition and metabolic risk factors in disabled stroke survivors. The time window for the effectiveness of exercise models extends many years beyond the index disabling stroke, long after completion of conventional care. Task-oriented exercise programmes that incorporate principles of motor learning provide the strongest evidence-base that structured physical activity can improve basic mobility function, including gait and balance in disabled stroke survivors. A proposed underlying mechanism is exercise-mediated brain plasticity, which involves activation of both cortical and subcortical midbrain-cerebellar networks that can be turned on by progressive locomotor-based exercise to improve walking in chronic stroke survivors (Luft *et al.* 2008; Enzinger *et al.* 2008; 2009). New evidence also shows that structured physical activity programmes improve balance to a degree sufficient to reduce categorical fall-risk in stroke survivors (Michael *et al.* 2009). Taken together, these findings indicate that exercise that is designed with task-specificity to improve targeted outcomes appears to be most clinically important to the stroke survivor's functional independence. Larger trials are now underway to determine whether exercise interventions can prevent falls and improve mobility for community dwelling stroke survivors (Dean *et al.* 2009).

The many advances generated over the last 15 years provide a public health rationale for more broadly implementing exercise after stroke. However, there are many remaining questions regarding the practice and effects of exercise in this population. For example, it is still unclear which exercise modalities are best to improve function after stroke. Similarly, the optimal exercise dose-intensity needed to improve cardiometabolic outcomes is an area of active investigation. Little is known about the long-term health and functional benefits of the exercise programmes outlined in this chapter, and future study should be directed at understanding whether exercise can prevent the development of diabetes, as well as reduce the rate of recurrent stroke, cardiovascular events or cardiovascular mortality in stroke survivors.

The impact of exercise therapy on cognition after stroke represents a potentially promising area of inquiry in the coming years. A meta-analysis of studies in ageing revealed that exercise can improve elements of cognitive function, particularly those related to executive function (Colcombe and Kramer 2003). Thus, future research is needed to investigate the effects of exercise on cognitive-executive function, the natural history of vascular cognitive impairment, and development of dementia; all of which are alarmingly increased after stroke (Greenberg 2009; Rockwood et al. 2009; Tatemichi et al. 1994). A recent pilot study provides encouraging initial evidence that aerobic exercise training improves elements of cognitive function that generalize to enhance motor learning (Quaney et al. 2009). As such, future trials should focus on whether exercise can augment motor learning to enhance stroke recovery and instrumental ADL function via improvements in cognitive-executive domains.

References

Ainsworth BE, Haskell WL, Whitt MC, Irwin ML, Swartz AM, Strath SJ, O'Brien WL, Bassett DR, Schmitz KH, Emplaincourt PO, Jacobs DR, Leon AS. (2000) Compendium of physical activities: an update of activity codes and MET intensities. *Med Sci Sports Exerc*; 32(9 Suppl):S498-S504.

Alon G. (2009) Defining and measuring residual deficits of the upper extremity following stroke: a new perspective. *Top Stroke Rehabil*; 16(3):167–76.

ACSM (2006) *American College of Sports Medicine's guidelines for exercise testing and prescription*. 7th edn. Baltimore: Lippincott, Williams & Wilkins.

ACSM (2009) *American College of Sports Medicine's guidelines for exercise testing and prescription*. Baltimore: Lippincott, Williams & Wilkins.

Bale M, Strand LI. (2008) Does functional strength training of the leg in subacute stroke improve physical performance? A pilot randomized controlled trial. *Clin Rehabil*; 22(10):911–21.

Barbeau H, Rossignol S. (1987) Recovery of locomotion after chronic spinalization in the adult cat. *Brain Res*; May 26; 412(1):84–95.

Barbeau H, Visintin M. (2003) Optimal outcomes obtained with body-weight support combined with treadmill training in stroke subjects. *Arch Phys Med Rehabil*; 84(10):1458–65.

Billinger SA, Gajewski BJ, Guo LX, Kluding PM. (2009) Single limb exercise induces femoral artery remodeling and improves blood flow in the hemiparetic leg poststroke. *Stroke*; 40(9):3086–90.

Bruce RA, Kusumi F, Hosmer D. (1973) Maximal oxygen intake and nomographic assessment of functional aerobic impairment in cardiovascular disease. *Am Heart J*; 85:546–62.

Buyukyazi G. (2005) Differences in blood lipids and apolipoproteins between master athletes, recreational athletes and sedentary men. *J Sports Med Phys Fitness*; 45(1):112–20.

Cheng PT, Wu SH, Liaw MY, Wong AM, Tang FT. (2001) Symmetrical body-weight distribution training in stroke patients and its effect on fall prevention. *Arch Phys Med Rehabil*; 82(12):1650–4.

Chokroverty S, Reyes MG, Rubino FA, Barron KD. (1976) Hemiplegic amyotrophy. Muscle and motor point biopsy study. *Arch Neurol*; February; 33(2):104–10.

Chu KS, Eng JJ, Dawson AS, Harris JE, Oakaplan A. (2004) Water-based exercise for cardiovascular fitness in people with chronic stroke: a randomized controlled trial. *Arch Phys Med Rehabil*; 85: 870–4.

Colcombe S, Kramer A. (2003) Fitness effects on the cognitive function of older adults: a meta-analytic study. *American Psychological Society*; 14(2):125–30.

Corcoran PJ, Jebsen RH, Brengelmann GL, Simons BC. (1970) Effects of plastic and metal leg braces on speed and energy cost of hemiparetic ambulation. *Arch Phys Med Rehabil*; February; 51(2):69–77.

Danielsson A, Sunnerhagen KS. (2000) Oxygen consumption during treadmill walking with and without body weight support in patients with hemiparesis after stroke and in healthy subjects. *Arch Phys Med Rehabil*; 81(7):953–7.

Daugaard JR, Richter EA. (2001) Relationship between muscle fibre composition, glucose transporter protein 4 and exercise training: possible consequences in non-insulin-dependent diabetes mellitus. *Acta Physiol Scand*; 171:267–76.

de Alvaro C, Teruel T, Hernandez R, Lorenzo M. (2004) Tumor necrosis factor alpha produces insulin resistance in skeletal muscle by activation of inhibitor kappaB kinase in a p38 MAPK-dependent manner. *J Biol Chem*; 279:17070–8.

De Deyne PG, Hafer-Macko CE, Ivey FM, Ryan AS, Macko RF. (2004) Muscle molecular phenotype after stroke is associated with gait speed. *Muscle and Nerve*; 30:209–15.

Dean CM, Rissel C, Sharkey M, Sherrington C, Cumming RG, Barker RN, Lord SR, O'Rourke SD, Kirkham C. (2009) Exercise intervention to prevent falls and enhance mobility in community dwellers after stroke: a protocol for a randomised controlled trial. *BMC Neurol*; 9:38.

Dobkin BH, Firestine A, West M, Saremi K, Woods R. (2007) Ankle dorsiflexion as an fMRI paradigm to assay motor control for walking during rehabilitation. *Neuroimage*; 23(1):370–81.

Dobrovolny CL, Ivey FM, Rogers MA, Sorkin JD, Macko RF. (2003) Reliability of treadmill exercise testing in older patients with chronic hemiparetic stroke. *Arch Phys Med Rehabil*; 84, 1308–12.

Duncan P, Richards L, Wallace D, Stoker-Yates J, Pohl P, Luchies C, Ogle A, Studenski S. (1998) A randomized, controlled pilot study of a home-based exercise program for individuals with mild and moderate stroke. *Stroke* October; 29(10):2055–60.

Duncan P, Studenski S, Richards L, Gollub S, Lai SM, Reker D, Perera S, Yates J, Koch V, Rigler S, Johnson D. (2003) Randomized clinical trial of therapeutic exercise in subacute stroke. *Stroke*; 34:2173–80.

Eich HJ, Mach H, Werner C, Hesse S. (2004) Aerobic treadmill plus Bobath walking training improves walking in subacute stroke: A randomized controlled trial. *Clin Rehabil*; 18:640–51.

Eng JJ, Chu KS, Kim CM, Dawson AS, Carswell A, Hepburn KE. (2003) A community-based group exercise program for persons with chronic stroke. *Med Sci Sports Exerc*; 35:1271–78.

Enzinger C, Dawes H, Johansen-Berg H, Wade D, Bogdanovic M, Collett J, Guy C, Kischka U, Ropele S, Fazekas F, Matthews PM. (2009) Brain activity changes associated with treadmill training after stroke. *Stroke*; 40(7):2460–7.

Enzinger C, Johansen-Berg H, Dawes H, Bogdanovic M, Collett J, Guy C, Ropele S, Kischka U, Wade D, Fazekas F, Matthews PM. (2008) Functional MRI correlates of lower limb function in stroke victims with gait impairment. *Stroke*; 39(5):1507–13.

Fisher SV, Gullickson G, Jr. (1978) Energy cost of ambulation in health and disability: a literature review. *Arch Phys Med Rehabil*; March; 59(3): 124–33.

Flansbjer UB, Miller M, Downham D, Lexell J. (2008) Progressive resistance training after stroke: effects on muscle strength, muscle tone, gait performance and perceived participation. *J Rehabil Med*; 40(1):42–8.

Forrester LW, Wheaton LA, Luft AR. (2008) Exercise-mediated locomoter recovery and lower-limb neuroplasticity after stroke. *J Rehabil Res Dev*; 45(2):205–20.

Frontera WR, Grimby L, Larsson L. (1997) Firing rate of the lower motoneuron and contractile properties of its muscle fibers after upper motoneuron lesion in man. *Muscle Nerve* August; 20(8):938–47.

Fujitani J, Ishikawa T, Akai M, Kakurai S. (1999) Influence of daily activity on changes in physical fitness and walking ability in subacute stroke patients. *Arch Phys Med Rehabil*; 78:540–44.

Gordon NF, Gulanic M, Costa F, Fletcher G, Franklin BA, Roth EJ, Shephard T. (2004) Physical activity and exercise recommendations for stroke survivors: An American Heart Association Scientific Statement. *Circulation*; 109:2031–41.

Green DJ, Maiorana A, O'Driscoll G., Taylor R. (2004) Effect of exercise training on endothelium-derived nitric oxide function in humans. *J Physiol*; 561(Pt 1):1–25.

Greenberg SM. (2009) Memory, executive function, and dementia. In: Stein J, Harvey R, Macko R.F., Winstein CJ, Zorowitz R, (eds) *Stroke Recovery & Rehabilitation*. 1st edn. New York: DemosMedical; p. 213–20.

Greiwe J, Cheng B, Rubin DC. (2001) Resistance exercise decreases skeletal muscle tumor necrosis factor alpha in frail elderly humans. *FASEB J*; 15:475–82.

Hachisuka K, Umezu Y, Ogata H. (1997) Disuse muscle atrophy of lower limbs in hemiplegic patients. *Arch Phys Med Rehabil*; January; 78(1):13–8.

Hafer-Macko CE, Ryan AS, Ivey FM, Macko RF. (2008) Skeletal muscle changes after hemiparetic stroke and potential beneficial effects of exercise intervention strategies. *J Rehabil Res Dev*; 45(2):261–72.

Hafer-Macko CE, Yu S, Ryan AS, Ivey FM, Macko RF. (2005) Elevated tumor necrosis factor-alpha in skeletal muscle after stroke. *Stroke*; 36(9):2021–3.

Harris-Love ML, Forrester LW, Macko RF, Silver KH, Smith GV. (2001) Hemiparetic gait parameters in overground versus treadmill walking. *Neurorehabil Neural Repair*; 15(2):105–12.

Hesse S. (2008) Treadmill training with partial body weight support after stroke: a review. *NeuroRehabilitation*; 23(1):55–65.

Hesse S, Bertelt C, Jahnke MT, Schaffrin A, Baake P, Malezic M, Mauritz KH. (1995) Treadmill training with partial body weight support compared with physiotherapy in nonambulatory hemiparetic patients. *Stroke*; 26(6):976–81.

Hesse S, Bertelt C, Schaffrin A, Malezic M, Mauritz KH. (1994) Restoration of gait in nonambulatory hemiparetic patients by treadmill training with partial body-weight support. *Arch Phys Med Rehabil*; October;75(10):1087–93.

Hesse S, Konrad M, Uhlenbrock D. (1999) Treadmill walking with partial body weight support versus floor walking in hemiparetic subjects. *Arch Phys Med Rehabil*; April; 80(4):421–7.

Hidler J, Hamm LF, Lichy A, Groah SL. (2008) Automating activity-based interventions: The role of robotics. *J Rehabil Res Dev*; 45(2):337–44.

Hidler J, Nichols D, Pelliccio M, Brady K, Campbell DD, Kahn JH, Hornby TG. (2009) Multicenter randomized clinical trial evaluating the effectiveness of the Lokomat in subacute stroke. *Neurorehabil Neural Repair*; 23(1):5–13.

Hjelstuen A, Anderssen SA, Holme I, Seljeflot I, Klemsdal TO. (2006) Markers of inflammation are inversely related to physical activity and fitness in sedentary men with treated hypertension. *Am J Hypertens*; 19(7):669–75.

Hjeltnes N. (1982) Capacity for physical work and training after spinal injuries and strokes. *Scand J Soc Med Suppl*; 29:245–51.

Holloszy JO. (2005) Exercise-induced increase in muscle insulin sensitivity. *J Appl Physiol*; 99(1):338–43.

Hooker SP, Sui X, Colabianchi N, Vena J, Ladtika J, Lamonte MJ, Blair SN. (2008) Cardiorespiratory fitness as a predictor of fatal and nonfatal stroke in asymptomatic women and men. *Stroke*; 39(11):2950–7.

Hornby TG, Campbell DD, Kahn JH, Demott T, Moore JL, Roth HR. (2008) Enhanced gait-related improvements after therapist versus robotic-assisted locomotor training in subjects with chronic stroke: a randomized controlled study. *Stroke*; 39(6):1786–92.

Huey KA, Roy RR, Baldwin KM, Edgerton VR. (2001) Temporal effects of inactivty on myosin heavy chain gene expression in rat slow muscle. *Muscle Nerve*; 24:517–26.

Hunter RB, Stevenson E, Koncarevic A, Mitchell-Felton H, Essig DA, Kandarian SC. (2002) Activation of an alternative NF-kappaB pathway in skeletal muscle during disuase atrophy. *FASEB J*; 16:529–38.

Ivey FM, Gardner AW, Dobrovolny CL, Macko RF. (2004) Unilateral Impairment of leg blood flow in chronic stroke patients. *Cerebrovasc Dis*; 18(4):283–9.

Ivey FM, Hafer-Macko CE, Macko RF. (2006a) Exercise rehabilitation after stroke. *NeuroRx*; 3(4):439–50.

Ivey FM, Hafer-Macko CE, Macko RF. (2008) Task-oriented treadmill exercise training in chronic hemiparetic stroke. *J Rehabil Res Dev*; 45(2):249–59.

Ivey FM, Macko R.F. (2009) Prevention of Deconditioning after Stroke. In: Stein J, Harvey R, Macko R.F., Winstein CJ, Zorowitz R, (eds). *Stroke Recovery & Rehabilitation*. 1st edn. New York: DemosMedical;. p. 387–404.

Ivey FM, Macko R.F., Ryan A.S., Hafer-Macko CE. (2005) Cardiovscular health and fitness after stroke. *Top Stroke Rehabil*; 12(1):1–16.

Ivey FM, Ryan A.S., Hafer-Macko CE, Garrity BM, Sorkin JD, Goldberg AP, Macko RF. (2006b) High prevalence of abnormal glucose metabolism and poor sensitivity of fasting plasma glucose in the chronic phase of stroke. *Cerebrovasc Dis*; 22(5):368–71.

Ivey FM, Ryan AS, Hafer-Macko CE, Goldberg AP, Macko RF. (2007) Treadmill aerobic training improves glucose tolerance and indices of insulin sensitivity in disabled stroke survivors: A preliminary report. *Stroke*; 38(10):2752–8.

Jakobsson F, Edstrom L, Grimby L, Thornell LE. (1991) Disuse of anterior tibial muscle during locomotion and increased proportion of type II fibres in hemiplegia. *J Neurol Sci*; September; 105(1):49–56.

Jette M, Sidney K, Blumchen G. (1990) Metabolic equivalents (METS) in exercise testing, exercise prescription, and evaluation of functional capacity. *Clin Cardiol*; 13(8):555–65.

Jorgensen HS, Nakayama H, Raaschou HO, Olsen TS. (1995) Recovery of walking function in stroke patients: the Copenhagen Stroke Study. *Arch Phys Med Rehabil*; January; 76(1):27–32.

Jorgensen HS, Nakayama H, Raaschou HO, Vive-Larsen J, Stoier M, Olsen TS. (1995) Outcome and time course of recovery in stroke. Part II: Time course of recovery. The Copenhagen Stroke Study. *Arch Phys Med Rehabil*; 76(5):406–12.

Kandarian SC, Stevenson EJ. (2002)Molecular events in skeletal muscle during disuse atrophy. *Exerc Sport Sci Rev*; 30:111–6.

Katz-Leurer M, Shochina M, Carmeli E, Friedlander Y. (2003) The influence of early aerobic training on the functional capacity in patients with cerebrovascular accident at the subacute stage. *Arch Phys Med Rehabil*; 84:1609–14.

Kelly JO, Kilbreath SL, Davis GM, Zeman B, Raymond J. (2003) Cardiorespiratory fitness and walking ability in subacute stroke patients. *Arch Phys Med Rehabil*; 84:1780–85.

Kernan WN, Inzucchi SE, Viscoli CM, Brass LM, Bravata DM, Shulman GI, McVeety JC, Horwitz RI. (2003) Impaired insulin sensitivity among nondiabetic patients with a recent TIA or ischemic stroke. *Neurology*; 60(9):1447–51.

Kim CM, Eng JJ, MacIntyre DL, Dawson AS. (2001) Effects of isokinetic strength training on walking in persons with stroke: a double-blind controlled pilot study. *J Stroke and Cerebrovasc Dis*; 10(6):265–73.

Kopunek SP, Michael KM, Shaughnessy M, Resnick B, Nahm ES, Whitall J, Goldberg A, Macko RF. (2007) Cardiovascular risk in survivors of stroke. *Am J Prev Med*; 32(5):408–12.

Krebs HI, Mernoff S, Fasoli SE, Hughes R, Stein J, Hogan N. (2008) A comparison of functional and impairment-based robotic training in severe to moderate chronic stroke: a pilot study. *NeuroRehabilitation*; 23(1): 81–7.

Kryger AI, Andersen JL. (2007) Resistance training in the oldest old: consequences for muscle strength, fiber types, fiber size, and MHC isoforms. *Scand J Med Sci Sports*; 17(4):422–30.

Landin S, Hagenfeldt L, Saltin B, Wahren J. (1977) Muscle metabolism during exercise in hemiparetic patients. *Clin Sci Mol Med*; September; 53(3):257–69.

Laukanen JA, Kurl S, Salonen R, Rauramaa R, Salonen JT. (2004) The predictive value of cardiorespiratory fitness for cardiovascular events in men with various risk profiles: a prospective population-based cohort study. *Eur Heart J*; 25(16):1428–37.

Lee MJ, Kilbreath SL, Singh MF, Zeman B, Lord SR, Raymond J, Davis GM. (2008) Comparison of effect of aerobic cycle training and progressive resistance training on walking ability after stroke: a randomized sham exercise-controlled study. *J Am Geriatr Soc*; 56(6):976–85.

Lewek MD, Cruz TH, Moore JL, Roth HR, Dhaher YY, Hornby TG. (2009) Allowing intralimb kinematic vaiability during locomotor training poststroke improves linematic consistency: a subgroup analysis from a randomized clinical trial. *Phys Ther*; 89(8):829–39.

Lexell J, Flansbjer UB. (2008)Muscle strength training, gait performance and physiotherapy after stroke. *Minerva Med*; 99(4):353–68.

Liang W, Lee AH, Binns CW, Zhou Q, Huang R, Hu D. (2009) Habitual physical activity reduces the risk of ischemic stroke: a case-control study in southern China. *Cerebrovasc Dis*; 28(5):454–9.

Luft AR, Macko RF, Forrester LW, Villarga F, Ivey F, Sorkin JD, Whitall J, McCombe-Waller S, Katzel L, Goldberg AP, Hanley DF. (2008) Treadmill exercise activates subcortical neural networks and improves walking after stroke: a randomized controlled trial. *Stroke*; 39(12):3341–50.

Luft AR, McCombe-Waller S, Whitall J, Forrester LW, Macko R, Sorkin JD, Schulz JB, Goldberg AP, Hanley DF. (2004) Repetitive bilateral arm training and motor cortex activation in chronic stroke: a randomized controlled trial. *JAMA*; 292(15):1853–61.

Lum PS, Mulroy S, Amdur RL, Requejo P, Prilutsky BI, Dromerick AW. (2009) Gains in upper extremity function after stroke via recovery or compensation: potential differential effects on amount of real-world limb use. *Top Stroke Rehabil*; 16(4):237–53.

MacKay-Lyons MJ, Makrides L. (2002a) Cardiovascular stress during a contemporary stroke rehabilitation program: is the intensity adequate to induce a training effect? *Arch Phys Med Rehabil*; October; 83(10):1378–83.

MacKay-Lyons MJ, Makrides L. (2002b) Exercise capacity early after stroke. *Arch Phys Med Rehabil*; December; 83(12):1697–702.

Macko RF, Benvenuti F, Stanhope S, Macellari V, Taviani A, Nesi B, Weinrich M, Stuart M. (2008) Adaptive physical activity improves mobility function and quality of life in chronic hemiparesis. *J Rehab Res Dev*; 45(2):249–61.

Macko RF, DeSouza CA, Tretter LD, Silver KH, Smith GV, Anderson PA, Tomoyasu N, Gorman P, Dengel DR. (1997a) Treadmill aerobic exercise training reduces the energy expenditure and cardiovascular demands of hemiparetic gait in chronic stroke patients. A preliminary report. *Stroke* February; 28(2):326–30.

Macko RF, Ivey FM, Forrester LW. (2005a) Task-oriented aerobic exercise in chronic hemiparetic stroke: training protocols and treatment effects. *Top Stroke Rehabil*; 12(1):45–57.

Macko RF, Ivey FM, Forrester LW, Hanley D, Sorkin JD, Katzel LI, Silver KH, Goldberg AP. (2005b) Treadmill exercise rehabilitation improves ambulatory function and cardiovascular fitness in patients with chronic stroke: a randomized, controlled trial. *Stroke*; 36(10):2206–11.

Macko RF, Katzel LI, Yataco A, Tretter LD, DeSouza CA, Dengel DR, Smith GV, Silver KH. (1997b) Low-velocity graded treadmill stress testing in hemiparetic stroke patients. *Stroke* May; 28(5):988–92.

Macko RF, Smith GV, Dobrovolny CL, Sorkin JD, Goldberg AP, Silver KH. (2001) Treadmill training improves fitness reserve in chronic stroke patients. *Arch Phys Med Rehabil*; July; 82(7):879–84.

Marigold DS, Eng JJ, Dawson AS, Inglis JT, Harris JE, Gylfadottir S. (2005) Exercise leads to faster postural reflexes, improved balance and mobility, and fewer falls in older persons with chronic stroke. *J Am Geriatr Soc*; 53(3):416–23.

Martel GF, Roth SM, Ivey FM, Lemmer JT, Tracy BL, Hurlbut DE, Metter EJ, Hurley BF, Rogers MA. (2005) Age and sex affect human muscle fiber adaptations to heavy-resistance strength training. *Exp Physiol*; 91(2):457–64.

McCain KJ, Pollo FE, Baum BS, Coleman SC, Baker S, Smith PS. (2008) Locomotor treadmill training with partial body-weight support before overground gait in adults with acute stroke: a pilot study. *Arch Phys Med Rehabil*; 89(4):684–91.

McGuigan MR, Bronks R, Newton RU, Sharman MJ, Graham JC, Cody DV, Kraemer WJ. (2001) Resistance training in patients with peripheral arterial disease: effects on myosin isoforms, fiber type distribution, and capillary supply to skeletal muscle. *J Gerontol A Biol Sci Med Sci*; 56(7):B302–B310.

Michael K. (2002) Fatigue and stroke. *Rehabil Nurs* May; 27(3): 89–94, 103.

Michael K, Goldberg A, Treuth M, Beans J, Normandt P, Macko R.F. (2009) Progressive Adaptive Physical Activity in Stroke Improves Balance, Gait, and Fitness: Preliminary Results. *Top Stroke Rehabil*; 16, 133–9.

Michael KM, Allen JK, Macko RF. (2006) Fatigue after stroke: relationship to mobility, fitness, ambulatory activity, social support, and falls efficacy. *Rehabil Nurs*; 31(5): 210–7.

Mosely AM, Stark A, Cameron ID, Pollock A. (2004) *Treadmill raining and body weight support for walking after stroke* (Cochrane Review). Chichester, UK: John Wiley & Sons, Ltd.

Nilsson L, Carlsson J, Danielsson A, Fugl-Meyer A, Hellstrom K, Kristensen L, Sjolund B, Sunnerhagen KS, Grimby G. (2001) Walking training of patients with hemiparesis at an early stage after stroke: a comparison of walking training on a treadmill with body weight support and walking training on the ground. *Clin Rehabil*; 15(5):515–27.

NINDS (2006) National Institute of Neurological Disorders and Stroke: Report of the Stroke Progress Review Group, September. Available at: http://www.ninds.nih.gov/find_people/ groups/stroke_prg/09_2006_stroke_prg_report.htm. [Accessed 9 October 2009].

Noh DK, Lim JY, Shin HI, Paik NJ. (2008) The effect of aquatic therapy on postural balance and muscle strength in stroke survivors-a randomized controlled pilot trial. *Clin Rehabil*; 22(10):966–76.

Olney SJ, Monga TN, Costigan PA. (1986) Mechanical energy of walking of stroke patients. *Arch Phys Med Rehabil* February; 67(2):92–8.

Ouellette MM, LeBrasseur NK, Bean JF, Phillips E, Stein J, Frontera WR, Fielding RA. (2004) High-intensity resistance training improves muscle strength, self-reported function, and disability in long-term stroke survivors. *Stroke*; 35:1404.

Pak S, Patten C. (2008) Strengthening to promote functional recovery poststroke: an evidence-based review. *Top Stroke Rehabil*; 15(3):177–99.

Pang MY, Eng JJ, Dawson AS, McHay HA, Harris JE. (2005) A community-based fitness and mobility exercise program for older adults with chronic stroke. *J Am Geriatr Soc*; 53:1667–74.

Pang MY, Harris JE, Eng JJ. (2006) A community-based upper-extremity group exercise program improves motor function and performance of functional activities in chronic stroke: a randomized controlled trial. *Arch Phys Med Rehabil*; 87:1–9.

Paolucci S, Grasso MG, Antonucci G, Bragoni M, Troisi E, Morelli D, Coiro P, De Angelis D. (2001) Mobility status after inpatient stroke rehabilitation: 1-year follow-up and prognostic factors. *Arch Phys Med Rehabil*; 82(1):2–8.

Patten C, Lexell J, Brown HE. (2004) Weakness and strength training in persons with poststroke hemiplegia: Rationale, method, and efficacy. *J Rehabil Res Dev*; 41(3A):293–312.

Patterson SL, Rodgers MM, Macko RF, Forrester LW. (2008) Effect of treadmill exercise training on spatial and temporal gait parameters in subjects with chronic stroke: A preliminary report. *J Rehabil Res Dev*; 45(2):221–8.

Potempa K, Lopez M, Braun LT, Szidon JP, Fogg L, Tincknell T. (1995) Physiological outcomes of aerobic exercise training in hemiparetic stroke patients. *Stroke* January; 26(1):101–5.

Quaney B, Boyd L, McDowd J, Zahner L, He J, Mayo M, Macko R. (2009) Aerobic exercise improves cognition and motor function post-stroke. *Neurorehabilitation and Neural Repair*; 23, 879–885.

Resnick B, Michael K, Shaughnessy M, Kopunek S, Nahm ES, Macko RF. (2008) Motivators for treadmill exercise after stroke. *Top Stroke Rehabil*; 15(5):494–502.

Richards CL, Malouin F, Wood-Dauphinee S, Williams JL, Bouchard JP, Brunet D. (1993) Task specific physical therapy for optimization of gait recovery in acute stroke patients. *Archives of Physical Medicine and Rehabilitation*; 74:612–20.

Rimmer JH, Rauworth AE, Wang EC, Nicola TL, Hill B. (2009) A preliminary study to examine the effects of aerobic and therapeutic (nonaerobic) exercise on cardiorespiratory fitness and coronary risk reduction in stroke survivors. *Arch Phys Med Rehabil*; 90(3):407–12.

Rimmer JH, Riley B, Creviston T, Nicola T. (2000) Exercise training in a predominantly African-American group of stroke survivors. *Med Sci Sports Exerc*; December; 32(12):1990–6.

Rimmer JH, Wang E, Smith D. (2008) Barriers associated with exercise and community access for individuals with stroke. *J Rehabil Res Dev*; 45(2):315–22.

Rockwood K, Wentzel C, Hachinski V. (2009) Prevalence and outcomes of vascular cognitive impairment: Vascular Cognitive Impairment Investigators of the Canadian Study of Health and Aging. *Neurology*; 54(2):447–51.

Rosenwinkel ET, Bloomfield DM, Arwady MA, Goldsmith RL. (2001) Exercise and autonomic function in health and cardiovascular disease. *Cardiol Clin*; 19(3): 369–87.

Roth EJ. (1993)Heart disease in patients with stroke: incidence, impact, and implications for rehabilitation. Part 1: Classification and prevalence. *Arch Phys Med Rehabil*; 74:752–60.

Roth EJ. (1994) Heart disease in patients with stroke. Part II: Impact and implications for rehabilitation. *Arch Phys Med Rehabil*; 75:94–101.

Ryan A.S., Dobrovolny L., Silver KH, Smith GV, Macko R.F. (2000) Cardiovascular fitness after stroke: role of muscle mass and gait deficit severity. *J Stroke Cerebrovasc Disorders*; 9:1–8.

Ryan AS, Dobrovolny CL, Smith GV, Silver KH, Macko RF. (2002) Hemiparetic muscle atrophy and increased intramuscular fat in stroke patients. *Arch Phys Med Rehabil*; December; 83(12):1703–7.

Saghizadeh M, Ong JM, Garvey WT, Henry RR, Kern PA. (1996) The expression of TNF alpha by human muscle: Relationship to insulin resistance. *J Clin Invest*; 97:1111–6.

Scelsi R, Lotta S, Lommi G, Poggi P, Marchetti C. (1984) Hemiplegic atrophy. Morphological findings in the anterior tibial muscle of patients with cerebral vascular accidents. *Acta Neuropathol*; 62:324–31.

Schmidt RA, Lee TD. (1999) *Motor control and learning: A behavioral emphasis*. 3rd edn. Champaign, IL: Human Kinetics.

Shaughnessy M, Resnick BM. (2009) Using theory to develop an exercise intervention for patients post stroke. *Top Stroke Rehabil*; 16(2):140–6.

Silver KH, Macko RF, Forrester LW, Goldberg AP, Smith GV. (2000) Effects of aerobic treadmill training on gait velocity, cadence, and gait symmetry in chronic hemiparetic stroke: a preliminary report. *Neurorehabil Neural Repair*; 14(1):65–71.

Sims J, Galea M, Taylor N, Dodd K, Jespersen S, Joubert L, Joubert J. (2009) Assessing the feasibility of a strength-training program to enhance the physical and mental health of chronic post stroke patients with depression. *Int J Geriatr Psychiatry*; 24(1):76–83.

States RA, Pappas E, Salem Y. (2009) Overground physical therapy gait training for chronic stroke patients with mobility deficits. *Cochrane Database Syst Rev*;3: CD006075.

Stroud N, Mazwi TM, Case LD, Brown RD, Brott TG, Worall BB, Meschia JF, Ischemic Stroke Genetics Study Investigators. (2009) Prestroke physical activity and early functional status after stroke. *J Neurol Neurosurg Psychiatry*; 80(9):1019–22.

Stuart M, Benvenuti F, Macko R, Taviani A, Segenni L, Mayer F, Sorkin JD, Stanhope SJ, Macellari V, Weinrich M. (2009) Community-based adaptive physical activity program for chronic stroke: feasibility, safety, and efficacy of the Empoli model. *Neurorehabil Neural Repair*; 23(7):726–34.

Sullivan KJ, Brown DA, Klassen T, Mulroy S, Ge T, Azen SP, Winstein CJ. (2007) Effects of task-specific locomoter and strength training in adults who were ambulatory after stroke: results of the STEPS randomized clinical trial. *Phys Ther*; 87(12):1580–602.

Sullivan KJ, Knowlton BJ, Dobkin BH. (2002) Step training with body weight support: Effect of treadmill speed and practice paradigms on poststroke locomotor recovery. *Arch Phys Med Rehabil*; May; 83(5):683–91.

Tang A, Sibley KM, Thomas SG, Bayley MT, Richardson D, McIlroy WE, Brooks D. (2009) Effects of an aerobic exercise program on aerobic capacity, spatiotemporal gait parameters, and functional capacity in subacute stroke. *Neurorehabilitation and Neural Repair*; 23(4):398–406.

Tatemichi TK, Paik M, Bagiella E. (1994) Risk of dementia after stroke in a hospitalized cohort: Results of a longitudinal study. *Neurology*; 44(10):1885–91.

Teixeira-Salmela L, Olney SJ, Nadeau S, Brouwer B. (1999) Muscle strengthening and physical conditioning to reduce impairment and disability in chronic stroke survivors. *Arch Phys Med Rehabil*; 80:1211–8.

Timmermans AA, Seelen HA, Willmann RD, Kingma H. (2009) Technology-assisted training of arm-hand skills in stroke: concepts on reacquisition of motor control and therapist guidelines for rehabilitation technology design. *J Neuroeng Rehabil*; 6:1.

USDHHS. (1995). *Post-Stroke Rehabilitation: Clinical Practice Guideline*. AHCPR; Report No.: 95–0662.

Vearrier LA, Langan J, Shumway-Cook A, Woollacott M. (2005) An intensive massed practice approach to retraining balance post-stroke. *Gait Posture*; 22(2):154–63.

Vermeer SE, Sandee W, Algra A, Koudstaal PJ, Kappelle LJ, Dippel DW, Dutch TIA Trial Study Group. (2006) Impaired glucose tolerance increases stroke risk in nondiabetic patients with transient ischemic attack or minor ischemic stroke. *Stroke*; 37(6):1413–7.

Visintin M, Barbeau H, Korner-Bitensky N, Mayo NE. (1998) A new approach to retrain gait in stroke patients through body weight support and treadmill stimulation. *Stroke*; 29:1122–8.

Winstein CJ, Wolf SL. (2009) Task-oriented training to promote upper extremity recovery. In: Stein J, Harvey R, Macko R.F., Winstein CJ, Zorowitz R, (eds) *Stroke Recovery & Rehabilitation*. 1st edn. New York: DemosMedical; p. 267–90.

Wolf SL, Winstein CJ, Miller JP, Taub E, Uswatte G, Morris D, Giuliani C, Light KE, Nichols-Larsen D. (2006) Effect of constraint-induced movement therapy on upper extremity function 3 to 9 months after stroke: the EXCITE randomized clinical trial. *JAMA*; 296(17):2095–104.

Womack CJ, Nagelkirk PR, Coughlin AM. (2003) Exercise-induced changes in coagulation and fibrinolysis in healthy populations and patients with cardiovascular disease. *Sports Med*; 33(11):795–807.

5

PERIPHERAL ARTERIAL DISEASE/ INTERMITTENT CLAUDICATION

Garry Tew and Irena Zwierska

Introduction

Peripheral arterial disease (PAD) is a common circulatory problem character-ised by obstruction of blood flow in the arteries outside of the heart and brain. It is usually caused by atherosclerosis, a hardening and narrowing of the arteries. As atherosclerosis is a systemic disease process, many patients with PAD also have coronary artery and cerebrovascular disease (Norgren *et al.*, 2007). For the purpose of this chapter, PAD refers to advanced arterial atherosclerosis of the lower-limbs.

PAD comprises a wide clinical spectrum ranging from individuals with asymptomatic arterial narrowing to those with the common symptom of inter-mittent claudication and, at the severe end of the spectrum, those with critical limb ischaemia. The ankle-to-brachial systolic blood pressure index (ABPI) is commonly used to help diagnose PAD. An ABPI of 0.7–0.9 is considered mild disease, 0.5–0.69 moderate, and <0.5 severe. Intermittent claudication is a cramp-like leg pain that occurs during walking (and is relieved by rest), when the ability to deliver and utilise oxygen is inadequate to meet the metabolic requirement of the active skeletal muscles. It causes a marked reduction in functional capacity (Regensteiner and Hiatt, 1995) and quality of life (Regensteiner *et al.*, 2008).

Among patients with intermittent claudication, most (~75 per cent) show no change in symptoms or an improvement in functional status, presumably due to development of collateral blood flow (Fowkes, 2001). Symptoms worsen in 25 per cent of patients, with about 5 per cent requiring amputation within 5 years and about 5 to 10 per cent developing critical limb ischaemia (Dormandy and Murray, 1991). Patients with intermittent claudication have a 5-year mortality rate of 15–30 per cent, with 75 per cent of these deaths attributed to cardiovascular causes (Weitz *et al.*, 1996). A further 20 per cent of claudicants will have a non-fatal cardiovascular event within 5 years (Weitz *et al.*, 1996).

For patients with intermittent claudication, conservative, non-operative therapy, including exercise training, cardiovascular risk factor modificaton and/or pharmacotherapy (e.g. cilostazol) is generally the treatment of choice. This approach is based on the fact that many patients have diffuse disease and the marginal long-term benefits of surgery in relation to risk of limb loss (Taylor *et al.*, 2008). Revascularisation procedures (e.g. angioplasty or bypass surgery) are thought to be necessary in <10 per cent of patients with intermittent claudication (Rowlands and Donnelly, 2007), and is generally reserved for those with proximal (aorto-iliac) disease, lifestyle/occupation limiting symptoms and/ or for those where conservative management has failed (Norgren *et al.*, 2007).

Objective assessment of walking performance in intermittent claudication

Treadmill walking tests are often used to assess functional capacity in patients with PAD. Following a transatlantic conference on clinical trials guidelines in PAD (Labs *et al.*, 1999), two internationally accepted treadmill protocols were recommended: (i) constant-pace treadmill protocol (constant walking speed of 3.2 km·h^{-1} at 12 per cent gradient) and (ii) graded (incremental) treadmill protocol (starting horizontally at a constant speed of 3.2 km·h^{-1}, but with the gradient increasing in pre-defined steps (e.g. 2 per cent) at pre-defined time intervals (e.g. every 2 minutes)). The main variables measured are (i) distance to the onset of claudication pain (CD) and (ii) maximum walking distance (MWD), at which point patients can no longer continue, usually because of intolerable claudication pain. The latter measure is used most frequently in clinical trials as the primary end-point. The 6-minute walk test is an alternative to treadmill testing, which is highly reproducible, valid and sensitive to change in patients with claudication (Gardner *et al.*, 1998; Montgomery and Gardner, 1998). Advantages of this test include the lack of need for special equipment and that it provides a better approximate of community walking compared to treadmill walking in older patients (McDermott *et al.*, 2008). Accelerometry data are also sometimes used to quantify physical activity in daily life.

Exercise rehabilitation

Functional capacity

Few studies have investigated the impact of exercise training on functional capacity in asymptomatic PAD. Nevertheless, the available evidence supports its efficacy. For example, a prospective study indicated that patients with asymptomatic PAD who walked for exercise ≥3 times per week had lower annual functional decline than those who walked less frequently (McDermott *et al.*, 2006). More recently, a randomised controlled trial conducted by McDermott *et al.* (2009) provided further evidence for clinicians to recommend exercise training for PAD patients, regardless of whether they have classic symptoms of intermittent claudication.

Exercise therapy to improve functional status in claudicants was first suggested by Erb in 1898 (cited in Gardner and Afaq, 2008), with the first randomised controlled trial published in 1966, demonstrating an improvement in treadmill walking ability (Larsen and Lassen, 1966). Data from several subsequent meta-analyses and systematic reviews support this finding (Gardner and Poehlman, 1995; Leng *et al.*, 2000; Bulmer and Coombes, 2004, Watson *et al.*, 2008). However, the magnitude of improvement appears to vary greatly and is largely dependent upon the frequency, intensity, duration and type of exercise training, and the method of assessment (e.g. incremental vs. constant-intensity tests). Indeed, the improvement in CD after exercise training has been reported to range from 44–746 per cent with MWD increasing by 25–765 per cent (Nehler *et al.*, 2003; Gardner and Afaq, 2008).

A meta-analysis of 21 randomised and non-randomised exercise rehabilitation studies from 1966–1993 revealed an mean improvement in CD of 179 per cent (126–351 m), and an mean improvement in MWD of 122 per cent (326–723 m) (Gardner and Poehlman, 1995). Similarly, a systematic review of 22 studies showed a median improvement of 119 per cent in CD and 83 per cent in MWD (Bulmer and Coombes, 2004). Consistent with these findings, a recent prospective study among patients with symptomatic PAD showed that self-directed walking exercise was associated with significantly less functional decline when performed ≥3 times versus 1–2 times per week (McDermott *et al.*, 2006). Higher baseline physical activity levels, as measured by a vertical accelerometer, also appear to be associated with a lower annual decline in 6-minute walk performance, fast-paced 4 m walking velocity and general physical performance in persons with PAD (Garg *et al.*, 2009). Exercise-induced improvements in walking performance appear to translate to enhanced community-based functional capacity (Regensteiner *et al.*, 1996).

Most of the studies described above involved walking exercise training. Although walking is the most specific exercise for treating patients' ambulatory dysfunction, there is evidence that other modes of exercise can also be beneficial, including stationary cycling (Walker *et al.*, 2000; Zwierska *et al.*, 2005), stair-climbing (Jones *et al.*, 1996) and arm-cranking (Walker *et al.*, 2000; Zwierska *et al.*, 2005; Tew *et al.*, 2009). The latter of these might be particularly useful for developing tolerance to exercise and overcoming barriers in patients who are initially unwilling or unable to perform lower-limb exercise, because of the pain experienced.

Cardiovascular morbidity and mortality

Compared to age-matched individuals without PAD, all-cause mortality of claudicants is increased by 3.1-fold and coronary artery disease mortality by 6.6-fold (Criqui *et al.*, 1992). The risk of stroke is increased by approximately 40 per cent

(Hirsch *et al.*, 2006). The annual mortality rate derived from epidemiological studies is 4–6 per cent for patients with intermittent claudication (Criqui *et al.*, 1992; McDermott *et al.*, 1994) and 25–45 per cent for those with critical limb ischaemia (Criqui *et al.*, 1992; Dormandy *et al.*, 1999). Therefore, a key goal of treatment for patients with intermittent claudication is cardiovascular risk reduction.

Despite it being well established that physically fit/active individuals have a reduced risk of developing cardiovascular disease (Blair *et al.*, 2001), few studies have investigated the effects of physical fitness/activity on cardiovascular morbidity and mortality in patients with intermittent claudication. A retrospective study by Sakamoto *et al.* (2009) indicated that patients who completed a 12-week supervised treadmill-walking programme had reduced cardiovascular mortality and morbidity compared with those who did not, at a follow-up of 5.7 ± 3.9 years. Garg *et al.* (2006) also reported a 3.5-fold increased risk of mortality in patients in the lowest quartile of physical activity. Gardner *et al.* (2008) also reported that patients who engaged in any amount of weekly physical activity beyond light intensity at baseline had a lower mortality rate than their more-sedentary counterparts when followed for a median of 64-months. Therefore, the available evidence suggests that exercise training reduces cardiovascular morbidity and mortality in patients with intermittent claudication.

There are several potential mechanisms by which exercise training could reduce cardiovascular risk in patients with intermittent claudication. First, exercise training has the potential to reduce the risk of cardiovascular ischaemic events via modification of traditional cardiovascular risk factors, such as hypertension and hypercholesteroloaemia. Second, it might reduce cardiovascular risk via an improvement in coronary-artery endothelial function. Indeed, exercise training has been shown to improve brachial-artery flow-mediated dilatation (a surrogate measure of coronary artery endothelial function) in patients with intermittent claudication (Brendle *et al.*, 2001; Andreozzi *et al.*, 2007; McDermott *et al.*, 2009). Third, there is evidence that exercise training can reduce cardiovascular risk by lowering inflammatory and thrombogenic factors that are implicated in the pathogenesis of acute cardiovascular events (Tisi *et al.*, 1997). Finally, other less established cardiovascular risk factors that can impact on patients with intermittent claudication, such as autonomic function, depression and psychosocial stress (Smith *et al.*, 2004), have also been shown to be favourably modified in patients undergoing cardiac rehabilitation (Milani *et al.*, 1996; Lucini *et al.*, 2002; Lavie and Milani, 2006).

Atherosclerosis progression

Atherosclerosis progression is also a useful surrogate marker for predicting future cardiovascular events (Revkin *et al.*, 2007). Unfortunately, data from human exercise studies are inconsistent with some studies demonstrating regression of coronary-artery atherosclerotic lesions (Schuler *et al.*, 1992; Hambrecht *et al.*, 1993), and others reporting no change in carotid-artery atherosclerosis (Rauramaa *et al.*, 2004; Meyer *et al.*, 2006). These discordant findings might be explained by differences in study populations and methods used. Furthermore, neither coronary angiography nor intima-media thickness measurements provide comprehensive assessment of atherosclerotic plaque burden in the lower-limbs.

Plausible mechanisms underpinning the regression of atherosclerosis with exercise training include glucose regulation, weight loss, fat redistribution/loss, amelioration of endothelial dysfunction and improvement of insulin sensitivity and cardiopulmonary fitness (Kadoglou *et al.*, 2008). Other potential mechanisms include lipid lowering, anti-thrombotic/fibrinolytic effects, suppression of elevated blood pressure levels and modification of novel cardiovascular risk factors (e.g. inflammatory cytokines) (Kadoglou *et al.*, 2008).

Claudication symptoms

Exercise training promotes symptomatic relief, as reflected by large improvements in walking performance. However, the mechanisms by which exercise training reduces claudication symptoms are not fully understood. Potential mechanisms can be sub-divided into those that improve blood flow and oxygen delivery to active skeletal muscles, those that improve skeletal muscle metabolism, and those that reduce the metabolic demands of ambulation.

Changes in blood flow and oxygen delivery to active skeletal muscles

Chronic exercise training can stimulate various physiological adaptations that would enhance muscle blood flow during walking in patients with intermittent claudication. These adaptations include enhanced cardiac function, capillarisation, collateralisation, improved endothelial function, and changes in blood volume and rheology. Therefore, an improved muscle blood supply is a plausible contributory mechanism for the reduction in claudication symptoms after exercise training.

Few studies have investigated the importance of improved cardiac function and adjustments to total peripheral resistance in relation to exercise intolerance in claudicants or the effects of exercise training on this variable. Hodges and colleagues demonstrated that cardiac function is impaired in patients with intermittent claudication (Hodges *et al.*, 2006) and unaffected by exercise training (Hodges *et al.*, 2008). This is in contrast to studies that have reported reductions in sub-maximal exercise heart rate after exercise training (Tan *et al.*, 2000; Walker *et al.*, 2000), which is indicative of enhanced cardiac stroke volume. Therefore, further research is needed to clarify the role of central adaptations in symptomatic improvement with exercise training.

Increases in muscle capillary density and capillary-to-fibre ratio should facilitate improved oxygen and nutrient exchange within the tissue by providing an increased blood transit time, a larger surface area and shorter diffusion distance. Although muscle capillarisation is a well-known physiological adaptation to exercise training in healthy older adults (Rogers and Evans, 1993), data for patients with intermittent claudication is sparse and inconclusive (Wang *et al.*, 2009).

An increase in muscle blood flow, secondary to the development of an effective collateral circuit that bypasses areas of arterial stenosis/occlusion is a further potential mechanism. While there is compelling evidence from animal models of peripheral arterial disease that collateral blood flow can be increased by exercise training (Weiss *et al.*, 1992, Yang *et al.*, 1995), this adaptation does not appear to be widespread among claudicants who participate in an exercise programme (Leng *et al.*, 2000; Tan *et al.*, 2000). This apparent contradiction might be explained by the fact that, unlike in animal models, human intermittent claudication often involves multiple levels of obstruction. This presents exceptional demands for the development of an effective collateral circuit, since it must accommodate successive obstructions with increasingly poorer perfusion pressure at each level. Alternatively, it is possible that improvements in collateral blood flow have been induced by exercise training, but not appropriately measured. It remains difficult to accurately measure collateral blood flow in humans.

Other researchers have proposed the concept of enhanced blood redistribution after exercise training (Sorlie and Myhre, 1978). This change could possibly occur via improved endothelium-dependent vasodilator function of the peripheral arteries and arterioles. Patients with PAD have decreased peripheral-artery endothelial function compared to age-matched healthy controls (Yataco *et al.*, 1999), and this appears to be due, at least in part, to increased oxidative stress (Loffredo *et al.*, 2007). While acute high-intensity exercise worsens endothelial function (Rossi *et al.*, 2002; Andreozzi *et al.*, 2007), chronic exercise training improves it (Brendle *et al.*, 2001; Andreozzi *et al.*, 2007; McDermott *et al.*, 2009). The mechanisms underpinning this observation are not fully understood, although it has been suggested that they could be nitric oxide (NO)-dependent. Regular exercise participation could improve NO-mediated vasodilator function through a shear stress-mediated increase in endothelial NO synthase expression (Green *et al.*, 2004) and/or an upregulation of antioxidant defence capacity (Franzoni *et al.*, 2004). Exercise training-induced increases in skeletal muscle blood flow might also occur due to an improvement in vascular smooth muscle responsiveness to NO (Colleran *et al.*, 2010).

Finally, aerobic exercise training is well known to increase blood volume, primarily through an increase in blood plasma volume (Wilmore and Costill, 1999). This results in a relative increase in the fluid portion of the blood, which reduces the blood's viscosity and facilitates the movement of blood through blood vessels. However, the exact contribution of this change to the reduction in claudication symptoms after exercise training is unclear.

Changes in skeletal muscle metabolism

Factors distal to the arterial obstruction, such as skeletal muscle metabolic abnormalities, also appear to contribute to exercise intolerance in intermittent claudication (Brass and Hiatt, 2000). Skeletal muscle metabolic abnormalities include altered mitochondrial expression, accumulation of metabolic intermediates (e.g. acylcarnitine), altered control of mitochondrial respiration, mitochondrial electron transport chain dysfunction and increased oxidative stress (Brass and Hiatt, 2000; Pipinos et al., 2007). These changes are likely to be the result of the inflammatory and reactive oxygen species production cascade, associated with walking-induced ischaemia and reperfusion (Pipinos et al., 2008).

Exercise training is a potent regulator of metabolic enzymes in normal individuals (Holloszy and Coyle, 1984). Supporting the concept that exercise rehabilitation modifies muscle metabolism in intermittent claudication, plasma acylcarnitine concentrations (intermediates of oxidative metabolism) decrease with training and this decrease is correlated with the magnitude of improved function (Hiatt et al., 1990; Hiatt et al., 1996). Whilst cause and effect cannot be determined in this relationship, this observation suggests that localised skeletal muscle adaptations might contribute to the improvement in claudication symptoms after lower-limb exercise training.

Changes in the metabolic demands of ambulation

Patients with intermittent claudication have an altered walking gait that favours stability over speed (Gardner et al., 2001a; McDermott et al., 2001). This causes an increase in the oxygen cost of walking (decreased economy), which contributes to the development of claudication pain at slow walking speeds. Regular walking exercise appears to improve walking economy in patients with intermittent claudication (Gardner et al., 2001b, 2002), and this might contribute to the reduction in claudication symptoms. Although improvements in walking economy are probably due to alterations in walking biomechanics, the available evidence suggests that walking gait is unchanged after long-term exercise training (Crowther et al., 2008). An increase in the proportion of oxidative muscle fibres might also be implicated; however, further research is needed to investigate this in patients with intermittent claudication.

In summary, the exact mechanisms of symptomatic improvement with exercise training are not fully understood, but probably include changes in muscle blood flow, muscle metabolism and walking economy.

Quality of life

Quality of life assessment tools

An important goal of healthcare is improvement in quality of life. Research tools that are commonly used to evaluate quality of life in these patients may be generic or disease-specific. Generic measures include the Medical Outcomes Study Short-Form 36 (SF-36) questionnaire, EuroQol Health Assessment, Nottingham Health Profile, Sickness Impact Profile, Quality of Well-Being Scale and World Health

Organization Quality of Life instrument. PAD-specific measures include the Walking Impairment Questionnaire (WIQ) and the Edinburgh Claudication, San Diego Claudication, Vascular Quality of Life and Claudication Scale questionnaires.

In PAD, the most commonly used generic questionnaire is the SF-36 *v2*, since it is both reliable and valid (Wann-Hansson *et al.*, 2004). This instrument encompasses eight quality of life domains; four specifically relating to physical health (general health, physical functioning, role limitation physical and bodily pain) and four relating to mental status (mental health, energy and vitality, role limitation emotional and social functioning). Most of the eight domains have been shown to be associated with objective measures of disease severity, such as ABPI, in patients with intermittent claudication (Izquierdo-Porrera *et al.*, 2005).

It has been suggested that when using the SF-36, a disease-specific measure should also be administered (Brazier *et al.*, 1992). The most commonly-used disease-specific measure is the WIQ, which assesses the ability of individuals to walk defined distances and speeds, and climb stairs (Hiatt *et al.*, 1995). It also evaluates symptoms (e.g. calf pain, shortness of breath, chest pain, joint pain) that could limit ambulation. A further instrument specifically developed for use in patients with lower-limb ischaemia is the Vascular Quality of Life questionnaire. It encompasses five domains (activity, symptom, pain, emotion and social functioning) and has been shown to be suitable for measuring the effects of interventions on quality of life in these patients (Morgan *et al.*, 2001).

Impact of intermittent claudication on quality of life

The loss of walking ability and the experience of pain with ambulation result in the deterioration of physical and emotional well-being in patients with intermittent claudication (Spronk *et al.*, 2007). Indeed, Pell (1995) reported that, compared with population norms, all health-related quality-of-life scores were lower in claudicants. Khaira *et al.* (1996) reported that patients with claudication have greater perceived problems in the areas of energy, pain, emotional reactions, sleep and physical mobility than healthy controls. Patients with claudication have also reported significant limitations in physical and social functioning, feelings of uncertainty and fear, and a sense of compromise of self (Nehler *et al.*, 2003). Therefore, intermittent claudication appears to impact adversely on quality of life. However, the magnitude of impairment can vary widely, depending on factors such as the patient's lifestyle, severity of claudication symptoms and co-morbidities (Binnie *et al.*, 1999).

Effects of exercise training on quality of life

Changes in physical health

Improvements in the range of 38–67 per cent in the physical functioning (Regensteiner *et al.*, 1996, 1997) and bodily pain (Patterson *et al.*, 1997;

Gardner *et al.*, 2004) domains of generic quality of life instruments have been reported after 12–24 weeks of supervised walking exercise training in claudicants. Improvements in the physical functioning and role-limitation physical domains of the SF-36 have also been seen after 6 weeks of supervised upper-limb aerobic exercise training (Walker *et al.*, 2000). In contrast, there were no changes in the physical health components of the SF-36 survey after 6-month (Gardner *et al.*, 2001b) and 12-month (Currie *et al.*, 1995) programmes of walking exercise. Several factors might explain these discrepant findings, including differences in study populations and exercise prescription characteristics.

Changes in mental health

Changes in mental health status are not usually apparent after exercise training in patients with intermittent claudication (Regensteiner *et al.*, 1996; Tsai *et al.*, 2002). This might be because the physical dimensions of quality of life, such as physical functioning and bodily pain, are the most relevant dimensions to intermittent claudication (Spronk *et al.*, 2007). Alternatively, improvements in mental health status might lag behind the improvements in functional capacity after exercise training (Tsai *et al.*, 2002).

Recommendations for exercise prescription

Exercise prescription should be developed with careful consideration of the individual's health status (including medications), risk factor profile, behavioural characteristics, personal goals and exercise preferences. The effectiveness of an exercise programme depends upon the mode(s), intensity, duration, frequency and progression of physical activity and the optimal exercise prescription will vary between different patients. The exercise guidelines described below are for patients with mild-to-moderate intermittent claudication, although they might also be useful for asymptomatic patients with PAD and those with atypical leg symptoms.

General recommendations

Exercise mode

The meta-analysis of Gardner and Poehlman (1995) demonstrated that programmes consisting of walking exercise were about twice as effective at improving walking performance compared to those that included other exercise modalities. This is probably because the specific muscles that become ischaemic during exercise (e.g. the calf muscles) are recruited during walking exercise, enabling favourable adaptations to occur. This is not to say that other modalities are not useful. Indeed, studies have demonstrated improved cardiopulmonary fitness and/or improved walking performance after programmes of stationary cycling (Walker *et al.*, 2000; Zwierska *et al.*, 2005), pole-striding (Collins *et al.*, 2005), stair-climbing (Jones *et al.*, 1996) and arm-cranking (Walker *et al.*, 2000; Zwierska *et al.*, 2005; Tew *et al.*, 2009). These alternative modalities might be prescribed to patients who are unwilling or unable to perform walking exercise because of the pain encountered. They might also be used to provide variety to help overcome other barriers. Resistance training can also serve as an adjunct treatment for improving muscular strength and endurance; however, it should not be used as a substitute for aerobic exercise.

Exercise intensity

For treadmill walking exercise, the evidence suggests that patients should walk at a speed and grade that evokes moderate claudication pain within 3–5 minutes (Hirsch *et al.*, 2006), at which time they rest until the pain subsides. Intermittent exercise is strongly recommended, as poor fitness and claudication pain make continuous exercise difficult. The speed or grade should be progressed if the patient can walk continuously for ≥10 minutes without moderate claudication pain. A goal should be to increase walking speed up to 4.8 $km \cdot h^{-1}$ (3 $miles \cdot h^{-1}$) from the average patient walking speed of 2.4–3.2 $km \cdot h^{-1}$ (1.5–2 $miles \cdot h^{-1}$) (Norgren *et al.*, 2007).

Improvements in walking distances have been reported to be >3 times greater when patients walk to near-maximal claudication pain versus the onset of claudication pain (Gardner and Poehlman 1995). In contrast, Gardner *et al.* (2005) reported that walking at 40 per cent maximum exercise capacity was equally as effective as 80 per cent maximum exercise capacity for improving walking performance, providing that a few additional minutes of exercise is accomplished in the lower-intensity sessions to accumulate a similar volume of exercise. Similarly, programmes of pain-free walking exercise have been shown to elicit clinically meaningful improvements in walking performance (Barak *et al.*, 2009; Martinez *et al.*, 2009). Therefore, it appears that development of claudication pain during exercise is not obligatory for improvements in walking performance to occur and this is also supported by arm cranking studies (Walker *et al.* 2005; Zwierska *et al.* 2005; Tew *et al.* 2009).

Exercise duration (min per session) and frequency (sessions per week) of exercise

The improvement in maximum walking distance appears to be much greater when exercise is performed for >30 min per session and ≥3 sessions per week compared to ≤30 minutes per session and <3 sessions per week (Gardner and Poehlman, 1995). As the patient adapts to the exercise programme and muscle fatigue becomes minimal 24 hours after exercise, the frequency should gradually increase from three times per week to an additional day every one to two weeks. The initial duration should be 35 minutes of aerobic exercise, and ideally increasing by 5 minutes each week until 50 to 60 minutes can be accomplished. Ideally, the goal for patients with PAD would be to exercise daily for at least 30 minutes.

Length of programme (weeks/months)

Exercise-induced functional benefits have been observed as early as six weeks after the start of an exercise training programme (Walker *et al.* 2000; Sanderson *et al.* 2006) and appear to continue to improve over six months of participation (Manfredini *et al.*, 2008). Few studies have extended beyond six months. Gardner *et al.* (2002) reported that improvements in walking distances after six months of supervised exercise rehabilitation were sustained when patients continued in an exercise maintenance programme for an additional twelve months. The key elements of an exercise programme for patients with mild-to-moderate PAD are summarised in Table 5.1.

Exercise adherence considerations

Cognitive factors such as stress, motivation to participate in exercise training and the belief that the therapy is beneficial appear to relate to improvements in walking distances (Rosfors *et al.*, 1990). An individualised, progressive and structured exercise training programme is recommended, since this affords the lowest possible risks of complications and takes into account the patient's comorbidities and medications that might necessitate close supervision by the patient's general practitioner or vascular surgeon.

Exercise training should ideally be supervised, since this elicits greater improvements in pain-free and maximum walking distances (Bendermacher *et al.*, 2006). However, adherence to supervised walking exercise can be difficult for many patients with claudication. This is reflected in the high drop-out rates of about 30 per cent from walking programmes (Womack *et al.*, 1997), due mainly to fear that claudication pain might cause some damage and/or the perception that going for a walk is not possible (Binnie *et al.*, 1999). Therefore, patients need to be assured that walking with claudication pain will not cause harm and will ultimately result in better physical function.

Exercise safety issues

Adverse cardiovascular and physiological responses during exercise training are possible in these patients, and this risk should be evaluated clinically before initiation of an exercise programme. Patients should ideally perform a standard treadmill exercise test with 12–lead electrocardiographic monitoring if available, before a therapeutic exercise programme is initiated (Hirsch *et al.*, 2006), to determine that there are no untoward cardiovascular responses during exercise. It will also provide information about claudication thresholds and heart rate and blood pressure responses for establishing an exercise prescription. In best practice it is generally recommended that heart rate, exertion and ischaemic symptoms are always monitored, given that an improvement in exercise tolerance might unmask myocardial ischaemia.

TABLE 5.1 Key elements of an exercise training programme for patients with mild-to-moderate PAD (adapted from Hirsch *et al.*, 2006)

Primary clinician role

Establish patient history and the clinical diagnosis of PAD
Determine that claudication is the major symptom limiting exercise
Discuss risk/benefit of claudication therapeutic alternatives, including pharmacological, percutaneous and surgical interventions
Initiate systemic atherosclerosis risk modification
Perform treadmill stress testing
Provide formal referral to a claudication exercise rehabilitation programme

---

Exercise guidelines for claudication*

Warm-up and cool-down period of five to 10 minutes each
Mode
  Walking is the most effective exercise for reducing claudication pain
  Other forms of aerobic exercise (e.g. cycling, stepping, arm-cranking) might be useful
  for patients who are unwilling or unable to perform walking exercise, or for variety
  Resistance training has conferred benefit to individuals with other forms of
  cardiovascular disease, and its use, as tolerated, for general fitness is complementary
  to, but not a substitute for walking
Intensity
  Commence at 50, with a gradual increase to 70 to 80% of heart rate reserve (as
  determined using the Karvonen formula)
Speed
  The speed and/or grade of walking should be set to elicit claudication symptoms
  within three to five minutes, at which point brief rest is recommended to let symptoms
  subside, after which walking should be recommenced and this cycle repeated
Duration
  The exercise–rest–exercise pattern should be repeated throughout the exercise session
  The initial duration will usually include 35 min of intermittent walking and should
  be increased by 5 min per week until 50 to 60 minutes of intermittent walking can be
  accomplished
Frequency
  Two or three exercise sessions per week up to daily activity for optimal benefits

---

Role of direct supervision

As patients improve their walking ability, the intensity of exercise should be increased
by modifying the treadmill grade or speed (or both) to ensure that there is always the
stimulus of claudication pain during the workout
As patients increase their walking ability, there is the possibility that cardiac signs and
symptoms might appear (e.g. dysrhythmia, angina, or ST-segment depression). These
events should prompt clinical re-evaluation

---

* These general guidelines should be individualised and based on the results of treadmill stress testing
and the clinical status of the patient.

Proper foot care is important, especially in those with diabetes mellitus, to prevent blisters and possible infections. Daily inspection of the toes and plantar surfaces of the feet is essential for early detection of any abnormality. Patients should be advised to return to their physician/general practitioner immediately if any changes occur in their feet.

Summary and conclusions

PAD is a common but under-recognised form of cardiovascular disease, which is associated with diminished functional capacity, reduced quality of life, and increased all-cause and cardiovascular mortality. Exercise training is a useful adjunct therapy for most patients with PAD, because it can reduce cardiovascular risk and enhance functional capacity and quality of life. Exercise training might also reduce atherosclerosis progression. Therefore, exercise training should be recommended for most patients with intermittent claudication.

References

Andreozzi, G.M., Leone, A., Laudani, R., Deinite, G. and Martini, R., 2007. Acute impairment of the endothelial function by maximal treadmill exercise in patients with intermittent claudication, and its improvement after supervised physical training. *International Angiology*, 26(1), 12–17.

Barak, S., Stopka, C.B., Martinez, C.A. and Carmeli, E., 2009. Benefits of low-intensity pain-free treadmill exercise for individuals presenting with intermittent claudication due to peripheral arterial disease. *Angiology*, 60(4), 477–86.

Bendermacher, B.L., Willigendael, E.M., Teijink, J.A. and Prins, M.H., 2006. Supervised exercise therapy versus non-supervised exercise therapy for intermittent claudication. *Cochrane Database of Systematic Reviews (Online)*, (2)(2), CD005263.

Binnie, A., Perkins, J. and Hands, L., 1999. Exercise and nursing therapy for patients with intermittent claudication. *Journal of Clinical Nursing*, 8(2), 190–200.

Blair, S.N., Cheng, Y. and Holder, J.S., 2001. Is physical activity or physical fitness more important in defining health benefits? *Medicine and Science in Sports and Exercise*, 33(6 Suppl), S379–99; discussion S419–20.

Brass, E.P. and Hiatt, W.R., 2000. Acquired skeletal muscle metabolic myopathy in atherosclerotic peripheral arterial disease. *Vascular Medicine*, 5(1), 55–59.

Brazier, J.E., Jones, N.B.M., O'Cathain, A., Thomas, K.J., Usherwood, T. and Westlake, L., 1992. Validating the SF 36 health survey questionnaire, a new outcome measure for primary care. *BMJ*, 305(6846), 160–164.

Brendle, D.C., Joseph, L.J., Corretti, M.C., Gardner, A.W. and Katzel, L.I., 2001. Effects of exercise rehabilitation on endothelial reactivity in older patients with peripheral arterial disease. *The American Journal of Cardiology*, 87(3), 324–329.

Bulmer, A.C. and Coombes, J.S., 2004. Optimising exercise training in peripheral arterial disease. *Sports Medicine*, 34(14), 983–1003.

Colleran, P.N., Li, Z., Yang, H.T., Laughlin, H.M. and Terjung, R.L., 2010. Vasoresponsiveness of collateral vessels in the rat hindlimb: influence of training. *The Journal of Physiology*, 588(8), 1293–1307.

Collins, E.G., Langbein, W.E., Orebaugh, C., Bammert, C., Hanson, K., Reda, D., Edwards, L.C. and Littooy, F.N., 2005. Cardiovascular training effect associated with polestriding exercise in patients with peripheral arterial disease. *The Journal of Cardiovascular Nursing*, 20(3), 177–185.

Criqui, M.H., Langer, R.D., Fronek, A., Feigelson, H.S., Klauber, M.R., Mccann, T.J. and Browner, D., 1992. Mortality over a period of 10 years in patients with peripheral arterial disease. *The New England Journal of Medicine*, 326(6), 381–386.

Crowther, R.G., Spinks, W.L., Leicht, A.S., Sangla, K., Quigley, F. and Golledge, J., 2008. Effects of a long-term exercise program on lower limb mobility, physiological responses, walking performance, and physical activity levels in patients with peripheral arterial disease. *Journal of Vascular Surgery*, 47(2), 303–309.

Currie, I.C., Wilson, Y.G., Baird, R.N. and Lamont, P.M., 1995. Treatment of intermittent claudication: the impact on quality of life. *European Journal of Vascular and Endovascular Surgery*, 10(3), 356–361.

Dormandy, J., Heeck, L. and Vig, S., 1999. The fate of patients with critical leg ischemia. *Seminars in Vascular Surgery*, 12(2), 142–147.

Dormandy, J.A. and Murray, G.D., 1991. The fate of the claudicant –a prospective study of 1969 claudicants. *European Journal of Vascular Surgery*, 5(2), 131–133.

Fowkes, F.G., 2001. Epidemiological research on peripheral vascular disease. *Journal of Clinical Epidemiology*, 54(9), 863–868.

Franzoni, F., Plantinga, Y., Femia, F.R., Bartolomucci, F., Gaudio, C., Regoli, F., Carpi, A., Santoro, G. and Galetta, F., 2004. Plasma antioxidant activity and cutaneous microvascular endothelial function in athletes and sedentary controls. *Biomedicine and Pharmacotherapy*, 58(8), 432–436.

Gardner, A.W. and Afaq, A., 2008. Management of lower extremity peripheral arterial disease. *Journal of Cardiopulmonary Rehabilitation and Prevention*, 28(6), 349–357.

Gardner, A.W., Montgomery, P.S. and Parker, D.E., 2008. Physical activity is a predictor of all-cause mortality in patients with intermittent claudication. *Journal of Vascular Surgery*, 47(1), 117–122.

Gardner, A.W., Montgomery, P.S., Flinn, W.R. and Katzel, L.I., 2005. The effect of exercise intensity on the response to exercise rehabilitation in patients with intermittent claudication. *Journal of Vascular Surgery*, 42(4), 702–709.

Gardner, A.W., Killewich, L.A., Montgomery, M.S. and Katzel, L.I., 2004. Response to exercise rehabilitation in smoking and nonsmoking patients with intermittent claudication. *Journal of Vascular Surgery*, 39(3), 531–538.

Gardner, A.W., Katzel, L.I., Sorkin, J.D. and Goldberg, A.P., 2002. Effects of long-term exercise rehabilitation on claudication distances in patients with peripheral arterial disease: a randomized controlled trial. *Journal of Cardiopulmonary Rehabilitation*, 22(3), 192–198.

Gardner, A.W., Forrester, L. and Smith, G.V., 2001a. Altered gait profile in subjects with peripheral arterial disease. *Vascular Medicine*, 6(1), 31–34.

Gardner, A.W., Katzel, L.I., Sorkin, J.D., Bradham, D.D., Hochberg, M.C., Flinn, W.R. and Goldberg, A.P., 2001b. Exercise rehabilitation improves functional outcomes and peripheral circulation in patients with intermittent claudication: a randomized controlled trial. *Journal of the American Geriatrics Society*, 49(6), 755–762.

Gardner, A.W., Womack, C.J., Sieminski, D.J., Montgomery, P.S., Killewich, L.A. and Fonong, T., 1998. Relationship between free-living daily physical activity and ambulatory measures in older claudicants. *Angiology*, 49(5), 327–337.

Gardner, A.W. and Poehlman, E.T., 1995. Exercise rehabilitation programs for the treatment of claudication pain. A meta-analysis. *JAMA*, 274(12), 975–980.

Garg, P.K., Liu, K., Tian, L., Guralnik, J.M., Ferrucci, L., Criqui, M.H., Tan, J. and McDermott, M.M., 2009. Physical activity during daily life and functional decline in peripheral arterial disease. *Circulation*, 119(2), 251–260.

Garg, P.K., Tian, L., Criqui, M.H., Liu, K., Ferrucci, L., Guralnik, J.M., Tan, J. and Mcdermott, M.M., 2006. Physical activity during daily life and mortality in patients with peripheral arterial disease. *Circulation*, 114(3), 242–248.

Green, D.J., Maiorana, A., O'Driscoll, G. and Taylor, R., 2004. Effect of exercise training on endothelium-derived nitric oxide function in humans. *The Journal of Physiology*, 561(Pt 1), 1–25.

Hambrecht, R., Niebauer, J., Marburger, C., Grunze, M., Kalberer, B., Hauer, K., Schlierf, G., Kubler, W. and Schuler, G., 1993. Various intensities of leisure time physical activity in patients with coronary artery disease: effects on cardiorespiratory fitness and progression of coronary atherosclerotic lesions. *Journal of the American College of Cardiology*, 22(2), 468–477.

Hiatt, W.R., Regensteiner, J.G., Wolfel, E.E., Carry, M.R. and Brass, E.P., 1996. Effect of exercise training on skeletal muscle histology and metabolism in peripheral arterial disease. *Journal of Applied Physiology*, 81(2), 780–788.

Hiatt, W.R., Hirsch, A.T., Regensteiner, J.G. and Brass, E.P., 1995. Clinical trials for claudication. Assessment of exercise performance, functional status, and clinical end points. Vascular Clinical Trialists. *Circulation*, 92(3), 614–621.

Hiatt, W.R., Regensteiner, J.G., Hargarten, M.E., Wolfel, E.E. and Brass, E.P., 1990. Benefit of exercise conditioning for patients with peripheral arterial disease. *Circulation*, 81(2), 602–609.

Hirsch, A.T., Haskal, Z.J., Hertzer, N.R., Bakal, C.W., Creager, M.A., Halperin, J.L., Hiratzka, L.F., Murphy, W.R., Olin, J.W., Puschett, J.B., Rosenfield, K.A., Sacks, D., Stanley, J.C., Taylor, L.M.,JR, White, C.J., White, J. and White, R.A., 2006. ACC/AHA 2005 Practice Guidelines for the management of patients with peripheral arterial disease (lower extremity, renal, mesenteric, and abdominal aortic). *Circulation*, 113(11), e463–654.

Hodges, L.D., Sandercock, G.R., Das, S.K. and Brodie, D.A., 2008. Randomized controlled trial of supervised exercise to evaluate changes in cardiac function in patients with peripheral atherosclerotic disease. *Clinical Physiology and Functional Imaging*, 28(1), 32–37.

Hodges, L.D., Sandercock, G.R., Das, S.K. and Brodie, D.A., 2006. Cardiac pumping capability in patients with peripheral vascular disease. *Clinical Physiology and Functional Imaging*, 26(3), 185–190.

Holloszy, J.O. and Coyle, E.F., 1984. Adaptations of skeletal muscle to endurance exercise and their metabolic consequences. *Journal of Applied Physiology*, 56(4), 831–838.

Izquierdo-Porrera, A.M., Gardner, A.W., Bradham, D.D., Montgomery, P.S., Sorkin, J.D., Powell, C.C. and Katzel, L.I., 2005. Relationship between objective measures of peripheral arterial disease severity to self-reported quality of life in older adults with intermittent claudication. *Journal of Vascular Surgery*, 41(4), 625–630.

Jones, P.P., Skinner, J.S., Smith, L.K., John, F.M. and Bryant, C.X., 1996. Functional improvements following StairMaster vs. treadmill exercise training for patients with intermittent claudication. *Journal of Cardiopulmonary Rehabilitation*, 16(1), 47–55.

Kadoglou, N.P., Iliadis, F. and Liapis, C.D., 2008. Exercise and carotid atherosclerosis. *European Journal of Vascular and Endovascular Surgery*, 35(3), 264–272.

Khaira, H.S., Hanger, R. and Shearman, C.P., 1996. Quality of life in patients with intermittent claudication. *European Journal of Vascular and Endovascular Surgery*, 11(1), 65–69.

Labs, K.H., Dormandy, J.A., Jaeger, K.A., Stuerzebecher, C.S. and Hiatt, W.R., 1999. Transatlantic Conference on Clinical Trial Guidelines in Peripheral Arterial Disease: clinical trial methodology. Basel PAD Clinical Trial Methodology Group. *Circulation*, 100(17), e75–81.

Larsen, O.A. and Lassen, N.A., 1966. Effect of daily muscular exercise in patients with intermittent claudication. *Lancet*, 2(7473), 1093–1096.

Lavie, C.J. and Milani, R.V., 2006. Adverse psychological and coronary risk profiles in young patients with coronary artery disease and benefits of formal cardiac rehabilitation. *Archives of Internal Medicine*, 166(17), 1878–1883.

Leng, G.C., Fowler, B. and Ernst, E., 2000. Exercise for intermittent claudication. *Cochrane Database of Systematic Reviews (Online)*, 2(2), CD000990.

Loffredo, L., Marcoccia, A., Pignatelli, P., Andreozzi, P., Borgia, M.C., Cangemi, R., Chiarotti, F. and Violi, F., 2007. Oxidative-stress-mediated arterial dysfunction in patients with peripheral arterial disease. *European Heart Journal*, 28(5), 608–612.

Lucini, D., Milani, R.V., Costantino, G., Lavie, C.J., Porta, A. and Pagani, M., 2002. Effects of cardiac rehabilitation and exercise training on autonomic regulation in patients with coronary artery disease. *American Heart Journal*, 143(6), 977–983.

Manfredini, F., Malagoni, A.M., Mascoli, F., Mandini, S., Taddia, M.C., Basaglia, N., Manfredini, R., Conconi, F. and Zamboni, P., 2008. Training rather than walking: the test in -train out program for home-based rehabilitation in peripheral arteriopathy. *Circulation Journal*, 72(6), 946–952.

Martinez, C.A., Carmeli, E., Barak, S. and Stopka, C.B., 2009. Changes in pain-free walking based on time in accommodating pain-free exercise therapy for peripheral arterial disease. *Journal of Vascular Nursing*, 27(1), 2–7.

McDermott, M.M., Ades, P., Guralnik, J.M., Dyer, A., Ferrucci, L., Liu, K., Nelson, M., Lloyd-Jones, D., Van Horn, L., Garside, D., Kibbe, M., Domanchuk, K., Stein, J.H., Liao, Y., Tao, H., Green, D., Pearce, W.H., Schneider, J.R., Mcpherson, D., Laing, S.T., Mccarthy, W.J., Shroff, A. and Criqui, M.H., 2009. Treadmill exercise and resistance training in patients with peripheral arterial disease with and without intermittent claudication: a randomized controlled trial. *JAMA*, 301(2), 165–174.

McDermott, M.M., Ades, P.A., Dyer, A., Guralnik, J.M., Kibbe, M. and Criqui, M.H., 2008. Corridor-based functional performance measures correlate better with physical activity during daily life than treadmill measures in persons with peripheral arterial disease. *Journal of Vascular Surgery*, 48(5), 1231–1237.

McDermott, M.M., Liu, K., Ferrucci, L., Criqui, M.H., Greenland, P., Guralnik, J.M., Tian, L., Schneider, J.R., Pearce, W.H., Tan, J. and Martin, G.J., 2006. Physical performance in peripheral arterial disease: a slower rate of decline in patients who walk more. *Annals of Internal Medicine*, 144(1), 10–20.

McDermott, M.M., Ohlmiller, S.M., Liu, K., Guralnik, J.M., Martin, G.J., Pearce, W.H. and Greenland, P., 2001. Gait alterations associated with walking impairment in people with peripheral arterial disease with and without intermittent claudication. *Journal of the American Geriatrics Society*, 49(6), 747–754.

McDermott, M.M., Feinglass, J., Slavensky, R. and Pearce, W.H., 1994. The ankle-brachial index as a predictor of survival in patients with peripheral vascular disease. *Journal of General Internal Medicine*, 9(8), 445–449.

Meyer, A.A., Kundt, G., Lenschow, U., Schuff-Werner, P. and Kienast, W., 2006. Improvement of early vascular changes and cardiovascular risk factors in obese children after a six-month exercise program. *Journal of the American College of Cardiology*, 48(9), 1865–1870.

Milani, R.V., Lavie, C.J. and Cassidy, M.M., 1996. Effects of cardiac rehabilitation and exercise training programs on depression in patients after major coronary events. *American Heart Journal*, 132(4), 726–732.

Montgomery, P.S. and Gardner, A.W., 1998. The clinical utility of a six-minute walk test in peripheral arterial occlusive disease patients. *Journal of the American Geriatrics Society*, 46(6), 706–711.

Morgan, M.B.F., Crayford, T., Murrin, B. and Fraser, S.C.A. 2001. Developing the Vascular Quality of Life Questionnaire: A new disease-specific quality of life measure for use in lower limb ischaemia. *Journal of Vascular Surgery*, 33(4), 679–687.

Nehler, M.R., McDermott, M.M., Treat-Jacobson, D., Chetter, I. and Regensteiner, J.G., 2003. Functional outcomes and quality of life in peripheral arterial disease: current status. *Vascular Medicine*, 8(2), 115–126.

Norgren, L., Hiatt, W.R., Dormandy, J.A., Nehler, M.R., Harris, K.A., Fowkes, F.G., TASC II Working Group, Bell, K., Caporusso, J., Durand-Zaleski, I., Komori, K., Lammer, J., Liapis, C., Novo, S., Razavi, M., Robbs, J., Schaper, N., Shigematsu, H., Sapoval, M., White, C., White, J., Clement, D., Creager, M., Jaff, M., Mohler, E.,3rd, Rutherford, R.B., Sheehan, P., Sillesen, H. and Rosenfield, K., 2007. Inter-Society Consensus for the Management of Peripheral Arterial Disease (TASC II). *European Journal of Vascular and Endovascular Surgery*, 33(Suppl 1), S1–75.

Patterson, R.B., Pinto, B., Marcus, B., Colucci, A., Braun, T. and Roberts, M., 1997. Value of a supervised exercise program for the therapy of arterial claudication. *Journal of Vascular Surgery*, 25(2), 312–318.

Pell, J., 1995. Impact of intermittent claudication on quality of life: the Scottish Vascular Audit Group. *European Journal of Vascular and Endovascular Surgery*, 9(4), 469–472.

Pipinos, I.I., Judge, A.R., Selsby, J.T., Zhu, Z., Swanson, S.A., Nella, A.A. and Dodd, S.L., 2008. The myopathy of peripheral arterial occlusive disease: Part 2. Oxidative stress, neuropathy, and shift in muscle fiber type. *Vascular and Endovascular Surgery*, 42(2), 101–112.

Pipinos, I.I., Judge, A.R., Selsby, J.T., Zhu, Z., Swanson, S.A., Nella, A.A. and Dodd, S.L., 2007. The myopathy of peripheral arterial occlusive disease: part 1. Functional and histomorphological changes and evidence for mitochondrial dysfunction. *Vascular and Endovascular Surgery*, 41(6), 481–489.

Rauramaa, R., Halonen, P., Vaisanen, S.B., Lakka, T.A., Schmidt-Trucksass, A., Berg, A., Penttila, I.M., Rankinen, T. and Bouchard, C., 2004. Effects of aerobic physical exercise on inflammation and atherosclerosis in men: the DNASCO Study: a six-year randomized, controlled trial. *Annals of Internal Medicine*, 140(12), 1007–1014.

Regensteiner, J.G., Hiatt, W.R., Coll, J.R., Criqui, M.H., Treat-Jacobson, D., Mcdermott, M.M. and Hirsch, A.T., 2008. The impact of peripheral arterial disease on health-related quality of life in the Peripheral Arterial Disease Awareness, Risk, and Treatment: New Resources for Survival (PARTNERS) Program. *Vascular Medicine*, 13(1), 15–24.

Regensteiner, J.G., Gardner, A. and Hiatt, W.R., 1997. Exercise testing and exercise rehabilitation for patients with peripheral arterial disease: Status in 1997. *Vascular Medicine*, 2(2), 147–155.

Regensteiner, J.G., Steiner, J.F. and Hiatt, W.R., 1996. Exercise training improves functional status in patients with peripheral arterial disease. *Journal of Vascular Surgery*, 23(1), 104–115.

Regensteiner, J.G. and Hiatt, W.R., 1995. Exercise rehabilitation for patients with peripheral arterial disease. *Exercise and Sport Sciences Reviews*, 23, 1–24.

Revkin, J.H., Shear, C.L., Pouleur, H.G., Ryder, S.W. and Orloff, D.G., 2007. Biomarkers in the prevention and treatment of atherosclerosis: need, validation, and future. *Pharmacological Reviews*, 59(1), 40–53.

Rogers, M.A. and Evans, W.J., 1993. Changes in skeletal muscle with aging: effects of exercise training. *Exercise and Sport Sciences Reviews*, 21, 65–102.

Rosfors, S., Arnetz, B.B., Bygdeman, S., Skoldo, L., Lahnborg, G. and Eneroth, P., 1990. Important predictors of the outcome of physical training in patients with intermittent claudication. *Scandinavian Journal of Rehabilitation Medicine*, 22(3), 135–137.

Rossi, M., Cupisti, A., Perrone, L., Mariani, S. and Santoro, G., 2002. Acute effect of exercise-induced leg ischemia on cutaneous vasoreactivity in patients with stage II peripheral artery disease. *Microvascular Research*, 64(1), 14–20.

Rowlands, T.E. and Donnelly, R., 2007. Medical therapy for intermittent claudication. *European Journal of Vascular and Endovascular Surgery*, 34(3), 314–321.

Sakamoto, S., Yokoyama, N., Tamori, Y., Akutsu, K., Hashimoto, H. and Takeshita, S., 2009. Patients with peripheral artery disease who complete 12-week supervised exercise training program show reduced cardiovascular mortality and morbidity. *Circulation Journal*, 73(1), 167–173.

Sanderson, B., Askew, C., Stewart, I., Walker, P., Gibbs, H. and Green, S., 2006. Short-term effects of cycle and treadmill training on exercise tolerance in peripheral arterial disease. *Journal of Vascular Surgery*, 44(1), 119–127.

Schuler, G., Hambrecht, R., Schlierf, G., Grunze, M., Methfessel, S., Hauer, K. and Kubler, W., 1992. Myocardial perfusion and regression of coronary artery disease in patients on a regimen of intensive physical exercise and low fat diet. *Journal of the American College of Cardiology*, 19(1), 34–42.

Smith, S.C. Jr, Milani, R.V., Arnett, D.K., Crouse, J.R.,3rd, Mcdermott, M.M., Ridker, P.M., Rosenson, R.S., Taubert, K.A., Wilson, P.W. and American Heart Association, 2004. Atherosclerotic Vascular Disease Conference: Writing Group II: risk factors. *Circulation*, 109(21), 2613–2616.

Sorlie, D. and Myhre, K., 1978. Effects of physical training in intermittent claudication. *Scandinavian Journal of Clinical and Laboratory Investigation*, 38(3), 217–222.

Spronk, S., White, J.V., Bosch, J.L. and Hunink, M.G., 2007. Impact of claudication and its treatment on quality of life. *Seminars in Vascular Surgery*, 20(1), 3–9.

Tan, K.H., Cotterrell, D., Sykes, K., Sissons, G.R., De Cossart, L. and Edwards, P.R., 2000. Exercise training for claudicants: changes in blood flow, cardiorespiratory status, metabolic functions, blood rheology and lipid profile. *European Journal of Vascular and Endovascular Surgery*, 20(1), 72–78.

Taylor, S.M., Kalbaugh, C.A., Healy, M.G., Cass, A.L., Gray, B.H., Langan, E.M. 3rd, Cull, D.L., Carsten, C.G. 3rd, York, J.W., Snyder, B.A. and Youkey, J.R., 2008. Do current outcomes justify more liberal use of revascularization for vasculogenic claudication? A single center experience of 1,000 consecutively treated limbs. *Journal of the American College of Surgeons*, 206(5), 1053–62.

Tew, G., Nawaz, S., Zwierska, I. and Saxton, J.M., 2009. Limb-specific and cross-transfer effects of arm-crank exercise training in patients with symptomatic peripheral arterial disease. *Clinical Science*, 117(12), 405–413.

Tisi, P.V., Hulse, M., Chulakadabba, A., Gosling, P. and Shearman, C.P., 1997. Exercise training for intermittent claudication: does it adversely affect biochemical markers of the exercise-induced inflammatory response? *European Journal of Vascular and Endovascular Surgery*, 14(5), 344–350.

Tsai, J.C., Chan, P., Wang, C.H., Jeng, C., Hsieh, M.H., Kao, P.F., Chen, Y.J. and Liu, J.C., (2002). The effects of exercise training on walking function and perception of health status in elderly patients with peripheral arterial occlusive disease. *Journal of Internal Medicine*, 252(5), 448–455.

Walker, R.D., Nawaz, S., Wilkinson, C.H., Saxton, J.M., Pockley, A.G. and Wood, R.F., 2000. Influence of upper- and lower-limb exercise training on cardiovascular function and walking distances in patients with intermittent claudication. *Journal of Vascular Surgery*, 31(4), 662–669.

Wang, J., Zhou, S., Bronks, R., Graham, J. and Myers, S., 2009. Effects of supervised treadmill walking training on calf muscle capillarization in patients with intermittent claudication. *Angiology*, 60(1), 36–41.

Wann-Hansson, C., Hallberg, I.R., Risberg, B and Klevsgard, R., 2004. A comparison of the Nottingham Health Profile and the Short Form 36 Health Survey in patients with chronic lower limb ischaemia in a longitudinal perspective. *Health and Quality of Life Outcomes*, 2(9), PMC 385253.

Watson, L., Ellis, B. and Leng, G.C., 2008. Exercise for intermittent claudication. *Cochrane Database of Systematic Reviews*, 4(4), CD000990.

Weiss, T., Fujita, Y., Kreimeier, U. and Messmer, K., 1992. Effect of intensive walking exercise on skeletal muscle blood flow in intermittent claudication. *Angiology*, 43(1), 63–71.

Weitz, J.I., Byrne, J., Clagett, G.P., Farkouh, M.E., Porter, J.M., Sackett, D.L., Strandness, D.E.,Jr and Taylor, L.M., 1996. Diagnosis and treatment of chronic arterial insufficiency of the lower extremities: a critical review. *Circulation*, 94(11), 3026–3049.

Wilmore, J.H. and Costill, D.L. 1999. *Physiology of Sport and Exercise*. Human Kinetics, Leeds, UK.

Womack, C.J., Sieminski, D.J., Katzel, L.I., Yataco, A. and Gardner, A.W., 1997. Improved walking economy in patients with peripheral arterial occlusive disease. *Medicine and Science in Sports and Exercise*, 29(10), 1286–1290.

Yang, H.T., Ogilvie, R.W. and Terjung, R.L., 1995. Training increases collateral-dependent muscle blood flow in aged rats. *The American Journal of Physiology*, 268(3 Pt 2), H1174–80.

Yataco, A.R., Corretti, M.C., Gardner, A.W., Womack, C.J. and Katzel, L.I., 1999. Endothelial reactivity and cardiac risk factors in older patients with peripheral arterial disease. *The American Journal of Cardiology*, 83(5), 754–758.

Zwierska, I., Walker, R.D., Choksy, S.A., Male, J.S., Pockley, A.G. and Saxton, J.M., 2005. Upper- vs lower-limb aerobic exercise rehabilitation in patients with symptomatic peripheral arterial disease: a randomized controlled trial. *Journal of Vascular Surgery*, 42(6), 1122–1130.

6

CHRONIC OBSTRUCTIVE PULMONARY DISEASE

Rachel Garrod and Fábio Pitta

Introduction

Chronic obstructive pulmonary disease (COPD) refers to a collection of lung diseases, including chronic bronchitis, emphysema and chronic obstructive airways disease. Mortality and morbidity are high in people with COPD and severe disabling symptoms are common. These include distressed breathing, limited exercise tolerance and frequent exacerbations. Anxiety and depression are other common symptoms of COPD and may be exacerbated by sleep disturbances and dyspnoea. Exercise is crucial in the management of COPD as a way of breaking the spiral of inactivity associated with dyspnoea. Lung impairment leads to breathlessness during exertion, fear and avoidance of activities which leads to deconditioning of skeletal muscles, greater dyspnoea and increasing inactivity. COPD is a progressive disease, with lung impairment further declining over time and there are few disease modifying treatments available (Hanania *et al.*, 2005). In a synergistic manner inactivity, dyspnoea and lung impairment interact to cause significant systemic consequences for people with COPD (Agusti, 2005). It is only in the last decade that health professionals have begun to fully appreciate the extent of the problems experienced as a result of COPD, including increased fatigue (Lewko *et al.*, 2009), difficulty performing tasks of daily activity and dyspnoea. Other clinical manifestations include an increased risk of osteoporosis (Graat-Verboom *et al.*, 2009), diabetes, carcinomas (Turner *et al.*, 2007), cardiovascular co-morbidity and alterations in body, both high and low, mass index (Barnes and Celli, 2009).

Limitations in exercise tolerance

Research from the last decade has identified a number of factors associated with limitations in exercise capacity in COPD. Whilst ventilatory impairment, ventilation perfusion mismatching and dynamic hyperinflation obviously contribute to limitations in exercise tolerance, they are not the only cause of the significant reductions seen in functional ability. A significant body of literature now clearly shows that weakness of the peripheral muscles contributes to limitations in exercise tolerance (Nici *et al.*, 2006). Patients with COPD enter a vicious downward spiral of disability; after an insidious start to the disease patients become increasingly aware of breathlessness, notable on exertion at first, but rapidly becoming significant with little or moderate activity. Inevitably (and especially in the context of fear or anxiety associated with breathlessness and poor understanding of the condition) patients become increasingly sedentary. In combination with raised systemic inflammatory levels that contribute to muscle cell apoptosis (Agusti, 2005; ATS/ERS 1999), reduced muscular contractions and general inactivity patients become further deconditioned, highly sensitive to dyspnoea and increasingly disabled. Pulmonary rehabilitation addresses these problems and attempts to break this cycle of dyspnoea via a number of mechanisms, importantly treatment of peripheral muscle weakness leads to improvements in exercise tolerance and quality of life. The focus of this chapter will be the peripheral muscles in patients with COPD although the effect of ventilatory, psychological and respiratory muscle impairments should also be considered as contributors to limitation in exercise tolerance (Marciniuk 2008; Marin *et al.*, 2001).

Skeletal muscle wasting in COPD

Skeletal muscle wasting and associated cachexia is well established as a major contributor to the limitations in exercise tolerance observed in COPD (ATS/ERS 1999). The nature of skeletal muscle wasting in COPD is complex and multi-factorial and only a brief overview will be provided here. One of the first major findings to be reported was the relative reduction in quadriceps cross-sectional area in people with COPD (Bernard *et al.*, 1998; Whittom *et al.*, 1998). Other studies have identified a reduction in the number of type I muscle fibres in the quadriceps and increase in type II fibres compared with healthy controls (Jakobsson *et al.*, 1990; Gosker *et al.*, 2002). Thus people with COPD suffer from a loss of fatigue resistant muscle fibres in the quadriceps leading to significant impairment in endurance output. Coronell and colleagues (Coronell *et al.*, 2004) reported convincing evidence of a reduction in skeletal muscle endurance performance by assessing task failure during a maximum voluntary contraction of the quadriceps against an external load. All the COPD subjects (with a mean FEV_1 of 36 per cent predicted) showed task failure whilst none of the age-matched healthy participants showed similar impairment. Furthermore, compared with the controls, COPD patients showed a decrease of 43 per cent in maximum voluntary contraction force. In this study, the decrease in performance was not specific to those with severe airflow limitation but also present in patients with relatively well-preserved lung function and physical activity profiles similar to that of the control participants. However, other authors contest this observation and argue that in stable COPD patients, without evidence of loss of fat-free mass, muscle strength does not differ from healthy individuals (Degens *et al.*, 2005). Furthermore, less is known about relative strength in the upper limbs, although one study suggests hand-grip strength is similar between patients with COPD and healthy individuals (Heijdra *et al.*, 2003). Whilst controversy persists surrounding the exact nature of skeletal muscle weakness in COPD, there is considerable support for the notion that for some patients, if not all, lower limb muscle weakness is a major contributor to limitations in exercise tolerance (Debigare and Maltais, 2008). For further consideration of muscle weakness in COPD, the reader is referred to a review article and statement published by the American Thoracic Society (ATS) and the European Respiratory Society (ERS) (ATS/ERS 1999).

Systemic inflammation in COPD and the effects of exercise

Increasingly it is recognised that COPD is a disease associated with increased inflammation. Data show that low grade systemic inflammation, as assessed by circulating levels of C-reactive protein (CRP), is negatively associated with FEV_1, supporting the premise that COPD is complicated by systemic abnormalities (Fogarty *et al.*, 2007; Gan *et al.*, 2004). In a cross-sectional study, CRP was shown to be higher amongst patients than a control group of smokers, after adjustment for age, gender, smoking history and body fat (Pinto-Plata *et al.*, 2006). It is possible that CRP may be associated with a faster decline in lung function over time in patients with COPD, although at present only trends have been identified (Fogarty *et al.*, 2007; Shaaban *et al.*, 2006). Inflammatory mediators have been shown to be predictive of both mortality (Dahl *et al.*, 2007), increased rates of hospitalisation (Dahl *et al.*, 2001) and respiratory symptoms at exacerbation (Perera *et al.*, 2007) in patients with COPD. Furthermore, skeletal muscle apoptosis is upregulated by elevated levels of TNF alpha in the skeletal muscle of COPD patients (Agusti, 2005; Wouters, 2002).

In healthy individuals, there is much evidence to suggest that exercise provides an anti-inflammatory effect (Fischer *et al.*, 2004; Petersen and Pedersen, 2005) and it has been hypothesised that this could also be relevant for individuals with COPD (Garrod *et al.*, 2007). Studies of patients with chronic heart failure (CHF) have shown convincing evidence of a reduction in local muscle inflammation after chronic exercise training. Significant reductions in the skeletal muscle production of Interlukin-6 (IL-6) and TNF-α were shown after six months of exercise training in one randomised controlled trial of CHF patients (Gielen *et al.*, 2003). Patients assigned to the exercise training group received two weeks of inpatient daily exercise training (cycle ergometry at 70 per cent of maximal oxygen consumption) with a continued unsupervised programme of 20 minutes cycle ergometry training and a once weekly group exercise training session. Using serum samples and muscle biopsies from the quadriceps, the authors showed that although baseline serum markers remained unchanged, local skeletal muscle TNF-α decreased from 1.9 ± 0.4 to 1.2 ± 0.3 relative units and IL-6 from 71.3 ± 16.5 to 41.3 ± 8.8 relative units. Whilst these statistically significant changes between the intervention and control groups suggest that the effect was due to the exercise intervention, the clinical relevance of these relatively small changes in inflammatory mediators is unclear. Another study which investigated the potential benefit of exercise on serum TNF-α in COPD patients showed no effect (Bolton *et al.*, 2007). In this study, the rehabilitation programme was provided twice weekly for only eight weeks and the skeletal muscle mass that had been accrued during the exercise training period was found to be reduced four weeks post-exercise training. Furthermore, in this study, only serum measures of TNF-α were monitored and no measures were obtained of local muscle inflammation.

The impact of exercise therapy on key health outcomes

Exercise as a therapeutic treatment for people with chronic obstructive pulmonary disease (COPD) is firmly established, with very strong evidence-based recommendations using data from numerous randomised controlled trials (1–3). Exercise for people with COPD is generally delivered in the context of a 7–12 week programme and combined with education and psychosocial support. This approach, where patients attend the hospital or primary care facility, is referred to as pulmonary rehabilitation.

Effects on quality of life

There is a compelling body of evidence supporting the role of pulmonary rehabilitation as a treatment that provides important clinical benefit to patients with COPD. A number of critically appraised guidelines and review documents are available. A recent update to the 2006 Cochrane airways meta-analysis on pulmonary rehabilitation (Lacasse, 2006) included a further eight randomised controlled trials (RCTs) to the original 23 RCTs.

In this updated review Lacasse and colleagues compared the effects of comprehensive rehabilitation (exercise and education components) to that of usual care (Lacasse, 2006). Studies were excluded where rehabilitation was compared to education only. In all domains of health-related quality of life (QoL), when measured using the valid and reliable Chronic Respiratory Disease Questionnaire (CRQ), statistically significant differences were shown between intervention patients and controls. Importantly, the domains of dyspnoea, fatigue, mastery and emotional function were also greater than the minimal clinically important difference in the CRQ, thus demonstrating clinical benefit. Similarly, when evaluating QoL using the St George's Respiratory Disease Questionnaire (SGRQ) all domains of the tool (Symptoms, Impact and Activity measures) showed common effect size changes that were greater than the minimum clinically important difference. All analyses were statistically significant with the exception of Symptoms. The updated guidelines from the American College of Chest Physicians (ACCP) and the American Association of Cardiovascular and Pulmonary Rehabilitation (ACCPR) unequivocally state that pulmonary rehabilitation leads to improvements in QoL in COPD and this is based on strong evidence (Ries *et al.*, 2007).

Effects of exercise on functional exercise tolerance

In general, in the clinical assessment of COPD, functional exercise tolerance is measured using one of two 'field' walking tests: the six-minute walk test (6MWT) (McGavin *et al.*, 1978) or the Incremental Shuttle Walk Test (ISWT) (Singh *et al.*, 1992). The ISWT is more properly considered a maximal walking test, as the results are closely correlated with maximum oxygen consumption ($\dot{V}O_{2max}$) in COPD patients (Singh *et al.*, 1994). Although the 6MWT is often cited as a measure of functional activity and the ISWT a measure of maximal ability, in reality relationships between distance walked and the $\dot{V}O_{2max}$, as measured in the lab, have been consistent and fairly high (Solway *et al.*, 2001). What must be remembered is that, on the whole, ventilatory impairment and/or skeletal muscle fatigue are the main limiting factors to exercise tolerance in COPD and, as such, a true measure of physiological $\dot{V}O_2$ is often unattainable. Hence, in COPD, the term $\dot{V}O_{2peak}$ is generally used for laboratory-based assessment of aerobic capacity, although this form of testing is probably more appropriate for early diagnosed patients with less severe disease.

In the most recent review of exercise in COPD, it is clear that a comprehensive package of exercise and education results in statistically significant improvements in functional exercise capacity (weighted mean difference of 48 metres). The distance a patient is required to walk to perceive an improvement in the 6MWT using patient recorded levels of benefit has been reported as 54 metres (Redelmeier *et al.*, 1996), using an alternative method depending on a threshold of clinical relevance greater than the standard error of as 35 metres (Puhan *et al.*, 2008). What has been clear for many years is that exercise as a component of comprehensive pulmonary rehabilitation is fundamental to achieving changes in exercise tolerance. Two early randomised controlled trials clearly demonstrated this; in the first, Ries and colleagues compared comprehensive rehabilitation (an eight-week programme of education, psychological support and exercise training) with that of education alone (Ries *et al.*, 1995) and in the second Wedzicha and colleagues compared exercise and education with that of education alone (Wedzicha *et al.*, 1998). In both studies the education group showed no effect on the outcomes of exercise tolerance, perception of dyspnoea, fatigue or QoL. An added arm to the Wedzicha study showed that individual home exercise for patients with severe COPD (housebound by breathlessness) was ineffective for all outcomes suggesting that some patients may be too severe to respond. This finding remains unqualified today although the absolute magnitude of the exercise training response is likely to be smaller in patients with very severe disease (Garrod *et al.*, 2006). In summary, a strong body of evidence reporting functional benefits in patients with COPD after programmes of exercise rehabilitation supports the statement that 'a programme of exercise training of the muscles of ambulation is recommended as a mandatory component of pulmonary rehabilitation' (Ries *et al.*, 2007).

Effects of exercise on cycle ergometry peak power output

In the Cochrane Airways review of pulmonary rehabilitation, 13 studies were considered that measured maximal exercise tolerance using cycle ergometry (Lacasse, 2006). A meta-analysis of these trials showed a statistically significant improvement of 8.4 watts but the clinical relevance of this in COPD is unknown. Furthermore, the lack of a strong association between maximal exercise tolerance and health-related QoL suggests that in COPD patients at least, maximal testing may be usefully employed to prescribe exercise intensity but should not be used to replace outcome measures of QoL and functional capacity.

Effects of exercise on muscle weakness

The role of skeletal muscle resistance exercise training and the importance of strong quadriceps in maintaining functional ability has been recognised in COPD for over a decade. The ATS and ERS statement on muscle dysfunction comprehensively describes a number of factors contributing to muscle impairment in COPD. However, the benefits of skeletal muscle training are clearly made and there is a significant body of evidence to support the notion that physiological resistance exercise training adaptations are achievable in COPD patients (ATS/ ERS 1999). In one early randomised controlled trial, COPD patients underwent eight weeks of resistance exercise training with weights, based on a percentage of the one repetition maximum strength, three times per week. Compared to a control group, the resistance exercise group showed a significant improvement in upper and lower limb skeletal muscle strength. Specifically, one repetition maximum strength increased by 33 per cent for the arm curl, by 44 per cent for leg extension and by 16 per cent for the leg press (Simpson *et al.*, 1992). Similarly, other authors have shown improvements in the cross-sectional area of skeletal muscle (Bernard *et al.*, 1999) and in knee extension and flexion forces following programmes of resistance exercise training (Spruit *et al.*, 2002).

More recently authors have explored the role of oxidative stress in muscle impairment in COPD patients and impact that resistance exercise might have (Bustamante *et al.*, 2008). Using magnetic stimulation to evoke contractions of the quadriceps and a healthy control group who received no treatment the authors compared the effects of the intervention on muscle protein carbonylation and nitration and antioxidant enzymes. They found that after eight weeks of magnetic stimulation, biopsies of the quadriceps in the intervention group showed an increase in the number of type I muscle fibres but redox status was still impaired in comparison to the control group.

Similarly, Rabinovich and colleagues showed that skeletal muscle anti-oxidation effects were impaired after high intensity resistance exercise training in COPD patients with low body mass index (BMI) compared to healthy individuals or those with COPD but normal BMI (Rabinovich *et al.*, 2006). In this study, oxidised glutathione was determined from muscle biopsies of the quadriceps before and after an eight-week high intensity cycle ergometry training programme. Exercise tolerance improved in all groups but skeletal muscle glutathione levels were unchanged in COPD with normal BMI, increased in healthy participants and decreased in low BMI COPD patients. Although, in this study, the sample size was relatively small (20 patients compared with 5 healthy participants) and the exercise training frequency unclear, the results supported previous work indicating impaired muscle redox status in patients with COPD and low BMI. Whilst there is compelling evidence that the skeletal muscles of patients with COPD can respond to resistance exercise training and achieve similar physiological changes to those observed in healthy individuals, it is not yet know whether this exercise modality in COPD patients can restore skeletal muscle physiology to that of healthy aged matched individuals, with respect to metabolic, oxidative and inflammatory markers. The interested reader is referred to a comprehensive review article by Benton and Swan (2006), which provides a thorough rationale for the importance of resistance exercise training in COPD.

Exercise prescription for COPD

Despite initial skepticism about the value of exercise training in patients with COPD, important scientific advances have occurred in the last two decades and, hence, recognition of the value of exercise in COPD has increased considerably. Nowadays, there is a strong body of evidence showing that exercise training by itself or as part of a pulmonary rehabilitation programme results in improvements in several adverse sequelae of the disease, such as dyspnoea, fatigue, exercise intolerance, muscle weakness and poor health-related QoL (Lacasse, 2006). In addition, it has also become clear that the magnitude (or even the occurrence) of exercise training effects depends on particular aspects of the exercise training programme, including exercise modality and the intensity, frequency and duration of exercise training.

Aerobic exercise prescription

Various training modalities have been used in the management of patients with COPD, all with generally good results. The majority of programmes use continuous (or aerobic) exercise training, incorporating an element of walking and/or cycling for 20–30 minutes per session. A more recent and alternative approach is interval training, i.e. the 30- or 40-minute exercise bout is divided into shorter bouts ranging from 30 seconds to 2–3 minutes, interspersed with periods of rest. When interval training was compared with continuous aerobic exercise training in COPD patients, it showed a different pattern of physiological response (Steiner *et al.*, 2005). Continuous exercise training resulted in improvements in maximal oxygen consumption, a reduction in minute ventilation and a more pronounced decrease in lactic acid production, whereas interval training resulted in improvements in peak work load and a decrease in leg pain. This difference in exercise training response might be a reflection of specific exercise training effects in either oxidative or glycolytic muscle metabolic pathways. On the other hand, a more recent study compared high intensity aerobic interval training (bouts of 30 s at 125 per cent maximal cycle ergometry power output and 30 s rest for 45 minutes), with equivalent constant load aerobic exercise (at 75 per cent of maximum power output for 30 minutes) three times per week for 10 weeks. Both groups showed significant exercise training effects; however, during the exercise sessions, symptoms of dyspnoea and leg discomfort were significantly lower for the interval training group (National Collaborating Centre for Chronic Conditions, 2004). These data suggest that in order to minimise discomfort associated with exercise training (and hence aid long-term adherence to exercise) patients may be advised to exercise in short, high intensity bursts of activity. Furthermore, interval training may enable more severe patients to achieve higher power outputs and to exercise longer with less symptoms due to lower dynamic hyperinflation (Sabapathy *et al.*, 2004; Vogiatzis *et al.*, 2002). However, total exercise time should not be compromised by interval training and rest times should be kept to the minimum necessary.

Intensity of aerobic exercise

Before considering an appropriate exercise intensity, it is necessary to revisit relevant assessment tools. Two common methods of prescribing intensity are used: symptom-limited exercise prescription and a prescription based on a percentage of various physiological measures, such as peak oxygen consumption, peak power output and peak heart rate, obtained during an incremental exercise test. In the first method, patients are instructed to exercise to a prescribed symptom level, for example 'moderately or somewhat short of breath' on the Borg breathlessness score (Borg, 1982) and usually scores of 4 to 6 on the Borg scale are useful targets (Horowitz *et al.*, 1996). Although this provides an effective exercise training stimulus for most patients, problems may occur when patients demonstrate very high levels of dyspnoea, thus limiting the intensity of exercise training. Dyspnoea is very much a subjective perception, meaning that fear and anxiety at the start of a exercise programme may heighten scores. Hence, when using this method it may be necessary to reassess the dyspnoea levels midway through the exercise programme with the aim of targeting a higher training level. Calculating aerobic exercise intensity from maximum oxygen consumption ($\dot{V}O_{2max}$) can be achieved using cycle ergometry or it can be predicted from a walking test, such as the ISWT (Singh *et al.*, 1994). However, it is worth remembering that for patients with COPD, a true $\dot{V}O_{2max}$ may be unattainable due to ventilatory limitations and the term peak $\dot{V}O_2$ should be used.

The initial intensity of aerobic exercise should ideally be set at 70–80 per cent of the peak $\dot{V}O_2$ (either measured or predicted from a walking test), with breathlessness scores being monitored during exercise training and used to inform adjustments to intensity (Mahler *et al.*, 2003). However, a more thorough discussion of optimal exercise intensity is presented below. Peak power output (measured during an incremental exercise test) has been used as an alternative approach to determine aerobic exercise training intensity, with an intensity of 60–80 per cent of the peak power output frequently shown to evoke positive results. Another option is to express aerobic exercise training intensity as a percentage of the maximal heart rate (using the prediction formula: 220 minus age). Caution is necessary using this approach though, as there is significant variability in heart rate measurements in patients with COPD and in the corresponding relationships with lactate threshold (Zacarias *et al.*, 2000). Furthermore heart rate is influenced by various medications commonly prescribed for COPD. Hence, individualised exercise prescription requires a flexible approach: for patients with mild COPD, not used to exercise, heart-rate based exercise prescription may result in significant cardiovascular benefits (Vallet *et al.*, 1994), with intensities of 80–85 per cent predicted maximum heart rate needed to achieve lactate threshold intensities (Zacarias *et al.*, 2000). Lower intensities can lead to less than expected change in functional outcomes (Pitta *et al.*, 2004). Clinical judgment is always required to determine the most appropriate aerobic exercise training prescription, with respect to optimising the exercise stimulus and encouraging long-term behaviour change.

What is the optimal intensity of aerobic exercise?

A number of studies have demonstrated greater physiological and cardiovascular benefits in patients who exercise at higher aerobic exercise intensities when compared with patients exercising at a lower intensity (Casaburi *et al.*, 1997; Puente-Maestu *et al.*, 2000). Other studies have also highlighted the positive effects of high-intensity aerobic exercise training (Gimenez *et al.*, 2000; Punzal *et al.*, 1991). These studies recommend exercise intensities of 60–80 per cent of peak power output or maximum (peak) oxygen consumption in order to achieve the greatest effects, although the rate of increase in work increment during the maximal incremental test is an important factor influencing whether a patient is able to achieve a target exercise training intensity of 80 per cent of the peak power output (Debigare *et al.*, 2000; Maltais *et al.*, 1997; Neder *et al.*, 2000). On the other hand, low-intensity aerobic exercise training also has been shown to result in significant improvements in symptoms, QoL (Normandin *et al.*, 2002) and exercise tolerance (Clark *et al.*, 1996; Roomi *et al.*, 1996). A recent systematic review suggested that in very severe patients, evidence that high intensity aerobic exercise is the ideal prescription is lacking (Puhan *et al.*, 2005). On this matter, the most recent consensus statement by the American Thoracic Society and European Respiratory Society states that:

although low-intensity [exercise] training results in improvements in symptoms, health related QoL and some aspects of performance in ADL, greater physiological training effects occur at higher intensity. Training programmes, in general, should attempt to achieve maximal physiologic training effects, but this approach may have to be modified because of disease severity, symptom limitation, co-morbidities and level of motivation. Furthermore, even though high intensity targets are advantageous for inducing physiologic changes in patients who can reach these levels, low intensity targets may be more important for long term adherence and health benefits for a wider population.

(Nici *et al.*, 2006)

In any case, should high-intensity aerobic exercise be proven to be effective in more symptomatic patients with severe COPD, interval training may be more appropriate and comfortable (Spruit *et al.*, 2002).

Duration and frequency of aerobic exercise training

The optimal duration of an exercise training programme for patients with COPD is not yet defined. Generally, exercise programmes that last at least 7 weeks (7–12 weeks) result in greater benefits than programmes shorter than that (Ries *et al.*, 2007). A well-designed meta-analysis showed strong trends for better results in functional exercise capacity where longer programmes with close supervision were applied (Lacasse, 2006). Programmes of six months duration may provide more sustainable benefits (Guell *et al.*, 2000; Troosters *et al.*, 2000) and there is evidence that patients are more active in daily life after such programmes (Pitta *et al.*, 2008); however, robust comparisons of programme duration on long-term exercise adherence need testing.

As with the duration of the programme, the optimal exercise training frequency is a topic which has been much debated but no unequivocal consensus has been made. General consensus is that patients should exercise at least three times per week with supervision at least twice weekly (Ries *et al.*, 2007). Short but more frequent programmes also yield positive results (Garrod *et al.*, 2000; Rossi *et al.*, 2005), suggesting that frequency and duration should not be considered in isolation.

Resistance exercise training

A number of recent studies have investigated the relative merits of other exercise training regimens in pulmonary rehabilitation, and it can be concluded that strength training exercises should be routinely incorporated into exercise rehabilitation programmes. Resistance exercise training (strength training) has potential to increase muscle mass and muscle force, which are common therapeutic aims in COPD patients. Strength training is generally performed as 2–4 sets of 6–12 repetitions at intensities ranging from 50–85 per cent of the one repetition maximum strength (O'Shea *et al.*, 2009) or peak muscle force (Probst *et al.*, 2006). A systematic review evaluating a number of comparative study designs concluded that strength training leads to larger improvements in health-related QoL than aerobic exercise training, although the benefits of strength over aerobic exercise are equivocal when considering the change in exercise tolerance (Wedzicha *et al.*, 1998). Interestingly, a randomised controlled trial showed that changes in muscle strength, distance walked and health-related QoL were no different between those who performed strength and aerobic exercise programmes (Garrod *et al.*, 2006). In addition, a major advantage of strength training is that cardiopulmonary stress is lower than during whole-body aerobic exercise and results in fewer symptoms (Probst *et al.*, 2006). As current data shows that skeletal muscle weakness contributes to the reductions in maximal walking performance but not to endurance walking performance, there appears to be a place for both types of exercise training (Man *et al.*, 2004). Guidelines for pulmonary rehabilitation in COPD patients currently recommend a combination of endurance and strength training as the latter has multiple beneficial effects and is well tolerated.

An interesting study by Sewell and co-workers investigated the relative benefit of generalised in comparison to individualised training programmes (Sewell *et al.*, 2005). General exercises consisted of three strength training activities for the lower limbs (step-ups, sit to standing and stationary cycling), thoracic exercises and upper limb activities (wall pushes, arm circling and shrugging). Individualised exercises were based on patient goals identified using the Canadian Occupational Performance Measure. After the seven-week programme there were no differences in any outcome measure between patients randomised to general or individualised training. The study had a large sample size and was adequately powered, which allows a solid conclusion to be drawn: that targeting exercises specifically to patient identified goals is unnecessary, assuming that both upper- and lower-limb exercises are included at an appropriate intensity.

Upper-limb exercise

Training the lower limbs has been the focus of most studies concerning exercise training in COPD patients. However, it has been shown that upper limbs are also affected, albeit to a lesser extent (Gosselink *et al.*, 2000) and upper limb activity increases dynamic hyperinflation and impairs pulmonary mechanics (Gigliotti *et al.*, 2005; McKeough *et al.*, 2003). As improvement in skeletal muscle function are limb specific, upper-limb activities should be included in exercise programmes for COPD patients (Ries *et al.*, 2007), especially exercises which reflect activities performed in daily life.

When exercise training the upper limbs, it is important to consider the principles of positioning during exercise. Exercise endurance is lower during unsupported upper limb activities compared with supported upper-limb exercise (Astrand *et al.*, 1968), especially when the arms are elevated above the head as in 'reaching' or 'arching the arms'. Stabilisation of the accessory muscles only occurs during movements where the shoulder girdle is fixed. These principles can be utilised during exercise training. Unsupported upper-limb exercise, by placing the thorax in a stretched position, effectively applies an increased load to breathing and the lack of stabilisation of upper thorax limits the ability of the accessory muscles to assist in ventilation. Training the upper limbs in unsupported positions enables patients to reduce sensitivity to dyspnoea during these activities and overall may achieve greater desensitisation of dyspnoea. However strength training of particular upper limb muscles is more effectively carried out in positions in which the upper thorax is fixed such as elbow supported by the knee for biceps curls. This in turn minimises dyspnoea enabling patients to maximise repetitions.

Summary and conclusions

NICE COPD guidelines state that 'pulmonary rehabilitation should be offered to all patients who consider themselves functionally disabled by COPD. Pulmonary rehabilitation is not suitable for patients who are unable to walk, have unstable angina or who have had a recent myocardial infarction' (National Collaborating Centre for Chronic Conditions, 2004). Access to rehabilitation, however, remains fairly low. Whilst there is increasing support for rehabilitation and increased service availability, local knowledge amongst health professionals remains poor and only a minority of patients with COPD receive exercise rehabilitation. As COPD and chronic health management in general receives greater attention, increasing numbers of patients will undergo a course of exercise therapy as part of their pulmonary rehabilitation.

The issue of who benefits the most from pulmonary rehabilitation is to some extent contentious, with ongoing debates about its relative efficacy in patients with severe end stage COPD in comparison to those with less severe disease. The importance of exercise rehabilitation early in the disease trajectory is increasingly being recognised, as is the role of exercise rehabilitation after exacerbation. A good rule of thumb would be referral to pulmonary rehabilitation early after the initial diagnosis (to provide patients with further education about the disease and to equip them with the skills to engage in and maintain healthy lifestyle behaviours), after an exacerbation (to facilitate a return to exercise participation) and at any stage when the patient complains of a worsening of the condition, even though optimisation of medical therapy has been established. Whilst studies are not yet available, it is possible that exercise rehabilitation provided early after the diagnosis of COPD might retard deterioration of the condition. The potential benefits of exercise rehabilitation on hospital admissions and the importance now being given to self-management of chronic conditions highlight the need for comprehensive holistic strategies which include exercise participation.

For exercise rehabilitation to be effective, optimising the exercise training intensity for each individual patient is very important. High-intensity aerobic exercise training (walking, cycling) generally produces greater physiologic benefit, although low-intensity aerobic exercise training can also be effective for more severe and symptomatic patients. In these patients, interval training (i.e. short bouts of high intensity exercise interspersed by rest) is recommended. Whilst longer aerobic exercise training programmes generally result in better long-term effects, shorter programmes will also yield significant improvements, particularly if sufficient exercise training sessions and adequate exercise training intensity are used. Patients also need to be instructed about the importance of exercising at home between supervised sessions, the importance of a long-term exercise routine and should be advised that walking on a daily basis remains an important therapeutic exercise. Strength training is also indicated for most patients. Providing additional strength training (particularly for the quadriceps) is likely to induce cumulative effects on exercise tolerance and muscle force. In summary, a combination of endurance and strength training (for both the lower and upper limbs) is highly recommended, particularly for patients with mild to moderate COPD.

References

ATS/ERS (1999). Skeletal muscle dysfunction in chronic obstructive pulmonary disease. A statement of the American Thoracic Society and European Respiratory Society, *Am J Respir Crit Care Med*, 159 (4) Pt 2, S1–40.

Agusti, A. G. (2005). Systemic effects of chronic obstructive pulmonary disease, *Proc Am Thorac Soc*, 2 (4), 367–370.

Astrand, I., Guharay, A. and Wahren, J. (1968). Circulatory responses to arm exercise with different arm positions, *J Appl Physiol*, 25 (5), 528–532.

Barnes, P. J. and Celli, B. R. (2009). Systemic manifestations and comorbidities of COPD, *European Respiratory Journal*, 33 (5), 1165–1185.

Benton, M. and Swan, P. (2006). Addition of resistance training to pulmonary rehabilitation programs: an evidence-based rationale and guidelines for use of resistance training with elderly patients with COPD, *Cardiopulmonary Physical Therapy Journal*, 17 (4), 127–133.

Bernard, S., LeBlanc, P., Whittom, F., Carrier, G., Jobin, J., Belleau, R., and Maltais, F. (1998). Peripheral muscle weakness in patients with chronic obstructive pulmonary disease, *Am J Respir Crit Care Med*, 158 (2), 629–634.

Bernard, S., Whittom, F., LeBlanc, P., Jobin, J., Belleau, R., Berube, C., Carrier, G. and Maltais, F. (1999), Aerobic and strength training in patients with chronic obstructive pulmonary disease, *Am J Respir Crit Care Med*, 159 (3), 896–901.

Bolton, C. E., Broekhuizen, R., Ionescu, A. A., Nixon, L. S., Wouters, E. F., Shale, D. J. and Schols, A. M. (2007). Cellular protein breakdown and systemic inflammation are unaffected by pulmonary rehabilitation in COPD, *Thorax*, 62 (2), 109–114.

Borg, C. (1982). Psychophysical basis of perceived exertion, *Medicine and Science in Sports Exercise*, 14, 377–381.

Bustamante, V., Casanova, J., Lopez de, S. E., Mas, S., Sellares, J., Gea, J., Galdiz, J. B. and Barreiro, E. (2008). Redox balance following magnetic stimulation training in the quadriceps of patients with severe COPD, *Free Radic Res*, 42 (11–12), 939–948.

Casaburi, R., Porszasz, J., Burns, M. R., Carithers, E. R., Chang, R. S. and Cooper, C. B. (1997). Physiologic benefits of exercise training in rehabilitation of patients with severe chronic obstructive pulmonary disease, *Am J Respir Crit Care Med*, 155 (5), 1541–1551.

Clark, C. J., Cochrane, L. and Mackay, E. (1996). Low intensity peripheral muscle conditioning improves exercise tolerance and breathlessness in COPD, *European Respiratory Journal*, 9 (12), 2590–2596.

Coronell, C., Orozco-Levi, M., Mendez, R., Ramirez-Sarmiento, A., Galdiz, J. B. and Gea, J. (2004). Relevance of assessing quadriceps endurance in patients with COPD, *Eur Respir J*, 24 (1), 129–136.

Dahl, M., Tybjaerg-Hansen, A., Vestbo, J., Lange, P. and Nordestgaard, B. G. (2001). Elevated plasma fibrinogen associated with reduced pulmonary function and increased risk of chronic obstructive pulmonary disease, *Am J Respir Crit Care Med*, 164 (6), 1008–1011.

Dahl, M., Vestbo, J., Lange, P., Bojesen, S. E., Tybjaerg-Hansen, A. and Nordestgaard, B. G. (2007). C-reactive protein as a predictor of prognosis in chronic obstructive pulmonary disease, *Am J Respir Crit Care Med*, 175 (3), 250–255.

Debigare, R. and Maltais, F. (2008). Last word on point: Counterpoint: The major limitation to exercise performance in COPD is 1) inadequate energy supply to the respiratory and locomotor muscles, 2) lower limb muscle dysfunction, 3) dynamic hyperinflation, *J Appl Physiol*, 105 (2), 764.

Debigare, R., Maltais, F., Mallet, M., Casaburi, R. and LeBlanc, P. (2000). Influence of work rate incremental rate on the exercise responses in patients with COPD, *Med Sci Sports Exerc*, 32 (8), 1365–1368.

Degens, H., Sanchez Horneros, J. M., Heijdra, Y. F., Dekhuijzen, P. N. and Hopman, M. T. (2005). Skeletal muscle contractility is preserved in COPD patients with normal fat-free mass, *Acta Physiol Scand*, 184 (3), 235–242.

Fischer, C. P., Plomgaard, P., Hansen, A. K., Pilegaard, H., Saltin, B. and Pedersen, B. K. (2004). Endurance training reduces the contraction-induced interleukin-6 mRNA expression in human skeletal muscle, *American Journal of Physiology – Endocrinology and Metabolism*, 287 (6), E1189–1194.

Fogarty, A. W., Jones, S., Britton, J. R., Lewis, S. A. and McKeever, T. M. (2007). Systemic inflammation and decline in lung function in a general population: a prospective study, *Thorax*, 62 (6), 515–520.

Gan, W. Q., Man, S. F., Senthilselvan, A. and Sin, D. D. (2004). Association between chronic obstructive pulmonary disease and systemic inflammation: a systematic review and a meta-analysis, *Thorax*, 59 (7), 574–580.

Garrod, R., Ansley, P., Canavan, J. and Jewell, A. (2007). Exercise and the inflammatory response in chronic obstructive pulmonary disease (COPD) – Does training confer anti-inflammatory properties in COPD?, *Med Hypotheses*, 68 (2), 291–298.

Garrod, R., Marshall, J., Barley, E. and Jones, P. W. (2006). Predictors of success and failure in pulmonary rehabilitation, *European Respiratory Journal*, 27 (4), 788–794.

Garrod, R., Paul, E. A. and Wedzicha, J. A. (2000). Supplemental oxygen during pulmonary rehabilitation in patients with COPD with exercise hypoxaemia, *Thorax*, 55 (7), 539–543.

Gielen, S., Adams, V., Mobius-Winkler, S., Linke, A., Erbs, S., Yu, J., Kempf, W., Schubert, A., Schuler, G. and Hambrecht, R. (2003). Anti-inflammatory effects of exercise training in the skeletal muscle of patients with chronic heart failure, *J Am Coll Cardiol*, 42 (5), 861–868.

Gigliotti, F., Coli, C., Bianchi, R., Grazzini, M., Stendardi, L., Castellani, C. and Scano, G. (2005). Arm exercise and hyperinflation in patients with COPD: effect of arm training, *Chest*, 128 (3), 1225–1232.

Gimenez, M., Servera, E., Vergara, P., Bach, J. R. and Polu, J. M. (2000). Endurance training in patients with chronic obstructive pulmonary disease: a comparison of high versus moderate intensity, *Archives of Physical Medicine and Rehabilitation*, 81(1), 102–109.

Gosker, H. R., van, M. H., van Dijk, P. J., Engelen, M. P., van, d., V, Wouters, E. F. and Schols, A. M. (2002). Skeletal muscle fibre-type shifting and metabolic profile in patients with chronic obstructive pulmonary disease, *Eur Respir J*, 19 (4), 617–625.

Gosselink, R., Troosters, T. and Decramer, M. (2000). Distribution of muscle weakness in patients with stable chronic obstructive pulmonary disease, *J Cardiopulm Rehabil*, 20 (6), 353–360.

Graat-Verboom, L., Wouters, E. F. M., Smeenk, F. W. J. M., van den Borne, B. E. E. M., Lunde, R. and Spruit, M. A. (2009). Current status of research on osteoporosis in COPD: a systematic review, *European Respiratory Journal*, 34, 1, 209–218.

Guell, R., Casan, P., Belda, J., Sangenis, M., Morante, F., Guyatt, G. H. and Sanchis, J. (2000). Long-term effects of outpatient rehabilitation of COPD: a randomized trial, *Chest*, 117 (4), 976–983.

Hanania, N. A., Ambrosino, N., Calverley, P., Cazzola, M., Donner, C. F. and Make, B. (2005). Treatments for COPD, *Respir Med*, 99 Suppl B, S28–S40.

Heijdra, Y. F., Pinto-Plata, V., Frants, R., Rassulo, J., Kenney, L. and Celli, B. R. (2003). Muscle strength and exercise kinetics in COPD patients with a normal fat-free mass index are comparable to control subjects, *Chest*, 124 (1), 75–82.

Horowitz, M. B., Littenberg, B. and Mahler, D. A. (1996). Dyspnea ratings for prescribing exercise intensity in patients with COPD, *Chest*, 109 (5), 1169–1175.

Jakobsson, P., Jorfeldt, L. and Brundin, A. (1990). Skeletal muscle metabolites and fibre types in patients with advanced chronic obstructive pulmonary disease (COPD), with and without chronic respiratory failure, *Eur Respir J*, 3 (2), 192–196.

Lacasse, Y., Goldstein, R., Lasserson, T J. and Martin, S. (2006). Pulmonary rehabilitation for chronic obstructive pulmonary disease. *Cochrane Database of Systematic Reviews*, Issue 4. Art. No.: CD003793. DOI: 10.1002/14651858.CD003793.pub2.

Lewko A., Bidgood P. and Garrod R. (2009). COPD related fatigue: evaluation of factors associated with fatigue in COPD and comparison with healthy elderly subjects. Open Access BMC Pulmonary Medicine. Unpublished work.

Mahler, D. A., Ward, J. and Mejia-Alfaro, R. (2003). Stability of dyspnea ratings after exercise training in patients with COPD, *Med Sci Sports Exerc*, 35 (7), 1083–1087.

Maltais, F., LeBlanc, P., Jobin, J., Berube, C., Bruneau, J., Carrier, L., Breton, M. J., Falardeau, G. and Belleau, R. (1997). Intensity of training and physiologic adaptation in patients with chronic obstructive pulmonary disease, *Am J Respir Crit Care Med*, 155 (2), 555–561.

Man, W. D., Polkey, M. I., Donaldson, N., Gray, B. J. and Moxham, J. (2004). Community pulmonary rehabilitation after hospitalisation for acute exacerbations of chronic obstructive pulmonary disease: randomised controlled study, *BMJ*, 329 (7476), 1209.

Marciniuk, D. D. (2008). The major limitation to exercise performance in COPD is inadequate energy supply to the respiratory and locomotor muscles vs. lower limb muscle dysfunction vs. dynamic hyperinflation. There is no magic bullet in COPD, *J Appl Physiol*, 105 (2), 762.

Marin, J. M., Carrizo, S. J., Gascon, M., Sanchez, A., Gallego, B., and Celli, B. R. (2001). Inspiratory capacity, dynamic hyperinflation, breathlessness, and exercise performance during the 6-minute-walk test in chronic obstructive pulmonary disease, *Am J Respir Crit Care Med*, 163 (6), 1395–1399.

McGavin, C. R., Artvinli, M., Naoe, H. and McHardy, G. J. (1978). Dyspnoea, disability, and distance walked: comparison of estimates of exercise performance in respiratory disease, *Br Med J*, 2, 6132, 241–243.

McKeough, Z. J., Alison, J. A. and Bye, P. T. (2003). Arm positioning alters lung volumes in subjects with COPD and healthy subjects, *Aust J Physiother.*, 49 (2), 133–137.

National Collaborating Centre for Chronic Conditions (2004). Chronic obstructive pulmonary disease. National clinical guideline on management of chronic obstructive pulmonary disease in adults in primary and secondary care, *Thorax*, 59 (Suppl 1), 1–232.

Neder, J. A., Jones, P. W., Nery, L. E. and Whipp, B. J. (2000). Determinants of the exercise endurance capacity in patients with chronic obstructive pulmonary disease. The power-duration relationship, *Am J Respir Crit Care Med*, 162 (2), Pt 1, 497–504.

Nici, L., Donner, C., Wouters, E., ZuWallack, R., Ambrosino, N., Bourbeau, J., Carone, M., Celli, B., Engelen, M., Fahy, B., Garvey, C., Goldstein, R., Gosselink, R., Lareau, S., MacIntyre, N., Maltais, F., Morgan, M., O'Donnell, D., Prefault, C., Reardon, J., Rochester, C., Schols, A., Singh, S. and Troosters, T. (2006). American Thoracic Society/European Respiratory Society statement on pulmonary rehabilitation, *Am J Respir Crit Care Med*, 173 (12), 1390–1413.

Normandin, E. A., McCusker, C., Connors, M., Vale, F., Gerardi, D. and ZuWallack, R. L. (2002). An evaluation of two approaches to exercise conditioning in pulmonary rehabilitation, *Chest*, 121 (4), 1085–1091.

O'Shea, S. D., Taylor, N. F. and Paratz, J. D. (2009). Progressive resistance exercise improves muscle strength and may improve elements of performance of daily activities for people with COPD: a systematic review, *Chest*, 136 (5), 1269–1283.

Perera, W. R., Hurst, J. R., Wilkinson, T. M., Sapsford, R. J., Mullerova, H., Donaldson, G. C. and Wedzicha, J. A. (2007). Inflammatory changes, recovery and recurrence at COPD exacerbation, *European Respiratory Journal*, 29 (3), 527–534.

Petersen, A. M. and Pedersen, B. K. (2005). The anti-inflammatory effect of exercise, *J Appl Physiol*, 98 (4), 1154–1162.

Pinto-Plata, V. M., Mullerova, H., Toso, J. F., Feudjo-Tepie, M., Soriano, J. B., Vessey, R. S. and Celli, B. R. (2006). C-reactive protein in patients with COPD, control smokers and non-smokers, *Thorax*, 61 (1), 23–28.

Pitta, F., Brunetto, A. F., Padovani, C. R. and Godoy, I. (2004). Effects of isolated cycle ergometer training on patients with moderate-to-severe chronic obstructive pulmonary disease, *Respiration*, 71 (5), 477–483.

Pitta, F., Troosters, T., Probst, V. S., Langer, D., Decramer, M. and Gosselink, R. (2008). Are patients with COPD more active after pulmonary rehabilitation?, *Chest*, 134 (2), 273–280.

Probst, V. S., Troosters, T., Pitta, F., Decramer, M. and Gosselink, R. (2006). Cardiopulmonary stress during exercise training in patients with COPD, *European Respiratory Journal*, 27 (6), 1110–1118.

Puente-Maestu, L., Sanz, M. L., Sanz, P., Cubillo, J. M., Mayol, J. and Casaburi, R. (2000). Comparison of effects of supervised versus self-monitored training programmes in patients with chronic obstructive pulmonary disease, *European Respiratory Journal*, 15 (3), 517–525.

Puhan, M. A., Mador, M. J., Held, U., Goldstein, R., Guyatt, G. H. and Schunemann, H. J. (2008). Interpretation of treatment changes in 6-minute walk distance in patients with COPD, *European Respiratory Journal*, 32 (3), 637–643.

Puhan, M. A., Schunemann, H. J., Frey, M., Scharplatz, M. and Bachmann, L. M. (2005). How should COPD patients exercise during respiratory rehabilitation? Comparison of exercise modalities and intensities to treat skeletal muscle dysfunction, *Thorax*, 60 (5), 367–375.

Punzal, P. A., Ries, A. L., Kaplan, R. M. and Prewitt, L. M. (1991). Maximum intensity exercise training in patients with chronic obstructive pulmonary disease, *Chest*, 100 (3), 618–623.

Rabinovich, R. A., Ardite, E., Mayer, A. M., Polo, M. F., Vilaro, J., Argiles, J. M. and Roca, J. (2006). Training depletes muscle glutathione in patients with chronic obstructive pulmonary disease and low body mass index, *Respiration*, 73 (6), 757–761.

Redelmeier, D. A., Guyatt, G. H. and Goldstein, R. S. (1996). Assessing the minimal important difference in symptoms: a comparison of two techniques, *J Clin Epidemiol*, 49 (11), 1215–1219.

Ries, A. L., Bauldoff, G. S., Carlin, B. W., Casaburi, R., Emery, C. F., Mahler, D. A., Make, B., Rochester, C. L., ZuWallack, R. and Herrerias, C. (2007). Pulmonary Rehabilitation: Joint ACCP/AACVPR Evidence-Based Clinical Practice Guidelines, *Chest*, 131 (5) Suppl, 4S–42S.

Ries, A. L., Kaplan, R. M., Limberg, T. M., and Prewitt, L. M. (1995). Effects of pulmonary rehabilitation on physiologic and psychosocial outcomes in patients with chronic obstructive pulmonary disease, *Ann Intern Med*, 122 (11), 823–832.

Roomi, J., Johnson, M. M., Waters, K., Yohannes, A., Helm, A. and Connolly, M. J. (1996). Respiratory rehabilitation, exercise capacity and quality of life in chronic airways disease in old age, *Age Ageing*, 25 (1), 12–16.

Rossi, G., Florini, F., Romagnoli, M., Bellantone, T., Lucic, S., Lugli, D. and Clini, E. (2005). Length and clinical effectiveness of pulmonary rehabilitation in outpatients with chronic airway obstruction, *Chest*, 127 (1), 105–109.

Sabapathy, S., Kingsley, R. A., Schneider, D. A., Adams, L. and Morris, N. R. (2004). Continuous and intermittent exercise responses in individuals with chronic obstructive pulmonary disease, *Thorax*, 59 (12), 1026–1031.

Sewell, L., Singh, S. J., Williams, J. E., Collier, R. and Morgan, M. D. (2005). Can individualized rehabilitation improve functional independence in elderly patients with COPD?, *Chest*, 128 (3), 1194–1200.

Shaaban, R., Kony, S., Driss, F., Leynaert, B., Soussan, D., Pin, I., Neukirch, F. and Zureik, M. (2006). Change in C-reactive protein levels and FEV_1 decline: a longitudinal population-based study, *Respir Med*, 100 (2), 2112–2120.

Simpson, K., Killian, K., McCartney, N., Stubbing, D. G. and Jones, N. L. (1992). Randomised controlled trial of weightlifting exercise in patients with chronic airflow limitation, *Thorax*, 47 (2), 70–75.

Singh, S. J., Morgan, M. D., Hardman, A. E., Rowe, C. and Bardsley, P. A. (1994). Comparison of oxygen uptake during a conventional treadmill test and the shuttle walking test in chronic airflow limitation, *Eur Respir J*, 7 (11), 2016–2020.

Singh, S. J., Morgan, M. D., Scott, S., Walters, D. and Hardman, A. E. (1992). Development of a shuttle walking test of disability in patients with chronic airways obstruction, *Thorax*, 47 (12), 1019–1024.

Solway, S., Brooks, D., Lacasse, Y. and Thomas, S. (2001). A qualitative systematic overview of the measurement properties of functional walk tests used in the cardiorespiratory domain, *Chest*, 119 (1), 256–270.

Spruit, M. A., Gosselink, R., Troosters, T., De Paepe, K. and Decramer, M. (2002). Resistance versus endurance training in patients with COPD and peripheral muscle weakness, *European Respiratory Journal*, 19 (6), 1072–1078.

Steiner, M. C., Singh, S. J. and Morgan, M. D. (2005). The contribution of peripheral muscle function to shuttle walking performance in patients with chronic obstructive pulmonary disease, *J Cardiopulm Rehabil*, 25 (1), 43–49.

Troosters, T., Gosselink, R. and Decramer, M. (2000). Short- and long-term effects of outpatient rehabilitation in patients with chronic obstructive pulmonary disease: a randomized trial, *Am J Med*, 109 (3), 207–212.

Turner, M. C., Chen, Y., Krewski, D., Calle, E. E. and Thun, M. J. (2007). Chronic obstructive pulmonary disease is associated with lung cancer mortality in a prospective study of never smokers, *Am J Respir Crit Care Med*, 176 (3), 285–290.

Vallet, G., Varray, A., Fontaine, J. L. and Prefaut, C. (1994). Value of individualized rehabilitation at the ventilatory threshold level in moderately severe chronic obstructive pulmonary disease, *Rev Mal Respir*, 11 (5), 493–501.

Vogiatzis, I., Nanas, S. and Roussos, C. (2002). Interval training as an alternative modality to continuous exercise in patients with COPD, *Eur Respir J*, 20 (1), 12–19.

Wedzicha, J. A., Bestall, J. C., Garrod, R., Garnham, R., Paul, E. A. and Jones, P. W. (1998). Randomized controlled trial of pulmonary rehabilitation in severe chronic obstructive pulmonary disease patients, stratified with the MRC dyspnoea scale, *European Respiratory Journal*, 12 (2), 363–369.

Whittom, F., Jobin, J., Simard, P. M., LeBlanc, P., Simard, C., Bernard, S., Belleau, R. and Maltais, F. (1998). Histochemical and morphological characteristics of the vastus lateralis muscle in patients with chronic obstructive pulmonary disease, *Med Sci Sports Exerc*, 30 (10), 1467–1474.

Wouters, E. F. M. (2002). Chronic obstructive pulmonary disease * 5: Systemic effects of COPD, *Thorax*, 57 (12), 1067–1070.

Zacarias, E. C., Neder, J. A., Cendom, S. P., Nery, L. E. and Jardim, J. R. (2000). Heart rate at the estimated lactate threshold in patients with chronic obstructive pulmonary disease: effects on the target intensity for dynamic exercise training, *J Cardiopulm Rehabil*, 20 (6), 369–376.

7

ASTHMA

Felix S. F. Ram and Elissa M. McDonald

Introduction

Characteristics of asthma

Key characteristics that define asthma are bronchial hyper-responsiveness, reversible airway obstruction and inflammation. Early definitions of asthma included the presence of airways obstruction that could reverse spontaneously or with treatment, and also the increased narrowing of the airways to stimuli (e.g. histamine, cold air, exercise, viral upper respiratory infection, cigarette smoke or respiratory allergens) causing bronchial hyper-responsiveness. Management of asthma has been enhanced by the recognition that the airways sub-mucosa of patients with asthma are chronically inflamed with a typical inflammatory infiltrate, and that inflammatory processes are important in causing the main characteristics of asthma of airways obstruction and bronchial hyper-responsiveness. As a result of inflammation, the airways are hyper-responsive and they narrow easily in response to a wide range of stimuli. This may result in coughing, wheezing, chest tightness and shortness of breath, with symptoms often worse at night. Narrowing of the airways is usually reversible with appropriate pharmacological intervention, but in patients with chronic inflammatory conditions it leads to irreversible airflow obstruction (BTS, 2008; Cressy and DeBoisblanc, 1998; EPR-3, 2007; Foggs, 2008; Levy *et al.*, 2009). Characteristic pathology of asthmatic airways displays lung hyperinflation, smooth muscle hypertrophy, mucosal edema, lamina thickening, epithelial cell sloughing, cilia disruption and mucus hyper-secretion. Its pathology is further characterized by the presence of increased numbers of eosinophils, neutrophils, lymphocytes and plasma cells in the bronchial tissues, bronchial secretions and mucus.

Physical exercise and asthma

The prevalence and severity of asthma is increasing and no one doubts that the cause of this increase is due to a multitude of factors. However, there is a growing body of evidence that implicates lifestyle changes, specifically decreased physical activity, as the single most important contributor to the increase in asthma prevalence and severity, seen globally. There has been a steady decrease in the levels of physical activity of adults and children over the years and this decrease corresponds in timecourse to the increased prevalence of asthma (Firrincieli *et al.*, 2005; Huovinen *et al.*, 2001; Rasmussen *et al.*, 2000). Furthermore, most studies have shown that asthmatic individuals have a lower aerobic fitness level than their non-asthmatic peers and that this limited fitness level in asthmatic participants seems not to be related to their degree of airway obstruction but rather to their decreased levels of habitual activity (Clark and Cochrane, 1988). Exercise has long been recognized as a possible method of improving subjective and objective asthma indices even though there is the potential for exercise-induced asthma (EIA) with physical exertion. However, it has been well documented that the incidence of EIA after proper medical (and pharmacological) prophylaxis is extremely low (Orenstein, 2002) and the benefits and safety of exercise in asthmatic individuals have been well demonstrated (Clark and Cochrane, 1988; Orenstein, 2002; Satta, 2000).

People with asthma have a unique response to exercise. In some, exercise can provoke an increase in airways resistance leading to EIA but regular exercise is also considered to be useful in the management of asthma, especially in children and adolescents (Orenstein, 1996). However, the fear of inducing an episode of breathlessness inhibits many people from taking part in exercise. A low level of regular exercise leads to a low level of physical fitness, so it is not surprising that a number of studies (Clark and Cochrane, 1988; Garfinkel *et al.*, 1992) have found that patients with asthma have lower cardiorespiratory fitness than their peers, although not every study has reported this finding (Santuz *et al.*, 1997).

Exercise programmes have been designed for people with asthma with the aim of improving physical fitness, neuromuscular co-ordination and self-confidence. Anecdotally, many patients report that they are symptomatically better when fit, but the physiological basis of this perceived benefit has not been consistently shown in studies published to date. A possible mechanism is that an increase in regular exercise of sufficient intensity to increase aerobic fitness will raise the ventilatory threshold, thereby lowering the minute ventilation during mild and moderate exercise. Consequently, breathlessness and the likelihood of provoking EIA will both be reduced. Exercise training may also reduce the perception of breathlessness through other mechanisms including strengthening of the respiratory muscles.

Systematic review

A systematic review of the literature was undertaken to gain a better understanding of the effects of regular exercise on the health of people with asthma.

This systematic review focused on the effects of exercise on resting pulmonary function, aerobic fitness, clinical status and quality of life (QoL) in people with asthma. With this systematic review explicit criteria were used to select studies for inclusion and to assess their quality. Various electronic medical databases were searched for suitable studies from their date of inception until August 2009. The reference lists of all studies obtained were reviewed to identify trials not captured by electronic and manual searches. In addition, authors of included studies were contacted when required for additional information or clarification and for any ongoing studies. This systematic review was originally published electronically (Ram *et al.*, 2000) in 2000 on the Cochrane Library and has since been updated to encompass literature search up to and including August 2009, which has resulted in 11 additional studies being included with a total of 650 participants (the original review published in 2000 had eight included studies with 226 participants). This current systematic review is therefore a substantial update of the original published in 2000.

Objectives

This systematic review was undertaken to gain a better understanding of the effects of regular exercise on the health of patients with asthma. The objective was to assess evidence from high quality randomized controlled clinical trials (RCTs) of the effects of regular exercise in the management of asthma.

Methods

Selection of studies and participants

Only studies that included participants with asthma who were randomized to regular exercise (intervention group) or no exercise (control group) were selected. Participants had to be aged 7 years and older and their asthma had to be diagnosed by a physician or by the use of objective criteria – for example bronchodilator reversibility. Participants with any degree of asthma severity were included. To qualify for inclusion regular exercise had to include whole body aerobic exercise for at least 20 minutes, two or more times a week, for a minimum of four weeks.

Database searches and trial retrieval

The following terms were used to search for studies: asthma AND (work capacity OR physical activity OR training OR rehabilitation OR physical fitness). The Cochrane Trials Database, CENTRAL, (August 2009) was searched for studies. Additional searches were carried out on Medline (1966–2009), Embase (1980–2009), SportDiscus (1949–2009), Current contents index (1995–2009) and Science Citation Index (1995–2009). The reference lists of all the papers that were obtained were reviewed to identify trials not captured by electronic and manual searches. Abstracts were reviewed without language restriction. When more data were required for the systematic review, authors of the study were contacted requesting additional information or clarification.

Data analysis

Following outcome measures were searched for:

- bronchodilator usage
- episodes of wheeze
- symptoms (recorded in diary cards)
- exercise endurance
- work capacity
- walking distance
- quality of life
- physiological measurements included the following:
    - PEFR: peak expiratory flow rate
    - FEV_1: forced expiratory volume in one second
    - FVC: forced vital capacity
    - VO_{2max}: maximum oxygen consumption or uptake
    - $V_E max$: maximum exercise ventilation
    - HR_{max}: maximum heart rate
    - MVV: maximum voluntary ventilation.

Two reviewers assessed the trials for inclusion by only looking at the methods section of each paper without reading the results of the study or conclusions; this is regarded as the most appropriate method of unbiased trial selection (Oxman et al., 1994). Each reviewer independently applied written inclusion/exclusion criteria to the methods section of each study. Disagreement about inclusion of a study was resolved whenever possible by consensus and an independent person was consulted if disagreement persisted. All trials that appeared potentially relevant were assessed, and if appropriate were included in the review. If an RCT was excluded on methodological grounds, the reason for exclusion was recorded.

The methodological quality of the included trials was assessed with particular emphasis on treatment allocation concealment, which was ranked using the following Cochrane Collaboration approach:

- Grade A: Adequate concealment
- Grade B: Uncertain
- Grade C: Clearly inadequate concealment
- Grade D: Not used (no attempt at concealment).

Two of the reviewers independently extracted data from the trials. The trials were combined for meta-analysis using Review Manager 4.3 (Nordic Cochrane Centre, 2003). Fixed effect model was used for statistical analysis. The outcomes of interest in this review were continuous data. Data from each of the continuous outcomes were analyzed as weighted mean difference (WMD) with 95 per cent confidence intervals (95% CI).

Results

The electronic search yielded 1,299 potential studies: 34 references were found in Embase, 343 in Medline, 79 in SportDiscus and 843 from the Cochrane Trials Database. An additional 35 references were added from bibliographic searching of relevant articles. Of a total of 1,334 abstracts, 109 dealt with physical training in asthma. The full text of each of the 109 papers was obtained and translated where necessary (one each from French, German and Chinese). Sixty-two studies were excluded as they were not relevant to the topic being reviewed, leaving 47 studies for potential inclusion in the review. Upon closer examination of the study methodology a further 28 studies were excluded (mostly due to not being an RCT) and the remaining 19 (Ahmaidi *et al.*, 1993; Arandelovic *et al.*, 2007; Basaran *et al.*, 2006; Cochrane and Clark, 1990; Counil *et al.*, 2003; Fanelli *et al.*, 2007; Fitch *et al.*, 1986; Girodo *et al.*, 1992; Huang *et al.*, 1989; King 1989; Matsumoto *et al.*, 1999; Moreira *et al.*, 2008; Sly *et al.*, 1972; Swann and Hanson, 1983; van Veldhoven *et al.*, 2001; Varray *et al.*, 1995; Varray *et al.*, 1991; Weisgerber *et al.*, 2003; Yuksel *et al.*, 2009) were included in this systematic review (Table 7.1).

These included studies involved a range of exercise which included: running on outdoor tracks, calisthenics, basketball, cycling, jogging, stretching, aerobics, treadmill, relaxation, soccer, netball, volleyball, sprints, swimming, team games, tumbling, parallel bars, rope climbing, squats thrusts, star jumps, sit-ups and press-ups. Exercises were completed 2–3 times a week over 6–13 weeks with each exercise session lasting between 20 to 120 minutes. Participants who took part in these exercises ranged from 7 to 33 years of age.

TABLE 7.1 Included randomized controlled trials characteristics

Study	Method of participant selection	Description of participants and duration of physical training	Type of physical training
Ahmaidi 1993	Participants were selected after performing incremental exercise test on a cycle ergometer and the 20 metre shuttle test	Children aged 12–17 years. Sessions were for one hour, three days a week for three months, 36 sessions in total	Running on an outdoor track
Arandelovic 2007	Participants were selected from those attending the Health Centre at University of Nis, Serbia	Participants mean age 33.07 years (exercise) and 33.55 years (control). Sessions were for one hour twice a week for six months	Swimming lessons
Basaran 2006	Participants were selected from those admitted to the pediatric allergy department for their follow-up visits	Children aged 7–15 years. During an 8-week training program, sessions were performed 3 times a week for one hour per session	Gymnasium session with warm-up and calisthenics followed by sub-maximal basketball training, cool-down and flexibility exercises
Cochrane 1990	Six week run-in period preceded patient selection	Participants aged 16–40 years. Sessions lasted 30 min, three days a week for 3 months	Warm-ups, cycling, jogging, light-calisthenics, stretching and aerobics
Counil 2003	One month of acclimatization to altitude (1400m), 6 weeks without any acute episode of wheezing, one year without emergency department visits for acute asthma and a baseline FEV_1 > 70% of predicted	Children aged 10–16 years (mean 13 years). Training group exercised three times weekly for 6 weeks with each session lasting 45 minutes	Continuous cycling activity

Study	Method of participant selection	Description of participants and duration of physical training	Type of physical training
Fanelli 2007	Participants were selected from patients attending a tertiary centre specialized in pediatric asthma	Children were aged 7–15 years. Physical training was performed twice a week for 90 minutes over 16 weeks	Warm up, stretching, cycle/treadmill, upper and lower limb and abdominal exercises, cooling down, stretching and relaxation
Fitch 1986	The 1962 American Thoracic Society definition of asthma was used for selection	Children aged 10–14 years. Physical training period was for 3 months	Jogging, calisthenics, soccer, netball, volleyball, sprints
Girodo 1992	Media solicitation was used to obtain volunteers	Participant age was 28–33 years. Subjects trained for one hour, three times a week for 16 weeks	No details provided in published paper, but the subjects were led by a person experienced in physical education
Huang 1989	A city-wide swimming programme for asthmatic children in Baltimore (USA)	Children aged 6–12 years. Subjects trained for one hour, three times a week for 2 months	Swimming training programme
King 1989	Children attending an allergy clinic in Cape Town (South Africa)	Boys aged 9–14 years. Subjects trained for 90 minutes twice a week for 3 months	Warm up, stretching, calisthenics, strengthening, breathing exercises, interval training, team games including soccer and swimming
Matsumoto 1999	Children with asthma diagnosed according to the ATS criteria who had been admitted to hospital	Children aged 9–12 years participated in the study. Subjects trained for 30 minutes a day for six days per week for six weeks	Swimming training programme
Moreira 2008	Participants were selected at the outpatient clinic at University Hospital, Sao Joalo (Porto, Portugal)	Participants were atopic school-aged children. Subjects trained for 50 minutes twice a week for 3 months	Warm up, aerobic exercises, strength training, balance and coordination exercises cool down, recreational games

Continued

TABLE 7.1 *continued*

Study	Method of participant selection	Description of participants and duration of physical training	Type of physical training
Sly 1972	Participants were selected from patients attending a pediatric allergy clinic at a hospital	Children aged 9–13 years. Sessions were for 2 hours three days a week, 39 sessions in total	Swimming, calisthenics, tumbling, parallel bars, rope climbing, abdominal strengthening, wall ladder and running
Swann 1983	Participants attending an asthma clinic with > 20% fall in FEV$_1$ were selected	Children aged 8–14 years. Sessions were twice a week and lasted for 3 months	Warm-ups, squat thrusts, star jumps, sit-ups and press-ups
van Veldhoven 2001	Children were recruited from an asthma centre, following an advertisement in the local paper and from a special school	Children aged 8–13 years (mean age 10.6). Physical training programme was done twice a week for one hour in a gymnasium and one 20 minute exercise session per week at home for a period of three months	Gymnastics with focus on improving and enhancing physical competence and learning asthma coping strategies in exercise situations
Varray 1991	Participants had to meet 3 of 4 criteria: clinical, allergic, immunological and functional (> 15% increase in FEV$_1$)	Children mean age 11.4 years. Sessions lasted for an hour each with 10 min on and 10 min off training	Indoor swimming pool training
Varray 1995	Participants selected if a 15% improvement in FEV$_1$ by inhaling a bronchodilator	Children mean age 10.3 years (exercise) and 11.7 years (control). Sessions lasted 30 min each, were twice a week for 3 months, 30 sessions in total	Indoor swimming pool used with individualized training intensity

Study	Method of participant selection	Description of participants and duration of physical training	Type of physical training
Weisgerber 2003	Subjects were recruited from the Medical College of Georgia Pediatric Pulmonary, Allergy/Immunology and General Pediatric clinics that had moderate persistent asthma according to symptoms criteria and a need for preventive daily asthma therapy	Children aged 7–14 years. Children met for physical training twice per week for five to six weeks for 45 minutes each time	Swimming lessons
Yuksel 2009	Subjects were recruited from the Department of Pediatric Allergy and Pulmonology Unit and were newly diagnosed, moderate asthmatics according to GINA guidelines	Children aged 8–13 years. Children met for physical exercise twice per week for eight weeks for one hour each time	Cycling

TABLE 7.2 Summarizing the quality of evidence

Outcome measure	Results	Level of evidence*
$\dot{V}O_{2max}$	9 RCTs (3 moderate, 6 small size)	A3
$\dot{V}_E$max	4 RCTs (2 moderate, 2 small size)	A3
Work Capacity	3 RCTs (3 moderate)	A3
Episodes of Wheeze	1 RCT of small size	A6
Asthma Quality of life	4 RCTs of moderate size	A3
6MWD	1 RCT of moderate size	A4
PEFR	6 RCTs (3 moderate, 3 small size)	A3
FEV_1	8 RCTs (5 moderate, 3 small size)	A3
FVC	7 RCTs (4 moderate, 3 small size)	A3
HR_{max}	5 RCTs (2 moderate, 3 small size)	A3

'A' grade level of evidence (randomized controlled trials only) has been shown in this review which has been graded as shown below. Arbitrarily, the following cut-off points for study size have been used; large study ³60 patients per study group; moderate study ³15 patients per study group; small study £ 15 patients in each study group.
* A1: evidence from two or more large sized RCTs.
A2: evidence from at least one large sized RCT.
A3: evidence from two or more moderate sized RCTs.
A4: evidence from at least one moderate sized RCT.
A5: evidence from two or more small sized RCTs.
A6: evidence from at least one small sized RCT.

Corresponding authors of included studies were contacted to clarify areas of uncertainty. Most of the trials did not describe the method of randomization and did not make any references to allocation concealment (method of blinding). All trials mentioned that participant allocation was carried out randomly but only four trials (Basaran et al., 2006; Fanelli et al., 2007; Moreira et al., 2008; Weisgerber et al., 2003) reported the method used. Using the Cochrane Collaboration approach for allocation concealment, these trials reporting method of allocation (using coded random numbers and drawing lots) were graded 'A' and all other trials included in this review were allocated a grade 'B' indicating that there was uncertainty as to the method of treatment allocation used by the authors in their trials. All outcomes were graded according to the quality of evidence obtained. This was based on the number and size of trial(s) contributing data towards any particular outcome (Table 7.2).

Figure 7.1 shows how the effect of physical training on $\dot{V}O_{2max}$ was assessed. The output from the statistical software used (RevMan 4.3) shows the mean and standard deviation for the exercise group and the control group (no exercise) for each of the nine studies where $\dot{V}O_{2max}$ was measured. On the right-hand side of Figure 7.1 the weighted mean difference (WMD) is shown. This is the difference between the exercise and control groups, weighted according to the precision of the study in estimating the effect (precision is calculated as the inverse of the variance). This method assumes that all of the trials have measured the outcome on the same scale and that for each study the baseline $\dot{V}O_{2max}$ was not significantly different between control and experimental groups. Where the WMD lies to the right of the line of zero effect it favours regular exercise. If the 95% CI (represented horizontal black lines) does not cross the line of zero effect, the result is statistically significant. The overall weighted mean difference (95% CI) for the nine studies was 5·12 (3.98 to 6.26) ml.kg^{-1}min^{-1}, represented by the diamond at the bottom of the figure – i.e. regular exercise resulted in an increase in $\dot{V}O_{2max}$ of 5·12 ml.kg^{-1}min^{-1}.

The Chi2 value (15.12) gives an indication of the heterogeneity of the studies. The test of heterogeneity shows whether or not the differences in the results of the nine studies are greater than would be expected by chance. In this instance the Chi2 value has to be greater than 15.51 (8 degrees of freedom and a = 0·05) before the studies would be considered heterogeneous. For $\dot{V}O_{2max}$ it is 15.12 and therefore it can be concluded that the RCTs contributing to this particular outcome were not heterogeneous. This is also denoted by the p value of 0.06 (i.e. non-significant heterogeneity).

Study or sub-category	N	Exercise group mean (SD)	N	Control group mean (SD)	WMD (fixed) 95% CI	Weight %	WMD (fixed) 95% CI
Ahmaidi 1993	10	51.20 (1.90)	10	45.80 (2.90)		28.03	5.40 [3.25, 7.55]
Cochrane 1990	18	28.40 (6.00)	18	25.00 (5.90)		8.57	3.40 [−0.49, 7.29]
Counil 2003	7	61.40 (1.10)	7	55.40 (2.30)		36.29	6.00 [4.11, 7.89]
Fanelli 2007	21	35.70 (8.17)	17	35.70 (7.90)		4.92	0.00 [−5.13, 5.13]
Fitch 1986	10	45.78 (8.08)	16	43.80 (6.65)		3.63	1.98 [−3.99, 7.95]
King 1989	6	54.00 (5.20)	6	49.70 (5.70)		3.40	4.30 [−1.87, 10.47]
van Veldhoven 2001	23	42.21 (6.87)	24	41.14 (8.83)		6.36	1.07 [−3.44, 5.58]
Varray 1991	7	48.75 (6.61)	7	39.06 (4.63)		3.62	9.69 [3.71, 15.67]
Varray 1995	9	48.50 (6.54)	9	38.84 (3.96)		5.19	9.66 [4.67, 14.65]
Total (95% CI)	111		114			100.00	5.12 [3.98, 6.26]

Test for heterogeneity: Chi^2 = 15.12, df = 8 (P = 0.06)
Test for overall effect: Z = 8.82 (P < 0.00001)

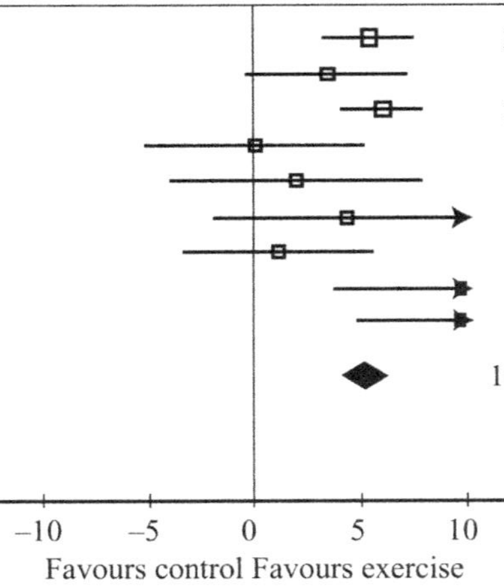

−10   −5   0   5   10

Favours control Favours exercise

FIGURE 7.1 Details of $\dot{V}O_{2max}$ (ml/kg/min) outcome. The mean value for each trial is indicated by a square box with the line through it representing the 95% confidence interval (CI). Mean values left of the zero effect line (0) favours control and values on the right favours exercise. The solid diamond indicates the overall mean effect exercise has on $\dot{V}O_{2max}$. A percentage weighting (Weight %), which is dependent on the precision and sample size of the estimation of the mean value for each RCT, is allocated to each study. The Chi$_2$ (15.12) and the degrees of freedom (df = 8) values at the bottom left gives a measure of heterogeneity of the combined results that contributed towards the overall mean result for $\dot{V}O_{2max}$. The Z statistic (8.82) indicates the level of significance for the overall result.

Study or sub-category	N	Exercise group mean (SD)	N	Control group mean (SD)	WMD (fixed) 95% CI	Weight %	WMD (fixed) 95% CI
Cochrane 1990	18	66.00 (16.00)	18	58.00 (14.00)		20.36	8.00 [−1.82, 17.82]
Counil 2003	7	102.10 (7.10)	7	87.30 (10.40)		21.97	14.80 [5.34, 24.26]
van Veldhoven 2001	23	62.58 (9.98)	24	60.06 (13.27)		43.82	2.52 [−4.17, 9.21]
Varray 1991	7	47.26 (12.80)	7	47.17 (9.73)		13.85	0.09 [−11.82, 12.00]
Total (95% CI)	55		56			100.00	6.00 [1.57, 10.43]

Test for heterogeneity: Chi² = 5.47, df = 3 (P = 0.14)
Test for overall effect: Z = 2.65 (P = 0.008)

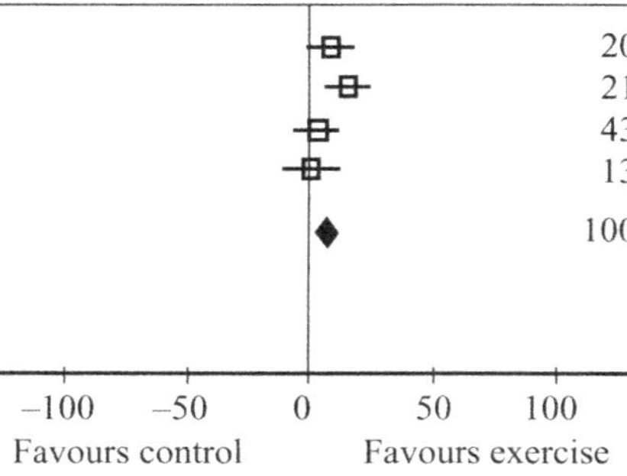

−100   −50   0   50   100

Favours control   Favours exercise

FIGURE 7.2 Details of $\dot{V}_E$max (l/min) outcome. The solid diamond is on the right-hand side of the line of no effect (favouring exercise) indicating that regular exercise increases $\dot{V}_E$max.

Study or sub-category	N	Exercise group mean (SD)	N	Control group mean (SD)	WMD (fixed) 95% CI	Weight %	WMD (fixed) 95% CI
01 PAQLQ activity							
Basaran 2006	30	5.93 (0.60)	28	5.28 (0.80)		64.59	0.65 [0.28, 1.02]
Faneli 2007	21	2.34 (1.63)	17	2.29 (1.70)		7.59	0.05 [−1.02, 1.12]
Morera 2008	16	5.72 (1.14)	15	5.69 (1.02)		14.95	0.03 [−0.73, 0.79]
Yuksel 2009	15	5.77 (1.12)	15	4.46 (1.17)		12.87	1.31 [0.49, 2.13]
Subtotal (95% CI)	82		75			100	0.60 [0.30, 0.89]

Test for heterogereity: Chi² = 6.13, df = 3 (P = 0.11)
Test for overall effect: Z = 3.98 (P < 0.0001)

02 PAQLQ emotion							
Basaran 2006	30	6.43 (0.50)	28	6.02 (0.90)		69.85	0.41 [0.03, 0.79]
Faneli 2007	21	3.40 (2.56)	17	3.46 (2.89)		3.24	−0.06 [−1.82, 1.70]
Morera 2008	16	6.42 (1.16)	15	6.23 (0.94)		18.20	0.19 [−0.55, 0.93]
Yuksel 2009	15	5.50 (1.41)	15	4.95 (1.58)		8.71	0.55 [−0.52, 1.62]
Subtotal (95% CI)	82		75			100	0.37 [0.05, 0.68]

Test for heterogereity: Chi² = 0.61, df = 3 (P = 0.89)
Test for overall effect: Z = 2.27 (P = 0.02)

FIGURE 7.2 *continued*

03 PAQLQ symptom

Study	N	Mean (SD)	N	Mean (SD)	Weight	SMD [95% CI]
Basaran 2006	30	6.23 (0.50)	28	5.73 (0.90)	73.05	0.50 [0.12, 0.88]
Faneli 2007	21	3.16 (2.52)	17	3.39 (2.98)	3.30	−0.23 [−2.01, 1.55]
Morera 2008	16	5.98 (0.99)	15	5.86 (1.33)	15.19	0.12 [−0.71, 0.95]
Yuksel 2009	15	5.50 (1.34)	15	4.51 (1.74)	8.46	0.99 [−0.12, 2.10]
Subtotal (95% CI)	82		75		100	0.46 [0.14, 0.78]

Subtotal for heterogereity: Chi^2 = 2.14, df = 3 (P = 0.54)
Test for overall effect: Z = 2.79 (P = 0.005)

04 PAQLQ total

Study	N	Mean (SD)	N	Mean (SD)	Weight	SMD [95% CI]
Basaran 2006	30	6.23 (0.40)	28	5.73 (0.80)	70.55	0.50 [0.17, 0.83]
Faneli 2007	21	2.97 (1.98)	17	3.04 (2.33)	3.93	−0.07 [−1.46, 1.32]
Morera 2008	16	6.07 (0.96)	15	5.95 (1.00)	16.01	0.12 [−0.57, 0.81]
Yuksel	15	5.58 (1.11)	15	4.65 (1.38)	9.51	0.93 [0.03, 1.83]
Subtotal (95% CI)	82		75		100.0	0.46 [0.18, 0.73]

Test for heterogereity: Chi^2 = 2.60, df = 3 (P = 0.46)
Test for overall effect: Z = 3.25 (P = 0.001)

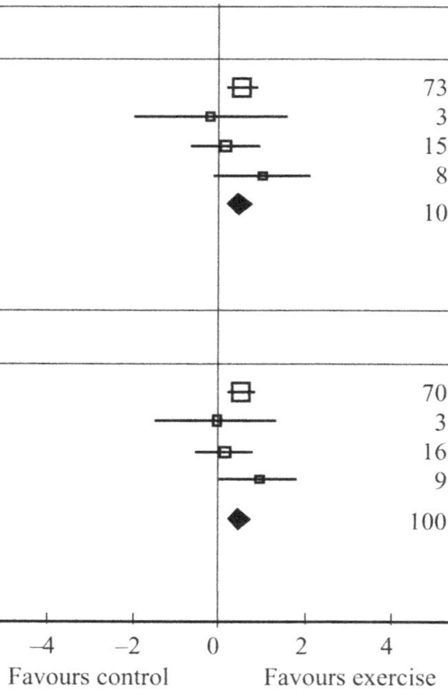

−4   −2   0   2   4

Favours control   Favours exercise

FIGURE 7.3 Details of Paediatric Asthma Quality of Life Questionnaire (PAQLQ). The solid diamond is on the right-hand side of the line of no effect (favouring exercise) indicating that regular exercise improves quality of life in people with asthma for all four components of the asthma quality of life questionnaire.

Study or sub-category	N	Exercise group mean (SD)	N	Control group mean (SD)	WMD (fixed) 95% CI	Weight %	WMD (fixed) 95% CI
Basaran 2006	30	84.60 (18.70)	28	70.30 (31.60)		33.57	14.30 [0.82, 27.78]
Fanelli 2007	21	129.90 (29.90)	17	110.50 (19.90)		24.12	19.40 [3.49, 35.31]
van Veldhoven 2001	23	116.90 (21.48)	24	113.96 (20.48)		42.32	2.94 [−9.07, 14.95]
Total (95% CI)	74		69			100.00	10.72 [2.91, 18.53]

Test for heterogeneity: Chi^2 = 3.03, df = 2 (P = 0.22)
Test for overall effect: Z = 2.69 (P = 0.007)

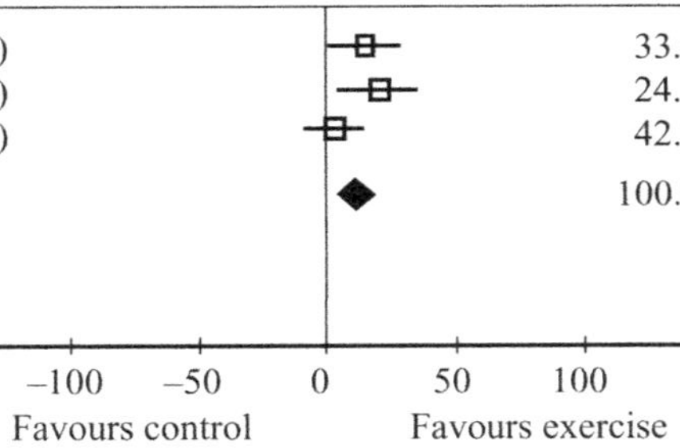

−100   −50   0   50   100

Favours control   Favours exercise

FIGURE 7.4 Details of Work capacity (W) outcome. The solid diamond is on the right-hand side of the line of no effect (favouring exercise) indicating that regular exercise increases work capacity in people with asthma.

Study or sub-category	N	Exercise group mean (SD)	N	Control group mean (SD)	WMD (fixed) 95% CI	Weight %	WMD (fixed) 95% CI
Arandelovic 2007	45	3.65 (0.86)	20	3.33 (0.84)		7.29	0.32 [−0.13, 0.77]
Basaran 2006	30	1.90 (0.70)	28	2.01 (0.50)		14.92	−0.11 [−0.42, 0.20]
Cochrane 1990	18	2.97 (0.69)	18	3.13 (0.80)		6.08	−0.16 [−0.65, 0.33]
Fanelli 2007	21	2.20 (0.59)	17	1.93 (0.53)		11.38	0.27 [−0.09, 0.63]
Sly 1972	12	0.99 (0.45)	12	1.26 (0.55)		8.95	−0.27 [−0.67, 0.13]
van Veldhoven 2001	23	2.16 (0.51)	24	2.18 (0.36)		22.55	−0.02 [−0.27, 0.23]
Varray 1991	7	1.66 (0.25)	7	1.74 (0.42)		11.04	−0.08 [−0.44, 0.28]
Weisgerber 2003	5	1.52 (0.18)	3	1.22 (0.21)		17.79	0.30 [0.01, 0.59]
Total (95% CI)	161		129			100.00	0.04 [−0.08, 0.16]

Test for heterogeneity: Chi^2 = 10.76, df = 7 (P = 0.15)

Test for overall effect: Z = 0.71 (P = 0.48)

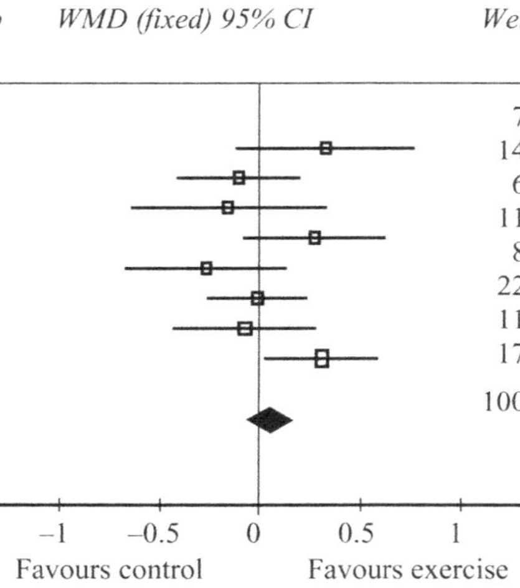

−1   −0.5   0   0.5   1

Favours control   Favours exercise

FIGURE 7.5 Details of FEV$_1$ (l/min) outcome. The solid diamond crosses the line of no effect therefore indicating that physical training does not alter FEV$_1$.

Study or sub-category	N	Exercise group mean (SD)	N	Control group mean (SD)	WMD (fixed) 95% CI	Weight %	WMD (fixed) 95% CI
Arandelovic 2007	45	4.37 (0.98)	20	4.01 (0.93)		9.69	0.36 [−0.14, 0.86]
Basaran 2006	30	2.03 (0.80)	28	2.19 (0.60)		18.31	−0.16 [−0.52, 0.20]
Fanelli 2007	21	2.70 (0.65)	17	2.32 (0.60)		15.16	0.38 [−0.02, 0.78]
Sly 1972	12	1.59 (0.68)	12	1.83 (0.74)		7.44	−0.24 [−0.81, 0.33]
van Veldhoven 2001	23	2.59 (0.57)	24	2.55 (0.48)		26.38	0.04 [−0.26 0.34]
Varray 1991	7	2.07 (0.87)	7	2.26 (0.55)		4.14	−0.19 [−0.95, 0.57]
Weisgerber 2003	5	1.89 (0.16)	3	1.54 (0.29)		18.88	0.35 [−0.01, 0.71]
Total (95% CI)	143		111			100.00	0.11 [−0.04, 0.27]

Test for heterogeneity: Chi² = 8.86, df = 6 (P = 0.18)
Test for overall effect: Z = 1.44 (P = 0.15)

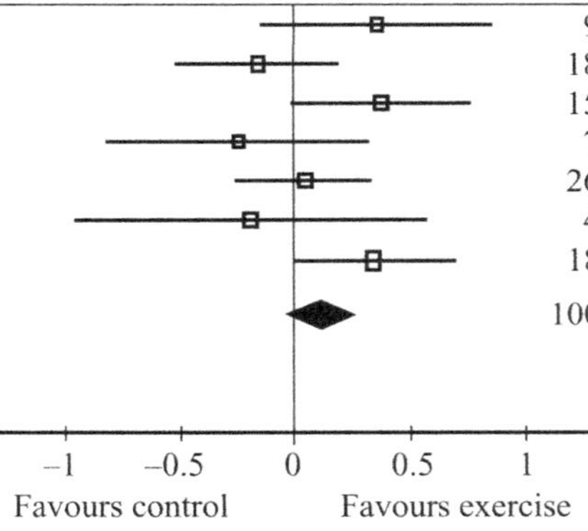

−1   −0.5   0   0.5   1

Favours control   Favours exercise

FIGURE 7.6 Details of FVC (l) outcome. The solid diamond crosses the line of no effect therefore indicating that physical training does not alter FVC.

Study or sub-category	N	Exercise group mean (SD)	N	Control group mean (SD)	WMD (fixed) 95% CI	Weight %	WMD (fixed) 95% CI
Arandelovic 2007	45	447.60 (100.20)	20	407.40 (87.00)		14.33	40.20 [−7.87, 88.27]
Basaran 2006	30	247.20 (84.00)	28	262.80 (84.00)		17.70	−15.60 [−58.86, 27.66]
Fitch 1986	10	298.70 (75.18)	16	319.60 (61.74)		10.73	−20.90 [−76.46, 34.66]
Sly 1972	11	217.00 (78.18)	11	196.00 (71.44)		8.46	21.00 [−41.58, 83.58]
van Veldhoven 2001	23	283.80 (57.00)	24	306.60 (49.20)		35.61	−22.80 [−53.30, 7.70]
Weisgerber 2003	5	193.32 (39.06)	3	156.40 (32.36)		13.18	36.92 [−13.21, 87.05]
Total (95% CI)	124		102			100.00	−0.72 [−18.92, 17.48]

Test for heterogeneity: Chi² = 8.39, df = 5 (P = 0.14)
Test for overall effect: Z = 0.08 (P = 0.94)

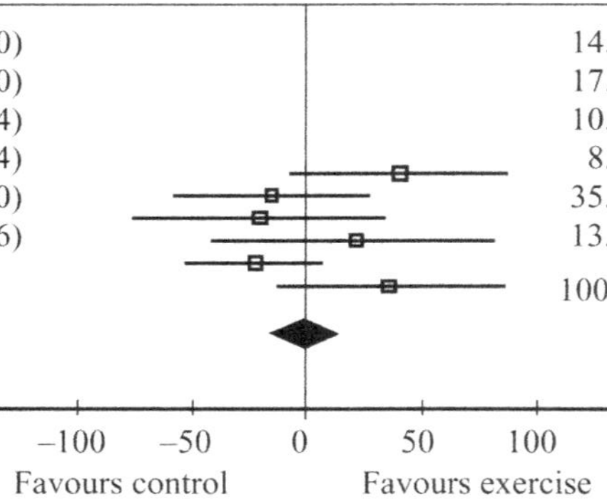

−100 −50 0 50 100

Favours control   Favours exercise

FIGURE 7.7 Details of PEFR (l/min) outcome. The solid diamond crosses the line of no effect indicating that physical training does not significantly alter PEFR in patients with asthma.

Table 7.3 provides a summary of the results. The overall WMD is shown for each of the outcome measure along with the 95 per cent confidence intervals. Regular exercise led to significant increase in $\dot{V}O_{2max}$ (Figure 7.1 with 9 studies), $\dot{V}_E max$ (Figure 7.2 with 4 studies) and peak exercise capacity (Figure 7.4 with 3 studies). Table 7.4 provides details of four studies reporting QoL (Basaran et al., 2006; Fanelli et al., 2007; Moreira et al., 2008; Yuksel et al., 2009) using the Pediatric Asthma Quality of Life Questionnaire (PAQLQ) which improved significantly with regular exercise for all components (activity, emotion, symptom and total) (Figure 7.3). 'Episodes of wheeze' as an outcome measure was reported in only one study (Sly et al., 1972). Although the number of episodes of wheeze was 7.5 days less in the exercise training group, this difference was not significant (p = 0.3). Six-minute walk distance, also reported by one study (Basaran et al., 2006), improved significantly with regular exercise. Exercise did not change FEV_1, FVC or PEFR (Figures 7.5, 7.6 and 7.7, respectively). Maximum heart rate showed a slight increase (3 beats/min) with regular exercise.

TABLE 7.3 Summary results for each outcome

Outcome measure	Weighted mean difference	95% confidence interval	Number of studies contributing to outcome	Study reference
$\dot{V}O_{2max}$ (ml.kg^{-1} min^{-1})	*5.12	3.98–6.26	9	(Ahmaidi et al., 1993, Cochrane and Clark, 1990, Counil et al., 2003, Fanelli et al., 2007, Fitch et al., 1986, King 1989, van Veldhoven et al., 2001, Varray et al., 1995, Varray et al., 1991)
$\dot{V}_E max$ (l/min)	*6.00	1.57 –10.43	4	(Cochrane and Clark, 1990, Counil et al., 2003, van Veldhoven et al., 2001, Varray et al., 1991)
Work capacity (W)	*10.72	2.91–18.53	3	(Basaran et al., 2006, Fanelli et al., 2007, van Veldhoven et al., 2001)
Episodes of wheeze (days)	–7.50	–22.42–7.42	1	(Sly et al., 1972)
6MWD (meters)	*47.90	14.79–81.01	1	(Basaran et al., 2006)

Outcome measure	Weighted mean difference	95% confidence interval	Number of studies contributing to outcome	Study reference
PEFR (l/min)	–0.72	–18.92–17.48	6	(Arandelovic *et al.*, 2007, Basaran *et al.*, 2006, Fitch *et al.*, 1986, Sly *et al.*, 1972, van Veldhoven *et al.*, 2001, Weisgerber *et al.*, 2003)
FEV$_1$ (l)	0.04	–0.08–0.16	8	(Arandelovic *et al.*, 2007, Basaran *et al.*, 2006, Cochrane and Clark, 1990, Fanelli *et al.*, 2007, Sly *et al.*, 1972, van Veldhoven *et al.*, 2001, Varray *et al.*, 1991, Weisgerber *et al.*, 2003)
FVC (l)	0.11	–0.04–0.27	7	(Arandelovic *et al.*, 2007, Basaran *et al.*, 2006, Fanelli *et al.*, 2007, Sly *et al.*, 1972, van Veldhoven *et al.*, 2001, Varray *et al.*, 1991, Weisgerber *et al.*, 2003)
HR$_{max}$ (bpm)	*3.71	0.65–5.70	4	(Ahmaidi *et al.*, 1993, Fitch *et al.*, 1986, van Veldhoven *et al.*, 2001, Varray *et al.*, 1991)

6MWD, 6 minute walk distance; PEFR, peak expiratory flow rate; FEV$_1$, forced expiratory volume in one second; FVC, forced vital capacity; HR$_{max}$, maximum heart rate; $\dot{V}_E$max, maximum expiratory flow.

* statistically significant outcome.

TABLE 7.4 Summary of Pediatric Asthma Quality of Life Questionnaire (PAQLQ) details

PAQLQ components	Weighted mean difference	95% confidence interval	P value	Number of studies (total number of subjects)
Activity	*0.60	0.30–0.89	<0.0001	4 (157)
Emotion	*0.37	0.05–0.68	0.02	4 (157)
Symptom	*0.46	0.14–0.78	0.005	4 (157)
Total	*0.46	0.18–0.73	0.0001	4 (157)

* statistically significant outcome with p<0.05.

No usable data were available for the following outcome measures: maximum voluntary ventilation, bronchodilator use, symptom diary scores, exercise endurance or walking distance. There were insufficient studies to justify subgroup analysis by gender, age or exercise intensity.

Discussion

The clearest finding of this systematic review was that cardiopulmonary fitness and QoL improved significantly with regular physical activity. This shows that the response of participants with asthma to regular exercise is similar to that of healthy people (Robinson *et al.*, 1992) and therefore, presumably, the benefits of improvements, in cardiorespiratory fitness and QoL are also accessible to them. In addition, exercise capacity (i.e. maximum exercise power output) also increased with regular exercise which is consistent with the observation that $\dot{V}O_{2max}$ and $\dot{V}_E max$ increased.

It is well known that asthma contributes significantly to morbidity among children and that it has significant impact on QoL and daily routines. Children with asthma have been shown to have significantly poorer health-related QoL, which is related to both disease and non-disease factors (Sawyer *et al.*, 2000). This review has shown that regular exercise significantly improves overall QoL score as well as each domain score (activity limitation, emotional function and symptom). The psychosocial benefits of participating in an exercise programme of team sport and sharing with other asthmatic children could have an additional effect on QoL besides the exercise programme itself. No significant correlations were observed between QoL and lung function parameters. Previous studies have also demonstrated that improvement in QoL seems to be independent of the physiological parameters (Fuchs-Climent *et al.*, 1999; Munzenberger and Vinuya, 2002).

This review has also convincingly showed that resting lung function does not change with regular exercise. This is not surprising as there is no obvious reason why regular exercise should alter PEFR, FEV_1 or FVC. It seems that any benefits of regular exercise in patients with asthma are unrelated to effects on lung function. On the other hand, evidence from this review suggests that regular exercise does not have any detrimental effect on lung function. This is reassuring for the continued promotion of exercise prescription by health professionals (Chakravarthy *et al.*, 2002), and this review provides evidence for further public health promotion of regular exercise for the management of asthma.

Typically chronic exercise training has no effect or slightly reduces the maximum heart rate whereas maximum stroke volume and, thus, maximum cardiac output, are increased (Brooks *et al.*, 1996; Haas *et al.*, 1987). In the studies which were included in this review, HR_{max} increased after physical training (Ahmaidi *et al.*, 1993; Fitch *et al.*, 1986; van Veldhoven *et al.*, 2001; Varray *et al.*, 1991), suggesting that cardiac factors did not limit maximum exercise capacity prior to training. It is likely that breathlessness or some other non-cardiac factor may have terminated the baseline tests before a true HR_{max} was achieved. The higher maximum heart rate following regular exercise may reflect the ability of participants to exercise for longer. An alternative explanation, which is improbable, is that the medication taken to prevent EIA caused the increased HR_{max}. Inhaled beta agonists can raise heart rate above resting levels but prophylactic medication was not changed during the study period and there is no evidence that physical training alters the cardiac response to b agonists. The effect of these agents on the exercise intensity–heart-rate relationship, and the possible consequences of this for exercise prescription (based on heart rate), is of potentially greater significance than the effect on maximum heart rate.

Unfortunately, there were no data available on a number of outcome measures of interest i.e. exercise endurance (as distinct from $\dot{V}O_{2max}$), diary symptoms (other than frequency of wheeze) and bronchodilator use. This review has revealed an important gap in our knowledge about the effects of regular exercise in the management of asthma. There is, however, evidence from one study (Cambach *et al.*, 1997) which was excluded from this review, suggesting that regular exercise may improve these outcomes. The study by Cambach *et al.* (1997) included participants with asthma, but was not included in our review because they also received education about their disease and breathing retraining. This means that any benefit could not be ascribed solely to physical training. Nonetheless, the intervention resulted in significant improvements in exercise endurance time and the total score for the Chronic Respiratory Disease Questionnaire increased by 17 points compared to the control group. In individuals with COPD, pulmonary rehabilitation does not lead to an improvement in these parameters unless the participants undertake exercise training (Ries *et al.*, 1995) and the same may be true of asthma. A study from Brazil (Neder *et al.*, 1999) allocated children to physical training or a control group. The study was not included in the review because the allocation of the participants was not truly random, but it did find that physical training led to significant reductions in the use of both inhaled and oral steroids.

Although there are a number of pitfalls when conducting a systematic review (e.g. incomplete electronic databases, bias in selection of relevant studies and quality of included studies), we believe these were adequately dealt with the methodology employed. Hand searching of journals was used, including a reference check of all studies obtained, two reviewers independently reviewed all studies obtained for inclusion and the review was restricted to randomized controlled trials only, thus eliminating a substantial source of lower quality study data.

Exercise recommendations

From studies included in this review the types of exercise that were beneficial for patients with asthma included whole body exercise with a minimum of two sessions per week, each session lasting at least 20 minutes. Exercises that were used most often included cycling, running, jogging or swimming. Most patients should notice an improvement in their cardiopulmonary fitness after six weeks of regular exercise.

Summary and conclusions

This review has shown that aerobic power, ventilation and QoL improve following regular exercise in patients with asthma. The evidence included in this review suggests that a minimum of 20 minutes of exercise, two or more times a week will lead to improvements in cardiorespiratory fitness and QoL in patients with asthma providing the same level of benefit afforded to people who do not have asthma. This appears to be a normal exercise training effect and is not due to an improvement in resting lung function. Examples of regular exercise that provided this benefit included whole body aerobic exercise (for example, running or jogging, gymnastics, basketball, cycling and swimming).

What is also clear from the evidence included in this review is that regular exercise should not be limited due to perceived (and unsubstantiated) limitations of asthma. Fear of inducing an episode of breathlessness inhibits many asthmatic patients from taking part in exercise. However, there was no evidence of any detrimental effect on lung function, deterioration or worsening symptoms in asthmatic patients included in this review. There is no reason to withhold regular physical exercise in patients with asthma. Therefore, it is recommended that children and adolescents with asthma should participate in regular exercise without the fear of asthma inhibiting their participation. This will not only improve asthma management and QoL but also provide associated general health benefits.

There still remains a need for further trials for assessment of the role of exercise in the management of asthma. It is particularly important to determine whether the improved exercise performance that follows regular exercise is translated into fewer symptoms. Further studies are required to confirm the improvements seen in six-minute walk distance reported by a single study to date that was included in this review. The majority of the studies included in this review investigated the effects of physical activity in children. Further randomized controlled trials need to be conducted in adults to confirm whether the benefits afforded to children with regular physical activity are also available to adults.

Acknowledgements

We would like to thank the following authors for their help in providing additional information and answering queries about their studies: S. Basaran (Adana, Turkey), C. Carvalho (Sao Paulo, Brazil), J. Neder (Sao Paulo, Brazil), I. Matsumoto (Fukuoka, Japan), A. Varray (Montpellier, France), H. Yuksel (Manisa, Turkey).

References

Ahmaidi, S. B., Varray, A. L., Savy-Pacaux, A. M. and Prefaut, C. G. (1993) Cardiorespiratory fitness evaluation by the shuttle test in asthmatic subjects during aerobic training. *Chest*, 103, 1135–41.

Arandelovic, M., Stankovic, I. and Nikolic, M. (2007) Swimming and persons with mild persistant asthma. *ScientificWorldJournal*, 7, 1182–8.

Basaran, S., Guler-Uysal, F., Ergen, N., Seydaoglu, G., Bingol-Karakoc, G. and Ufuk Altintas, D. (2006) Effects of physical exercise on quality of life, exercise capacity and pulmonary function in children with asthma. *J Rehabil Med*, 38, 130–5.

Brooks, G. A., Fahey, T. D. and White, T. P. (1996) *Exercise Physiology: Human Bioenergetics and its Applications*, Mountain View, Canada, Mayfield Publishing Co.

BTS (2008) British Guideline on the Management of Asthma. *Thorax*, 63, Suppl 4, 1–125.

Cambach, W., Chadwick-Straver, R. V., Wagenaar, R. C., Van Keimpema, A. R. and Kemper, H. C. (1997) The effects of a community-based pulmonary rehabilitation programme on exercise tolerance and quality of life: a randomized controlled trial. *Eur Respir J*, 10, 104–13.

Chakravarthy, M. V., Joyner, M. J. and Booth, F. W. (2002) An obligation for primary care physicians to prescribe physical activity to sedentary patients to reduce the risk of chronic health conditions. *Mayo Clin Proc*, 77, 165–73.

Clark, C. J. and Cochrane, L. M. (1988) Assessment of work performance in asthma for determination of cardiorespiratory fitness and training capacity. *Thorax*, 43, 745–9.

Cochrane, L. M. and Clark, C. J. (1990) Benefits and problems of a physical training programme for asthmatic patients. *Thorax*, 45, 345–51.

Counil, F. P., Varray, A., Matecki, S., Beurey, A., Marchal, P., Voisin, M. and Prefaut, C. (2003) Training of aerobic and anaerobic fitness in children with asthma. *J Pediatr*, 142, 179–84.

Cressy, D. S. and Deboisblanc, B. P. (1998) Diagnosis and management of asthma: a summary of the National Asthma Education and Prevention Program guidelines. National Institutes of Health. *J La State Med Soc*, 150, 611–17.

EPR-3 (2007) Expert Panel Report 3 (EPR-3): Guidelines for the Diagnosis and Management of Asthma-Summary Report 2007. *J Allergy Clin Immunol*, 120, S94–138.

Fanelli, A., Cabral, A. L., Neder, J. A., Martins, M. A. and Carvalho, C. R. (2007) Exercise training on disease control and quality of life in asthmatic children. *Med Sci Sports Exerc*, 39, 1474–80.

Firrincieli, V., Keller, A., Ehrensberger, R., Platts-Mills, J., Shufflebarger, C., Geldmaker, B. and Platts-Mills, T. (2005) Decreased physical activity among Head Start children with a history of wheezing: use of an accelerometer to measure activity. *Pediatr Pulmonol*, 40, 57–63.

Fitch, K. D., Blitvich, J. D. and Morton, A. R. (1986) The effect of running training on exercise-induced asthma. *Ann Allergy*, 57, 90–4.

Foggs, M. B. (2008) Guidelines management of asthma in a busy urban practice. *Curr Opin Pulm Med*, 14, 46–56.

Fuchs-Climent, D., Le Gallais, D., Varray, A., Desplan, J., Cadopi, M. and Prefaut, C. (1999) Quality of life and exercise tolerance in chronic obstructive pulmonary disease: effects of a short and intensive inpatient rehabilitation program. *Am J Phys Med Rehabil*, 78, 330–5.

Garfinkel, S., Kesten, S., Chapman, K. and Rebuck, A. S. (1992) Physiologic and nonphysiologic determinants of aerobic fitness in mild to moderate asthma. *Am Rev Respir Dis*, 145, 741–5.

Girodo, M., Ekstrand, K. A. and Metivier, G. J. (1992) Deep diaphragmatic breathing: rehabilitation exercises for the asthmatic patient. *Arch Phys Med Rehabil*, 73, 717–20.

Haas, F., Pasierski, S., Levine, N., Bishop, M., Axen, K., Pineda, H. and Haas, A. (1987) Effect of aerobic training on forced expiratory airflow in exercising asthmatic humans. *J Appl Physiol*, 63, 1230–5.

Huang, S. W., Veiga, R., Sila, U., Reed, E. and Hines, S. (1989) The effect of swimming in asthmatic children – participants in a swimming program in the city of Baltimore. *J Asthma*, 26, 117–21.

Huovinen, E., Kaprio, J., Laitinen, L. A. and Koskenvuo, M. (2001) Social predictors of adult asthma: a co-twin case-control study. *Thorax*, 56, 234–6.

King, M. (1989) Physiological effects of a physical training program in children with exercise-induced asthma. *Pediatric Exercise Science*, 1, 137–44

Levy, M. L., Thomas, M., Small, I., Pearce, L., Pinnock, H. and Stephenson, P. (2009) Summary of the 2008 BTS/SIGN British Guideline on the management of asthma. *Prim Care Respir J*, 18 Suppl 1, S1–16.

Matsumoto, I., Araki, H., Tsuda, K., Odajima, H., Nishima, S., Higaki, Y., Tanaka, H., Tanaka, M. and Shindo, M. (1999) Effects of swimming training on aerobic capacity and exercise induced bronchoconstriction in children with bronchial asthma. *Thorax*, 54, 196–201.

Moreira, A., Delgado, L., Haahtela, T., Fonseca, J., Moreira, P., Lopes, C., Mota, J., Santos, P., Rytila, P. and Castel-Branco, M. G. (2008) Physical training does not increase allergic inflammation in asthmatic children. *Eur Respir J*, 32, 1570–5.

Munzenberger, P. J. and Vinuya, R. Z. (2002) Impact of an asthma program on the quality of life of children in an urban setting. *Pharmacotherapy*, 22, 1055–62.

Neder, J. A., Nery, L. E., Silva, A. C., Cabral, A. L. and Fernandes, A. L. (1999) Short-term effects of aerobic training in the clinical management of moderate to severe asthma in children. *Thorax*, 54, 202–6.

Nordic Cochrane Centre, C. C. (2003) Review Manager (RevMan). 4.2.10 for Windows ed. Copenhagen.

Orenstein, D. M. (1996) The child and the adolescent athlete. In Bar-Or, O. (Ed.) *Asthma and Sports*. London, Blackwell.

Orenstein, D. M. (2002) Pulmonary problems and management concerns in youth sports. *Pediatr Clin North Am*, 49, 709–21, v–vi.

Oxman, A. D., Cook, D. J. and Guyatt, G. H. (1994) VI How to Use an Overview. *JAMA*, 17, 1367–71.

Ram, F. S., Robinson, S. M. and Black, P. N. (2000) Physical training for asthma. *Cochrane Database Syst Rev*, CD001116.

Rasmussen, F., Lambrechtsen, J., Siersted, H. C., Hansen, H. S. and Hansen, N. C. (2000) Low physical fitness in childhood is associated with the development of asthma in young adulthood: the Odense schoolchild study. *Eur Respir J*, 16, 866–70.

Ries, A. L., Kaplan, R. M., Limberg, T. M. and Prewitt, L. M. (1995) Effects of pulmonary rehabilitation on physiologic and psychosocial outcomes in patients with chronic obstructive pulmonary disease. *Ann Intern Med*, 122, 823–32.

Robinson, D. M., Egglestone, D. M., Hill, P. M., Rea, H. H., Richards, G. N. and Robinson, S. M. (1992) Effects of a physical conditioning programme on asthmatic patients. *N Z Med J*, 105, 253–6.

Santuz, P., Baraldi, E., Filippone, M. and Zacchello, F. (1997) Exercise performance in children with asthma: is it different from that of healthy controls? *Eur Respir J*, 10, 1254–60.

Satta, A. (2000) Exercise training in asthma. *J Sports Med Phys Fitness*, 40, 277–83.

Sawyer, M. G., Spurrier, N., Whaites, L., Kennedy, D., Martin, A. J. and Baghurst, P. (2000) The relationship between asthma severity, family functioning and the health-related quality of life of children with asthma. *Qual Life Res*, 9, 1105–15.

Sly, R. M., Harper, R. T. and Rosselot, I. (1972) The effect of physical conditioning upon asthmatic children. Ann Allergy, 30, 86–94.

Swann, I. L. and Hanson, C. A. (1983) Double-blind prospective study of the effect of physical training on childhood asthma. In Oseid, S. and Edwards, A. (Eds) *The Asthmatic Child – In Play and Sport*. London, Pitman Books Limited.

Van Veldhoven, N. H. M., Vermeer, A., Bogaard, J. M., Hessels, M. G., Wijnroks, L., Colland, V. T. and Van Essen-Zandvliet, E. E. (2001) Children with asthma and physical exercise: effects of an exercise programme. *Clinical Rehabilitation*, 15, 360–70.

Varray, A. L., Mercier, J. G. and Prefaut, C. G. (1995) Individualized training reduces excessive exercise hyperventilation in asthmatics. *Int J Rehabil Res*, 18, 297–312.

Varray, A. L., Mercier, J. G., Terral, C. M. and Prefaut, C. G. (1991) Individualized aerobic and high intensity training for asthmatic children in an exercise readaptation program. Is training always helpful for better adaptation to exercise? *Chest*, 99, 579–86.

Weisgerber, M. C., Guill, M., Weisgerber, J. M. and Butler, H. (2003) Benefits of swimming in asthma: effect of a session of swimming lessons on symptoms and PFTs with review of the literature. *J Asthma*, 40, 453–64.

Yuksel, H., Sogut, A., Yilmaz, O., Gunay, O., Tikiz, C., Dundar, P. and Onur, E. (2009) Effects of physical exercise on quality of life, pulmonary function and symptom score in children with asthma. *Asthma Allergy Immunology*, 7, 58–65.

8

OSTEOARTHRITIS

Marlene Fransen

Introduction

Overview

Osteoarthritis (OA), the most common form of arthritis, is a disease primarily affecting the articular cartilage and subchondral bone of a synovial joint, and ultimately resulting in joint failure. People with symptomatic OA complain of deep, aching pain around the joints. In early disease, pain is intermittent and mostly associated with joint use. For many people, symptomatic disease will progress, the pain becomes chronic and will then often present at rest and during the night. The daily functional activities required to remain independent become increasingly more difficult.

The pain and physical disability burden associated with OA is mostly attributable to disease of the large weight-bearing joints, i.e. the knees and the hips. In fact, knee OA is responsible for more disability in walking, stair climbing and housekeeping in non-institutionalised people aged 50 years and over than any other disease (Davis *et al.*, 1991; Guccione *et al.*, 1994). Symptomatic hip OA is similarly associated with physical disability and poor health status (Croft *et al.*, 2002; Dawson *et al.*, 2004). However, while progression between the onset of hip pain to severe symptoms and end-stage disease is variable, disease progression generally appears to be much more rapid than that observed in knee OA (Arden and Nevitt, 2006). More than 90 per cent of hip or knee total joint replacement surgery is conducted because of severe OA (Australian Orthopaedic Association, 2008).

Aetiology of osteoarthritis

The main functions of articular cartilage are to permit movement 'with low friction under high load' (Radin *et al.*, 1991a) and to attenuate stresses transmitted to the subchondral bone. Articular cartilage is a dynamic, hypocellular, macroscopically smooth tissue composed mostly of water (70–80 per cent), proteoglycan aggregates and Type II collagen (Bullough, 1992). The proteoglycan aggregates form a strongly hydrophilic matrix around the sparsely distributed chondrocytes. The chondrocytes are the cells that, through a 'synchronised balance between anabolism and catabolism', produce and assemble the collagen and proteoglycan matrix (Keuttner *et al.*, 1991). The load-bearing properties of cartilage, functioning to decrease stresses transmitted to the subchondral bone, are provided by the binding of water by proteoglycan 'retained and restrained by the collagen meshwork' (Bland and Cooper, 1984). Frictionless movement, functioning to reduce shear forces, is a result of the arrangement of the surface collagen fibres parallel to the axis of motion and load initiated lubrication of the joint with synovial fluid or fluid squeezed out of the cartilage (Bland and Cooper, 1984; Martin, 1994).

The initial pathology of OA results from an inadequate or inappropriate response to injury of the affected tissues (Pritzker, 1998). Early OA is characterised by a deterioration of the collagen meshwork resulting in an early increase in water content of the articular cartilage (Buckwalter and Mow, 1992). The chondrocytes react by increased synthesis of proteoglycan and type II collagen, but the process appears to be impaired resulting in less efficient aggregation of the proteoglycan (Malemud, 1991). If the attempted reparative process is inadequate, the cartilage then loses water, fragments and develops fissures. At some stage in the pathological process, a similar attempted reparative process in response to mechanical insults or biological imbalance occurs in the subchondral bone. Bone formation predominates over bone resorption resulting in the subchondral bone becoming less compliant and less able to dissipate forces impacting on the joint. Due to the dependence of the articular cartilage on the mechanical properties of the subchondral bone, it has been hypothesised that subchondral bone changes may precede changes in the articular cartilage.

Disease pathogenesis in most individuals is suspected to be initiated biomechanically and further mediated biochemically. Altered joint biomechanics lead to increased impulsive loading or localised stress, initiating matrix damage and biochemical changes in the articular cartilage (Radin *et al.*, 1991a). In addition, despite articular cartilage being a tissue functioning to resist shear and load-bearing forces, it has been argued that there is 'not enough of it to matter' according to Bland and Cooper (1984). The bone and the neuromuscular apparatus absorb most of the impact forces. It is hypothesised that with reduced lower-limb muscle strength and impaired proprioception during 'the ordinary activities of daily living, walking, sitting, stair climbing, relatively minor insults may become major ones' (Bland and Cooper, 1984). Both animal and human studies have demonstrated that loading rate rather than load magnitude is the critical factor for cartilage damage (Radin *et al.*, 1991a).

Knee OA

Adequate neuromuscular control is essential during ambulation to decelerate the limb prior to ground contact, attenuating the heel strike transient and thus reducing potentially damaging impulsive loading of the knee joint (Jefferson *et al.*, 1990). Higher loading rates at heel strike have been demonstrated among people with mild, activity-related, knee pain compared with controls (Radin *et al.*, 1991b). Radin *et al.* (1991b) speculated that the ineffective energy-absorbing function of the lower-limb muscles displayed by these individuals, who were free of pain during testing, was pathogenic for knee OA as walking is, for most people, a highly repetitive activity. Adequate and timely co-contraction of the knee extensor and flexors are required to decrease the high impact loading during ambulation.

Furthermore, large prospective studies have demonstrated that reduced relative knee extensor strength (adjusted for body weight) significantly increases the risk of incident symptomatic knee OA (Slemenda *et al.*, 1998; Segal *et al.*, 2009). Reduced lower-limb muscular strength is also a characteristic of established symptomatic knee OA (Hall *et al.*, 1993; Tan *et al.*, 1995; Wessel, 1996; Fisher and Pendergast,1997; Slemenda *et al.*, 1997; O'Reilly *et al.*, 1998) and there appears to be a threshold value below which knee extensor strength is critical for independent walking, standing balance and sit-stand function (Ferrucci *et al.*, 1997). Several large cross-sectional studies have established that reduced quadriceps strength in people with knee OA is strongly associated with increased pain and poor physical function (Hochberg *et al.*, 1989; Dekker *et al.*, 1993; McAlindon *et al.*, 1993; Slemenda *et al.*, 1997; O'Reilly *et al.*, 1998; van Baar *et al.*, 1998).

The level of knee adduction moment has also been related to OA progression in this joint (Andriacchi *et al.*, 2004). Even in normally aligned knees, the ground reaction force passes through the medial tibio-femoral compartment (adduction moment), resulting in this compartment bearing around 70 per cent of the weight-bearing load. Loss of medial compartment articular cartilage (the most commonly affected compartment for knee OA) results in varus mal-alignment and a further increased adduction moment. The protective role of the hip abductor and adductor muscles for knee biomechanics is increasingly being highlighted (Bennell *et al.*, 2008): the hip abductors resist pelvic drop during ambulation (pelvic drop shifting the ground reaction force medially) and the hip adductors restrain the varus shift by their attachment to the medial femoral condyl.

Hip OA

Risk factors for incident hip OA include a wide range of local and systemic factors (Arden and Nevitt, 2006; Lane, 2007; Moskositz *et al.*, 2007). While age, genetic disposition and many musculoskeletal comorbidities (Paget's Disease, developmental deformities of the hip joint, rheumatoid arthritis, etc) are arguably not modifiable risk factors, improving the mechanical environment of the hip joint and reducing joint loading has some face validity as a useful therapeutic intervention.

In support of this, it has been shown that hip OA is associated with markedly reduced lower limb muscle strength (Arokoski *et al.*, 2002; Suetta *et al.*, 2007). It appears logical that strategies designed to increase lower-limb muscle strength may have 'the potential to reduce a vast burden of disability, dependency and cost' (McAlindon *et al.*, 1993) associated with hip and knee OA.

Role of exercise in the management of OA

Regular moderate physical activity provides a wide range of health benefits for individuals with OA (Macera *et al.*, 2003). Unfortunately, many people with symptomatic OA involving the weight-bearing joints find themselves increasingly unable to participate in many popular leisure-time physical activity options for older people due to exacerbation of their joint pain. However, coupled with a sedentary lifestyle, chronic hip or knee OA often leads to decreasing lower limb muscle strength, reduced aerobic fitness and an increased risk of cardiovascular comorbidity (Minor *et al.*, 1988; Philbin *et al.*, 1995).

Currently, there is no known cure for OA or pharmaceutical agent for slowing down the rate of articular cartilage loss. People with symptomatic disease are usually recommended simple analgesics (paracetamol) or non-steroidal anti-inflammatory drugs (NSAIDs) to relieve their joint pain. However, important disease-related factors, such as impaired skeletal muscle function and reduced fitness levels, are potentially amenable to exercise regimens. In fact, most international clinical guidelines strongly advocate therapeutic exercise as the first line of effective disease management for people with hip or knee OA (Roddy *et al.*, 2005a; Zhang *et al.*, 2008). Ultimately, the long-term goal of therapeutic exercise programmes is self-management and the uptake of appropriate ongoing leisure-time physical activity to further increase or maintain improvements in pain, disability and quality of life (QoL) achieved with supervised therapeutic exercise programmes.

Evidence-base for the therapeutic effects of exercise

The highest level of scientific evidence for therapeutic effectiveness of exercise is provided by systemic reviews of well-conducted randomised controlled clinical trials (RCTs). For people with OA, therapeutic exercise can broadly be provided either as land-based or water-based (aquatic) programmes. Land-based exercise regimens include conventional exercise training modalities, such as aerobic exercise (cycle ergometry, treadmill walking, etc.) and resistance exercise (strength) training. Aquatic exercise (often termed hydrotherapy) involves exercising in a pool usually heated to around 32–36°C. Exercising in water provides buoyancy, reducing the impact loading on weight-bearing joints. Heating the water is suggested to relax the muscles and reduce joint stiffness, therefore allowing a more pain-free environment in which to exercise. Several systematic reviews of RCTs evaluating land-based and aquatic exercise programmes for people with symptomatic knee or hip OA, in terms of joint pain and self-reported physical function, have been published (Brosseau *et al.*, 2004; Pelland *et al.*, 2004; Roddy *et al.*, 2005b; Bartels *et al.*, 2007; Pisters *et al.*, 2007; Fransen and McConnell, 2008; Lange *et al.*, 2008; Fransen *et al.*, 2009; Fransen and McConnell, 2009).

There are various systems used to grade the level of evidence of therapeutic treatment benefit. In brief, the following grading system has been recommended by the Cochrane Musculoskeletal Review Group (Tugwell and Shea, 2004): Platinum: a published systematic review that has at least two rigorously conducted RCTs with at least 50 participants per allocation group; Gold: at least one rigorously conducted RCT with at least 50 participants per allocation group; Silver: RCTs that do not meet the above criteria.

Over the years, clinical studies conducted among people with OA have used a variety of questionnaires and measurement scales to quantify disease-related pain and physical function. To be able to combine these various continuous level scores in a meta-analysis requires a unitless measure of treatment effect size such as the standardized mean difference (SMD: mean difference/standard deviation). The SMD is derived either from the within allocation group change score (pre– post-treatment) or the end of treatment scores between groups, which is then divided by the respective standard deviation. This SMD is therefore a unitless quantification of treatment effect in terms of its variability. Generally, an effect size of 0.2–0.4 is rated small, 0.5–0.7 is rated moderate and ≥ 0.8 is rated large (Cohen, 1977).

In a meta-analysis of RCTs included in a systematic review, the results of the various studies are combined, or pooled, using either a fixed-effects or random-effects model. In a random-effects model, the overall effects are adjusted to include an estimate of the degree of variation between studies, or heterogeneity, in intervention effect (tau-squared) (Higgins and Green, 2008). A tau-squared value of 30–60 per cent represents moderate heterogeneity while >50 per cent is considered to represent substantial heterogeneity. However, even when marked heterogeneity is evident, a fixed effects model is often chosen as the primary method to pool results in order to avoid the potential influence of small sample bias introduced by the random-effects mode (Higgins and Green, 2008). The Chi-squared test assesses whether the differences in results between subgroups are beyond those that can be attributed to sampling error (chance).

Land-based and aquatic exercise programmes for knee OA

A recent systematic review evaluating land-based exercise programmes for knee OA (Fransen and McConnell, 2008) was able to combine knee pain and self-reported physical function data on almost 3,800 people participating in 32 different RCTs (Minor *et al.*, 1989; Kovar *et al.*, 1992; Schilke *et al.*, 1996; Bautch *et al.*, 1997; Ettinger *et al.*, 1997; Rogind *et al.*, 1998; van Baar *et al.*, 1998; Maurer *et al.*, 1999; O'Reilly *et al.*, 1999; Peloquin *et al.*, 1999; Deyle *et al.*, 2000;

Hopman-Rock and Westhoff, 2000; Petrella and Bartha, 2000; Baker *et al.*, 2001; Fransen *et al.*, 2001; Gür *et al.*, 2002; Thomas *et al.*, 2002; Topp *et al.*, 2002; Foley *et al.*, 2003; Huang *et al.*, 2003; Quilty *et al.*, 2003; Song *et al.*, 2003; Talbot *et al.*, 2003; Hughes *et al.*, 2004; Keefe *et al.*, 2004; Messier *et al.*, 2004; Bennell *et al.*, 2005; Huang *et al.*, 2005; Thorstensson *et al.*, 2005; Hay *et al.*, 2006; Mikesky *et al.*, 2006; Milkesky 2006; Fransen *et al.*, 2007). Combining the change scores (baseline – post treatment) demonstrated a statistically significant effect size (SMD) of 0.40 (95% confidence interval [CI]: 0.30 to 0.50) for knee pain and a SMD of 0.37 (95% CI: 0.25 to 0.49) for self-reported physical function (Table 8.1). Both these effect sizes would be considered small (Cohen, 1977). Interestingly, however, the demonstrated mean effect size for pain appears to be markedly larger than that reported for the effect of non-steroidal anti-inflammatory drugs (NSAIDs) (Bjordal *et al.*, 2004). The meta-analysis of RCTs evaluating the analgesic effect of NSAIDs for knee OA demonstrated a smaller effect size: SMD 0.23 (95% CI: 0.15 to 0.31). In addition, exercise is not associated with increased risk of serious gastro-intestinal or cardiovascular adverse events that is evident with the chronic use of NSAIDs in older people.

However, between-study heterogeneity was considerable for pain and physical function. It is known that small or poorly conducted RCTs are more likely to overestimate treatment benefit compared with larger or more rigorously conducted studies. Marked differences between the RCTs in methodological quality could account for some of the demonstrated between-study heterogeneity and including a lot of small or poorly conducted RCTs may be overestimating the benefit of exercise. To examine the influence of study methodology, the quality of each included RCT was evaluated according to the following three criteria (Schulz *et al.*, 1995; Jadad *et al.*, 1996): 1. Blinding of outcomes assessment; 2. Appropriate handling of withdrawals and dropouts; 3. Adequate allocation concealment. An overall assessment of bias risk was then assigned: low (all three criteria met); moderate (one or two criteria met); high (none of the criteria met). Differences in treatment effect size between the three bias risk stratifications were tested with Chi-squared distribution.

According to the above criteria, nine (28%) RCTs would be considered 'low', 14 (44%) 'moderate' and nine (28%) 'high' risk of bias. Each of the three groups (low, medium or high risk of bias) achieved significant mean treatment benefits in terms of pain and physical function. However, studies at low risk of bias demonstrated small mean treatment effects for pain and physical function while studies at high risk of bias demonstrated moderate to large treatment effect sizes (Table 8.1). The difference between the three sub-groups was significant for both outcome measures. When restricting the meta-analysis to rigorously conducted RCTs deemed to have a low risk of biased results, the mean effect size for pain was still a significant SMD 0.28 (95% CI: 0.15 to 0.42; Table 8.1), almost exactly the same treatment effect as demonstrated for NSAIDs versus placebo (Bjordal *et al.*, 2004).

TABLE 8.1 Exercise and knee OA (Fransen and McConnell, 2008). Effect size estimates for knee pain and physical function. Exploration of between-study heterogeneity

Outcome and Subgroup	RCTs n	Participants n	Effect estimate SMD (95% CI)	Chi dist (p)
KNEE PAIN				
Overall	*32*	*3616*	*0.40 (0.30 to 0.50)*	
Study methodology				
Low bias risk	10	2021	0.28 (0.15 to 0.42)	7.98 (0.02)
Moderate bias risk	13	972	0.48 (0.29 to 0.67)	
High bias risk	9	623	0.51 (0.30 to 0.72)	
Exercise programme				
Delivery mode				
Individual	10	849	0.55 (0.29 to 0.81)	Not significant
Classes	17	1608	0.37 (0.24 to 0.51)	
Home programme	6	1260	0.28 (0.16 to 0.39)	
Direct supervision				
Less than 10 occasions	9	1594	0.28 (0.16 to 0.40)	4.82 (0.03)
12 or more occasions	23	2022	0.46 (0.32 to 0.60)	
PHYSICAL FUNCTION				
Overall	*31*	*3820*	*0.36 (0.25 to 0.48)*	
Study Methodology				
Low bias risk	10	2024	0.25 (0.13 to 0.38)	8.98 (0.01)
Moderate bias risk	14	1140	0.39 (0.18 to 0.60)	
High bias risk	7	555	0.55 (0.21 to 0.90)	
Exercise programme				
Delivery mode				
Individual	10	849	0.52 (0.19 to 0.86)	Not significant
Classes	16	1563	0.35 (0.19 to 0.50)	
Home programme	6	1408	0.28 (0.17 to 0.38)	
Direct supervision				
Less than 10 occasions	9	1731	0.23 (0.09 to 0.37)	5.52 (0.02)
12 to more occasions	22	1988	0.45 (0.29 to 0.62)	

The systematic review evaluated the most immediate post-treatment outcomes reported but is there evidence for sustainability? Furthermore, how long do the benefits persist without ongoing participation in the evaluated exercise programmes? Another well-conducted systematic review aimed to evaluate the long-term effectiveness of exercise therapy for people with knee (or hip) OA (Pisters et al., 2007). One of the criteria for inclusion in this systematic review was a reporting of follow-up assessments at least six months after the exercise therapy had ended. In total, 11 RCTs (land-based and aquatic exercise programmes) were included in the meta-analysis but only five were considered to be 'high-quality' studies. Overall, the pooled results found no evidence for sustained benefit, in terms of either pain or physical function. Six months after the exercise programmes were completed, there was no difference in reported pain and physical function between participants allocated to the active exercise programme compared with the controls. The authors, however, commented that the two RCTs including a few 'booster' sessions after the end of the exercise programme, did achieve sustained benefits. The efficacy of 'booster' sessions is probably intuitive to the many allied health professionals who would consider it difficult for most people to maintain an adequate dosage of exercise without some form of formal monitoring or ongoing encouragement.

In summary, there is platinum level evidence that land-based therapeutic exercise has at least short-term benefit in terms of reduced knee pain and disability for people with knee OA. This statement is supported by the results of a meta-analysis that included at least two RCTs demonstrating benefit, each with sample sizes of at least 50 per group and satisfying methodological quality criteria (Tugwell and Shea, 2004). The magnitude of pain relief can be comparable to that achieved by currently available oral analgesics.

Land-based and aquatic exercise programmes for hip OA

In sharp contrast to knee OA, there have only been a small number of RCTs able to provide data for the evaluation of land-based exercise for people with OA hip. The very recent meta-analysis of land-based programmes could only identify five RCTs (van Baar et al., 1998; Hopman-Rock and Westhoff, 2000; Foley et al., 2003; Tak et al., 2005; Fransen et al., 2007), with only one RCT (Tak et al., 2005) restricting recruitment to people with symptomatic hip OA. The other four studies also recruited participants with knee OA. The five included studies provided data on only 204 and 187 hip OA participants for pain and physical function, respectively. Combining the results of the five included RCTs demonstrated a small post-treatment effect for pain: SMD 0.38 (95% CI: 0.09 to 0.67). Due to the small number of RCTs included in this meta-analysis, the confidence interval is very wide. Hence, the magnitude of treatment benefit could lie anywhere between 'imperceptible' to large. No significant benefit in terms of improved self-reported physical function was detected: SMD 0.02 (95% CI: −0.29 to 0.31). Between-study heterogeneity was also large in this meta-analysis of exercise for hip OA. However, using this criteria for blinding, handling of withdrawals and allocation concealment, none of the five included RCTs would be considered as providing a 'high risk of bias'. As all RCTs evaluating land-based exercise for hip OA have been small (less than 50 participants per allocation group), there is only silver level evidence of short-term benefit in terms of pain and physical function.

There has been one meta-analysis evaluating aquatic exercise specifically for people with knee or hip OA (Bartels *et al.*, 2007). This systematic review combined the effects of four RCTs with a total of more than 650 participants. Significant benefit in terms of pain reduction: SMD 0.19 (95% CI: 0.04 to 0.35) and improved physical function: SMD 0.26 (95% CI: 0.11 to 0.42) were demonstrated. However, these effect sizes are considerably smaller than those demonstrated by land-based therapeutic exercise programmes. Between-study heterogeneity was not demonstrated in these two meta-analyses. This study provides gold level evidence for a small short-term benefit of an aquatic exercise programme in terms of pain and physical function for people with OA of the hips or knees.

Mode, intensity, duration, frequency of land-based exercise

Knee OA

A wide range of therapeutic exercise programmes have been assessed in the various meta-analyses evaluating exercise for knee OA (Brosseau *et al.*, 2004; Pelland *et al.*, 2004; Roddy *et al.*, 2005; Fransen and McConnell, 2008; Lange *et al.*, 2008; Fransen and McConnell, 2009). Four of these meta-analyses have focused on either aerobic exercise programmes (Brosseau *et al.*, 2004), resistance exercise (strength) training programmes (Pelland *et al.*, 2004; Lange *et al.*, 2008) or a comparison of RCTs evaluating strengthening programmes with RCTs evaluating an aerobic walking programme (Roddy *et al.*, 2005) for people with knee or hip OA. To date, there has only been one large RCT allowing a direct randomised comparison between a strength training programme and an aerobic walking programme (Ettinger *et al.*, 1997). This RCT found that both class-based exercise programmes resulted in modest benefits in terms of pain and disability over an 18-month period above benefits achieved by a non-exercise control group, without superiority being demonstrated for either of the two exercise programmes. A weaker, indirect comparison of various studies evaluating either aerobic walking (3 RCTs, 449 participants) or home-based quadriceps strengthening exercises (9 RCTs, 2004 participants) in a recent meta-analysis (Roddy *et al.*, 2005) also concluded 'no difference' in the ability of the two forms of exercise to reduce pain or disability. A research group from the University of Ottawa conducted two separate systematic reviews of controlled clinical trials evaluating strengthening and aerobic exercises for OA (Brosseau *et al.*, 2004; Pelland *et al.*, 2004). They concluded that 'the most efficacious exercise regimen has yet to be determined'. This group of researchers concluded that aerobic exercise in general was at least equivalent to strengthening exercise (or even superior), and that strengthening exercise programmes were best when simple quadriceps exercises were supplemented with a more complete exercise programme, i.e. included range of motion, stretching, functional balance and aerobic exercises (Brosseau et al., 2004; Pelland et al., 2004).

In the recent Cochrane review restricted to RCTs evaluating exercise programmes for knee OA (Fransen and McConnell, 2009), the exercise programmes evaluated in 32 RCTs were categorised according to the treatment delivery mode: individual treatments provided by a physical therapist, class-based programmes or home-based programmes. It should be noted that this terminology is not exactly descriptive. Many home-based programmes incorporated home or clinic visits by a trained nurse or physiotherapist (O'Reilly et al., 1999; Baker et al., 2001; Thomas et al., 2002; Hay et al., 2006). Also, most individual treatments or class-based programmes included the provision of a structured home-exercise programme. Probably as a result of the lack of clear definition, the sub-group comparison could not detect a significant difference in treatment effect size between the three different modes of treatment delivery for either pain or physical function (Table 8.1). However, the number of directly supervised sessions within an exercise programme was significantly associated with treatment benefit. The total number of supervised exercise sessions provided by RCTs in the meta-analysis ranged from none (Petrella and Bartha, 2000; Talbot et al., 2003) to 36 or more (Minor et al., 1989; Bautch et al., 1997; Ettinger et al., 1997; Peloquin et al., 1999; Keefe et al., 2004; Messier et al., 2004). All-inclusive stratification was made as 10 or less monitored sessions (provided as individual treatments, exercise classes or home visits) versus 12 or more supervised exercise sessions. Programmes providing 10 or less monitored sessions achieved what would be considered small mean treatment effect sizes for pain and physical function; programmes providing at least 12 monitored sessions achieved larger effect sizes for these outcomes. The conclusion is that regardless of the delivery mode (individual or class-based, clinic or home visits), treatment effect size is significantly associated with the number of supervised exercise sessions provided.

In this same meta-analysis (Fransen and McConnell 2008), the authors describe treatment intensity in the various RCTs as ranging from 'maximum effort' muscle strengthening (Schilke et al., 1996; Gür et al., 2002) to low intensity aerobic walking (Bautch et al., 1997; Talbot et al., 2003; Messier et al., 2004). Treatment content varied from mostly aerobic walking programmes (Minor et al., 1989; Kovar et al., 1992; Ettinger et al., 1997; Talbot et al., 2003; Messier et al., 2004) to very complex, comprehensive programmes including manual therapy, upper-limb and/or truncal muscle strengthening and balance coordination (Rogind et al., 1998; van Baar et al., 1998; Peloquin et al., 1999; Deyle et al., 2000; Bennell et al., 2005) in addition to the more usual lower-limb muscle strengthening programmes. Two studies evaluated Tai Chi classes (Song et al., 2003; Fransen et al., 2007). The 32 included studies were categorised according to the main treatment focus: simple quadriceps strengthening, lower limb muscle strengthening (Theraband, cuff weights, isokinetics), strengthening and aerobic component (stationary bicycle or walking), walking programme only or 'other' (not specifically focused on lower limb muscle strengthening or increasing aerobic capacity). The simple quadriceps programmes achieved only borderline significance for both pain and physical function and the 'other' programmes resulted in an insignificant treatment effect for physical function. However, for both pain and physical function, no significant difference in effect size could be demonstrated between the groups of exercise programmes when testing the Chi^2 distribution. Between study heterogeneity was considerable within most of the study categories.

Only two relatively large RCTs have examined the influence of structural disease severity on the effectiveness of therapeutic exercise (Fransen *et al.*, 2001; Lim *et al.*, 2008). Both RCTs obtained standardised knee radiographs on study participants prior to randomisation. The first RCT conducted among 126 people with symptomatic knee OA (Fransen *et al.*, 2001) clearly demonstrated that the degree of tibio-femoral joint space narrowing modified responsiveness to the exercise-based interventions. Participants who had less severe disease achieved moderate to large effect sizes for reduced pain, improved physical function and increased lower-limb muscle strength, while those participants who had marked loss of tibio-femoral joint space achieved only small treatment effects. The more recent RCT (Lim *et al.*, 2008) stratified 107 participants by knee joint alignment (neutral or varus) before randomising to a quadriceps strengthening programme or control group. Among those participants allocated to the exercise programme, strength increased irrespective of knee alignment. However, knee pain improved only in the neutrally aligned (early structural disease) group.

There is as yet no strong evidence from clinical trials favouring one form of exercise over another when the goal is to decrease knee pain and disability among people with knee OA. However, it is apparent that restricting exercise programmes to simple quadriceps strengthening or providing less than 10 occasions of exercise supervision is likely to be less clinically effective than lengthier exercise programmes focusing on more comprehensive lower limb muscle strengthening and increasing general aerobic fitness. There is evidence that therapeutic exercise is more likely to be clinically beneficial in early disease, before OA has progressed to marked loss of joint space or structural mal-alignment.

Hip OA

There was large variability in treatment dosage and content in the five RCTs included in the systematic review of land-based exercise for people with hip OA (Fransen *et al.*, 2009). Two studies provided less than 10 supervised sessions (Hopman-Rock and Westhoff, 2000; Tak *et al.*, 2005), while the other three studies provided access to at least 18 sessions. Four of the five RCTs evaluated class-based programmes, while only one (van Baar *et al.*, 1998) provided treatments as individual sessions with a physical therapist. While one of the five RCTs evaluated a specific 'Tai Chi for Arthritis' programme (Fransen *et al.*, 2007), the other four provided more traditional exercise programmes. Due to the small number of RCTs conducted to date, it is not meaningful to try and explore the possible effect of treatment dosage (frequency, intensity or duration) or exercise programme content on the magnitude of treatment benefit.

Aquatic exercise

The content of the four aquatic exercise programmes for hip or knee OA evaluated in the published meta-analysis (Bartels *et al.*, 2007) were examined to try and clarify why the mean treatment benefits demonstrated for pain and physical disability were so much smaller than those achieved by land-based exercise programmes. The largest RCT (Cochrane *et al.*, 2005) in that analysis measured patient outcomes from a low to moderate intensity aqua-aerobics programme at 18 months. However, classes were only provided for 12 months and only 25 per cent of participants were still enrolled in aqua-aerobics (at own cost) at 18 months, the time of the outcomes assessment. Another two of the four RCTs evaluated an Arthritis Foundation certified aquatic programme (Patrick *et al.*, 2001; Wang *et al.*, 2007). These classes focus on whole body gentle movements and were originally designed for people with rheumatoid arthritis, therefore not necessarily targeting the physiological impairments specific to chronic hip and knee OA – reduced lower limb muscle strength and poor aerobic fitness. The lengthy period between end of treatment and outcomes assessment in one RCT and the mostly low intensity exercise programmes evaluated in another two RCTs may explain the disappointingly small treatment benefits demonstrated.

There have been three further RCTs comparing aquatic exercise classes with a non-exercise group among people with symptomatic hip or knee OA published after the above systematic review (Fransen *et al.*, 2007; Hinman *et al.*, 2007; Lund *et al.*, 2008) The two larger Australian studies (Fransen *et al.*, 2007; Hinman *et al.*, 2007) evaluated twice-weekly aquatic exercise programmes of progressive lower-limb muscle strengthening. The exercise classes were small (6–10 participants) and the exercises were rigorously progressed to ensure participants were at least exercising at a moderate intensity. These two studies demonstrated significant change scores for pain and physical function of a magnitude very comparable to those demonstrated by land-based exercise programmes. The smaller Swedish study (Lund *et al.*, 2008) also evaluated an aquatic exercise programme directed at muscle strengthening but could not demonstrate statistically significant benefits. The authors attribute the non-significant findings to inadequate study power to detect the small to moderate effect sizes feasibly anticipated for exercise programmes involving community samples of people with a chronic musculoskeletal disease. The development of aquatic exercise programmes, specifically directed at lower-limb muscle strengthening and aerobic fitness, are likely to provide greater clinical benefits for people with lower limb OA compared with more gentle programmes directed at overall joint flexibility.

Summary and conclusions

There is considerable scientific evidence supporting the benefit of graded therapeutic exercise for knee OA in terms of reducing pain and disability. In contrast, there is limited research regarding the symptomatic effectiveness of exercise for hip OA. Additionally, there is no evidence to date able to establish that lower limb muscle strengthening exercise will slow down the rate of cartilage loss. This hypothesis is based on biological plausibility, but has not yet been established in clinical research. This area of research (disease-modification) is suggested to have the most impact on disease burden.

There are some important caveats to the evidence presented in this chapter. The first concerns the responsiveness of self-reported pain and physical function. Many of the RCTs evaluating exercise for OA include mostly participants with early or mild symptomatic disease. Although people with early disease frequently demonstrate reduced muscle strength and aerobic capacity compared with their age- and gender-matched peers without symptomatic OA, these physiological impairments are often not yet large enough to translate into reportable difficulties on simple questionnaires. This lack of reportable difficulties would considerably reduce the potential range of improvement possible (ceiling effect) on self-report questionnaires in people with early or mild disease. One of the potential benefits of exercise in people with early OA, such as increasing 'physiological reserve capacity', will not be captured by these questionnaires. Second, regular exercise provides general health benefits beyond reducing joint symptoms. The outcomes of the various systematic reviews are therefore, likely to be underestimating the overall beneficial effect of exercise amongst people with OA.

References

Andriacchi, T. P., Mundermann, A., Lane Smith, R., Alexander, E. J., Dyrby, C. O. and Koo, S. (2004). A framework for the in vivo pathomechanics of osteoarthritis of the knee. *Ann Biomed Engineering* 32: 447–57.

Arden, N. and Nevitt, M. C. (2006). Osteoarthritis: Epidemiology. Best Pract Res Clin *Rheumatol* 20: 3–25.

Arokoski, M. H., Arokoski, J. P., Haas, M., Kankaanpas, M., Vesterinen, N. and Niemitukia, L. H. (2002). Hip muscle strength and muscle cross sectional area in men with and without hip osteoarthritis. *J Rheumatol* 29: 2185–95.

Australian Orthopaedic Association (2008). *National Joint Replacement Registry. Annual Report*. Adelaide, AOA.

Baker, K. R., Nelson, M. E., Felson, D. T., Layne, J. E., Sarno, R. and Roubenoff, R. (2001). The efficacy of home-based progressive strength training in older adults with knee osteoarthritis: a randomized controlled trial. *J Rheumatol* 28: 1655–1665.

Bartels, E. M., Lund, H., Hagen, K. B., Dagfinrud, H., Christensen, J. and Danneskiold-Samsoe, B. (2007). Aquatic exercise for the treatment of knee and hip osteoarthritis. Cochrane Database of Systematic Reviews Issue 4.

Bautch, J., Malone, D. and Vailas, A. (1997). Effects of exercise on knee joints with osteoarthritis: a pilot study of biologic markers. *Arthritis Care Res* 10: 48–55.

Bennell, K. L., Hinman, R. S., Metcalf, B. R., Buchbinder, R., McConnell, J., McColl, G., Green, S. and Crossley, K. M. (2005). Efficacy of physiotherapy management of knee joint osteoarthritis: a randomised, double blind, placebo controlled trial. *Ann Rheum Dis* 64: 906–12.

Bennell, K. L., Hunt, M. A., Wrigley, T. V., Lim, B.-W. and Hinman, R. S. (2008). Role of muscle in the genesis and management of knee osteoarthritis. *Rheum Dis Clin N Am* 34: 731–54.

Bjordal, J. M., Ljunggren, A. E., Klovning, A. and Slordal, L. (2004). Non-steroidal anti-inflammatory drugs, including cyclo-oxygenase-2 inhibitors, in osteoarthritic knee pain: meta-analysis of randomised placebo controlled trials. *BMJ* 329: 1317–20.

Bland, J. H. and Cooper, S. M. (1984). Osteoarthritis: a review of the cell biology involved and evidence for reversibility. Management rationally related to known genesis and pathophysiology. *Seminars Arthritis Rheum* 14: 106–133.

Brosseau, L., Pelland, L., Wells, G., Macleay, L., Lamothe, C., Michaud, G., Lambert, J., Robinson, V. and Tugwell, P. (2004). Efficacy of aerobic exercises for osteoarthritis (Part II): A meta-analysis. *Phys Ther Reviews* 9: 125–145.

Buckwalter, J. A. and Mow, V. C. (1992). Cartilage repair in osteoarthritis. *Osteoarthritis. Diagnosis and Medical/Surgical Management.* R. W. Moskowitz, D. S. Howell, V. M. Goldberg and H. J. Mankin. Philadelphia, W.B. Saunders Company.

Bullough, P. G. (1992). The pathology of osteoarthritis. *Osteoarthritis. Diagnosis and Medical/Surgical Management.* R. W. Moskowitz, D. S. Howell, V. M. Goldberg and H. J. Mankin. Philadelphia, W.B.Saunders Company.

Cochrane, T., Davey, R. C. and Matthes Edwards, S. M. (2005). Randomised controlled trail of the cost-effectiveness of water-based therapy for lower limb osteoarthritis. *Health Technol Assess* 9.

Cohen, J. (1977). *Statistical Power Analysis for the Behavioural Sciences*, New York: Academic.

Croft, P., Lewis, M., Wynn Jones, C., Coggon, D. and Cooper, C. (2002). Health status in patients awaiting hip replacement for osteoarthritis. *Rheumatol* 41: 1001–7.

Davis, M. A., Ettinger, W. H., Neuhaus, J. M. and Mallon, K. P. (1991). Knee osteoarthritis and physical functioning: evidence from the NHANES 1 epidemiologic followup study. *J Rheumatol* 18: 591–598.

Dawson, J., Linsell, L., Zondervan, K., Rose, P., Randall, T., Carr, A. and Fitzpatrick, R. (2004). Epidemiology of hip and knee pain and its impact on overall health status in older adults. *Rheumatol* 43: 497–504.

Dekker, J., Tola, P., Aufdemkampe, G. and Winckers, M. (1993). Negative affect, pain and disability in osteoarthritis patients: the mediating role of muscle weakness. *Behav Res Ther* 31: 203–206.

Deyle, G. D., Henderson, N. E., Matekel, R. L., Ryder, M. G., Garber, M. B. and Allison, S. C. (2000). Effectiveness of manual physical therapy and exercise in osteoarthritis of the knee. A randomized, controlled trial. *Ann Int Med* 132: 173–181.

Ettinger, W. H, Burns, R., Messier, S. P., Applegate, W., Rejeski, W. J., Morgan, T., Shumaker, S., Berry, M. J., O'Toole, M., Mau, J. and Craven, T. (1997). A randomized trial comparing aerobic exercise and resistance exercise with a health education program in older adults with knee osteoarthritis. The Fitness Arthritis and Seniors Trial (FAST). *JAMA* 277: 25–31.

Ferrucci, L., Guralnik, J. M., Buchner, D., Kasper, J., Lamb, S. E., Simonsick, E. M., Corti, M. C., Bandeen-Roche, K. and Fried, L. P. (1997). Departures from linearity in the relationship between measures of muscular strength and physical performance of the lower extremities: the Women's Health and Aging Study. *J Gerontol 52A*: M275–M285.

Fisher, N. M. and Pendergast, D. R. (1997). Reduced muscle function in patients with osteoarthritis. *Scand J Rehabil Med* 29: 213–221.

Foley, A., Halbert, J., Hewitt, T. and Crotty, M. (2003). Does hydrotherapy improve strength and physical function in patients with osteoarthritis – a randomised controlled trial comparing a gym based and a hydrotherapy based strengthening programme. *Ann Rheum Dis* 62: 1162–1167.

Fransen, M., Crosbie, J. and Edmonds, J. (2001). Physical therapy is effective for patients with osteoarthritis of the knee: a randomized controlled clinical trial. *J Rheumatol* 28: 156–164.

Fransen, M. and McConnell, S. (2008). Exercise for osteoarthritis of the knee. Cochrane Database of Systematic Reviews Issue 4.

Fransen, M. and McConnell, S. (2009). Land-based exercise for osteoarthritis of the knee: a metaanalysis of randomized controlled trials. *J Rheumatol* 36: 1109–17.

Fransen, M., McConnell, S., Hernandez-Molina, G. and Reichenbach, S. (2009). Exercise for osteoarthritis of the hip. Cochrane Database of Systematic Reviews Issue 3.

Fransen, M., Nairn, L., Winstanley, J., Lam, P. and Edmonds, J. (2007). The Physical Activity for Osteoarthritis Management (PAFORM) study. A randomised controlled clinical trial evaluating hydrotherapy and Tai Chi classes. *Arthritis Rheum* 57: 407–414.

Guccione, A. A., Felson, D. T., Anderson, J. J., Anthony, J. M., Zhang, Y., Wilson, P. W., Kelly-Hayes, M., Wolf, P. A., Kreger, B. E. and Kannel, W. B. (1994). The effects of specific medical conditions on the functional limitations of elders in the Framingham study. *Am J Public Health* 84: 351–358.

Gür, H., Cakin, N., Akova, B., Okay, E. and Kucukoglu, S. (2002). Concentric versus combined concentric-eccentric isokinetic training: effects on functional capacity and symptoms in patients with osteoarthrosis of the knee. *Arch Phys Med Rehabil* 83: 308–316.

Hall, K. D., Hayes, K. W. and Falconer, J. (1993). Differential strength decline in patients with osteoarthritis of the knee: revision of a hypothesis. *Arthritis Care Res* 6: 89–96.

Hay, E. M., FosterNadine, E., Thomas, E., Peat, G., Phelan, M., Yates, H. E. and Blenkisopp, A. (2006). Effectiveness of community physiotherapy and enhanced pharmacy review for knee pain in people aged over 55 presenting to primary care: pragmatic randomized trial. *BMJ* 333: 995.

Higgins, J. P. T. and Green, S. (2008). *Cochrane Handbook for Systematic Reviews of Interventions*. The Cochrane Collaboration.

Hinman, R. S., Heywood, S. E. and Day, A. R. (2007). Aquatic physical therapy for hip and knee osteoarthritis: results of a single-blind randomized controlled trial. *Physi Ther* 87: 32–43.

Hochberg, M. C., Lawrence, R. C., Everett, D. F. and Cornoni-Huntley, J. (1989). Epidemiologic associations of pain in osteoarthritis of the knee: data from the National Health and Nutrition Examination Survey and the National Health and Nutrition Examination-I epidemiologic followup survey. Seminars *Arthritis Rheum* 18: 4–9.

Hopman-Rock, M. and Westhoff, M. (2000). The effects of a health educational and exercise program for older adults with osteoarthritis of the hip or knee. *J Rheumatol* 27: 1947–54.

Huang, M.-H., Lin, Y.-S., Yang, R.-C. and Lee, C.-L. (2003). A comparison of various therapeutic exercises on the functional status of patients with knee osteoarthritis. *Semin Arthritis Rheum* 32: 398–406.

Huang, M.-H., Yang, R.-C., Lee, C.-L., Chen, T.-W. and Wang, M.-C. (2005). Preliminary results of integrated therapy for patients with knee osteoarthritis. *Arthritis Rheum* 53: 812–20.

Hughes, S. L., Seymour, R. B., Campbell, R., Pollak, N., Huber, G. and Sharma, L. (2004). Impact of the Fit and Strong intervention on older adults with osteoarthritis. *The Gerontologist* 44: 217–28.

Jadad, A. R., Moore, R. A., Carroll, D., Jenkinson, C., Reynolds, D. J., Gavaghan, D. J. and McQuay, H. J. (1996). Assessing the quality of reports of randomized clinical trials: is blinding necessary? *Controlled Clin Trials* 17: 1–12.

Jefferson, R. J., Collins, J. J., Whittle, M. W., Radin, E. L. and O'Connor, J. J. (1990). The role of the quadriceps in controlling impulsive forces around the heel. Proceedings of the Institution of Mechanical Engineers. Part H *J Engineer Med* 204: 21–28.

Keefe, F. J., Blumenthal, J., Baucom, D., Affleck, G., Waugh, R., Caldwell, D. S., Beaupre, P., Kashikar-Zuck, S., Wright, K., Egert, J. and Lefebvre, J. (2004). Effects of spouse-assisted coping skills and exercise training in patients with osteoarthritic knee pain: a randomized controlled study. *Pain* 110: 539–549.

Keuttner, K. E., Aydelotte, M. B. and Thonar, E. J. (1991). Articular cartilage matrix and structure: a minireview. *J Rheumatol* 18: 46–48.

Kovar, P. A., Allegrante, J. P., MacKenzie, C. R., Peterson, M. G., Gutin, B. and Charlson, M. E. (1992). Supervised fitness walking in patients with osteoarthritis of the knee. A randomized, controlled trial. *Ann Intern Med* 116: 529–34.

Lane, N. E. (2007). Osteoarthritis of the hip. *New Engl J Med* 357: 1413–21.

Lange, A. K., Vanwanseele, B. and Fiatarone Singh, M. A. (2008). Strength training for treatment of osteoarthritis of the knee: a systematic review. *Arthritis Rheum* 59: 1488–94.

Lim, B.-W., Hinman, R. S., Wrigley, T. V., Sharma, L. and Bennell, K. L. (2008). Does knee malalignment mediate the effects of quadriceps strengthening on knee adduction moment, pain, and function in medial knee osteoarthritis? A randomized controlled trial. *Arthritis Rheum* 59: 943–51.

Lund, H., Weile, U., Christensen, R., Rostock, B., Downey, A., Bartels, E. M., Danneskiold-Samsoe, B. and Bliddal, H. (2008). A randomized controlled trial of aquatic land land-based exercise in patients with knee osteoarthritis. *J Rehabil Med* 40: 137–44.

Macera, C. A., Hootman, J. M. and Sniezek, J. E. (2003). Major public health benefits of physical activity. *Arthritis Rheum.* 49: 122–8.

Malemud, C. (1991). Changes in proteoglycans in osteoarthritis: biochemistry, ultrastructure and biosynthetic processing. *J Rheumatol* 18: 60–2.

Martin, D. F. (1994). Pathomechanics of knee osteoarthritis. *Med Sci Sports Exerc* 26: 1429–34.

Maurer, B. T., Stern, A. G., Kinossian, B., Cook, K. D. and Schumacher, H. R. (1999). Osteoarthritis of the knee: isokinetic quadriceps exercise versus an educational intervention. *Arch Phys Med Rehabil* 80: 1293–1299.

McAlindon, T. E., Cooper, C., Kirwan, J. R. and Dieppe, P. A. (1993). Determinants of disability in osteoarthritis of the knee. *Ann Rheum Dis* 52: 258–262.

Messier, S. P., Loeser, R. F., Miller, G. D., Morgan, T. M., Rejeski, W. J., Sevick, M. A., Ettinger, W. H., Pahor, M. and Williamson, J. D. (2004). Exercise and dietary weight loss in overweight and obese older adults with knee osteoarthritis: The Arthritis, Diet and Activity Promotion Trial (ADAPT). *Arthritis Rheum* 50: 1501–10.

Mikesky, A. E., Mazzuca, S. A., Brandt, K. D., Perkins, S. M., Damush, T. and Lane, K. A. (2006). Effects of strength training on the incidence and progression of knee osteoaarthritis. *Arthritis Rheum* 55: 690–9.

Milkesky, A. E. (2006). Weight training does not increase strength but may slow progression in OA patients. *Arthritis Care* 55: 690–99.

Minor, M. A., Hewett, J. E., Webel, R. R., Anderson, S. K. and Kay, D. R. (1989). Efficacy of physical conditioning exercise in patients with rheumatoid arthritis and osteoarthritis. *Arthritis Rheum* 32: 1396–1405.

Minor, M. A., Hewett, J. E., Webel, R. R., Dreisinger, T. E. and Kay, D. R. (1988). Exercise tolerance and disease related measures in patients with rheumatoid arthritis and osteoarthritis. *J Rheumatol* 15: 905–11.

Moskositz, R. W., Altman, R. D., Hochberg, M. C., Buckwalter, J. A. and Goldberg, V. M. (2007). *Osteoarthritis: Diagnosis and medical/surgical management.* Philadelphia PA, Lippincott Williams & Wilkins.

O'Reilly, S. C., Jones, A., Muir, K. R. and Doherty, M. (1998). Quadriceps weakness in knee osteoarthritis: the effect on pain and disability. *Ann Rheum Dis* 57: 588–594.

O'Reilly, S. C., Muir, K. R. and Doherty, M. (1999). Effectiveness of home exercise on pain and disability from osteoarthritis of the knee: a randomised controlled trial. *Ann Rheum Dis* 58: 15–19.

Patrick, D. L., Ramsey, S. D., Spencer, A., Kinne, S., Belza, B. and Topolski, T. D. (2001). Economic evaluation of aquatic exercise for persons with osteoarthritis. *Med Care* 39: 413–424.

Pelland, L., Brosseau, L., Wells, G., Macleay, L., Lambert, J., Lamothe, C., Robinson, V. and Tugwell, P. (2004). Efficacy of strengthening exercises for osteoarthritis (Part I): A meta-analysis. *Phys Ther Reviews* 9: 77–108.

Peloquin, L., Bravo, G., Gauthier, P., Lacombe, G. and Billiard, J.-S. (1999). Effects of a cross-training exercise program in persons with osteoarthritis of the knee. A randomized controlled trial. *J Clin Rheumatol* 5: 126–36.

Petrella, R. J. and Bartha, C. (2000). Home based exercise therapy for older patients with knee osteoarthritis: a randomized clinical trial. *J Rheumatol* 27.

Philbin, E. F., Groff, G. D., Ries, M. D. and Miller, T. E. (1995). Cardiovascular fitness and health in patients with end-stage osteoarthritis. *Arthritis Rheum* 38: 799–805.

Pisters, M. F., Veenhof, C., Van Meeteren, N. L., Ostelo, R. W., de Bakker, D. H., Schellevis, F. G. and Dekker, J. (2007). Long-term effectiveness of exercise therapy in patients with osteoarthritis of the hip or knee: a systematic review. *Arthritis Rheum* 57: 1245–53.

Pritzker, K. P. (1998). Pathology of osteoarthritis. *Osteoarthritis.* K. D. Brandt, M. Doherty and L. S. Lohmander. Oxford, Oxford University Press.

Quilty, B., Tucker, M., Campbell, R. and Dieppe, P. (2003). Physiotherapy, including quadriceps exercises and patellar taping, for knee osteoarthritis with predominant patello-femoral joint involvement: randomized controlled trial. *J Rheumatol* 30: 1311–17.

Radin, E. L., Burr, D. B., Caterson, B., Fyhrie, D., Brown, T. D. and Boyd, R. D. (1991a). Mechanical determinants of osteoarthrosis. *Seminars Arthritis Rheum* 21: 12–21.

Radin, E. L., Yang, K. H., Riegger, C., Kish, V. L. and O'Connor, J. J. (1991b). Relationship between lower limb dynamics and knee joint pain. *J Orthop Res* 9: 398–405.

Roddy, E., Zhang, W. and Doherty, M. (2005a). Aerobic walking or strengthening exercise for osteoarthritis of the knee? A systematic review. *Ann Rheum Dis* 64: 544–8.

Roddy, E., Zhang, W., Doherty, M., Arden, N. K., Barlow, J., Birell, F., Carr, A., Chakravaty, K., Dickson, J., Hay, E., Hosie, G., Hurley, M., Jordan, K. M., McCarthy, C., Peat, G., Pendleton, A. and Richards, S. (2005b). Evidence- based recommendations for the role of excercise in the management of the hip or knee- The MOVE consensus. *Rheumatol* 44.

Rogind, H., Bibow-Nielsen, B., Jensen, B., Moller, H. C., Frimodt-Moller, H. and Bliddal, H. (1998). The effects of a physical training program on patients with osteoarthritis of the knees. *Arch Phys Med Rehabil* 79: 1421–7.

Schilke, J. M., Johnson, G. O., Housh, T. J. and O'Dell, J. R. (1996). Effects of muscle-strength training on the functional status of patients with osteoarthritis of the knee joint. *Nursing Research* 45: 68–72.

Schulz, K. F., Chalmers, I., hayes, R. J. and Altman, D. (1995). Empirical evidence of bias: dimensions of methodological quality associated with estimates of treatment effects in controlled trials. *JAMA* 273: 408–12.

Segal, N. A., Torner, J. C., Felson, D., Niu, J., Sharma, L., Lewis, C. E. and Nevitt, M. (2009). Effect of thigh strength on incident radiographic and symptomatic knee osteoarthritis in a longitudinal cohort. *Arthritis Rheum* 61: 1210–17.

Slemenda, C., Brandt, K. D., Heilman, D. K., Mazzuca, S., Braunstein, E. M., Katz, B. P. and F.D., W. (1997). Quadriceps weakness and osteoarthritis of the knee. *Ann Intern Med* 127: 97–104.

Slemenda, C., Heilman, D. K., Brandt, K. D., Katz, B. P., Mazzuca, S. A., Braunstein, E. M. and Byrd, D. (1998). Reduced quadriceps strength relative to body weight. A risk factor for knee osteoarthritis in women? *Arthritis Rheum* 41: 1951–9.

Song, R., Lee, E.-O., Lam, P. and Bae, S.-C. (2003). Effects of Tai Chi exercise on pain, balance, muscle strength, and perceived difficulties in physical functioning in older women with osteoarthritis: a randomized clinical trial. *J Rheumatol* 30: 2039–44.

Suetta, C., Aagaard, P., Magnusson, S. P., Andersen, L. L., Sipila, S., Rosted, A., Jakobsen, A. K., Duus, B. and Kjaer, M. (2007). Muscle size, neuromuscular activation, and rapid force characteristics in elderly men and women: effects of unilateral long-term disuse due to hip osteoarthritis. *J Appl Physiol* 102: 942–8.

Tak, E., Staats, P., van Hespen, A. and Hopman-Rock, M. (2005). The effects of an exercise program for older adults with osteoarthritis of the hip. *J Rheumatol* 32: 1106–13.

Talbot, L. A., Gaines, J. M., Huynh, T. N. and Metter, E. J. (2003). A home-based pedometer-driven walking program to increase physical activity in older adults with osteoarthritis of the knee: a preliminary study. *J Am Geriatr Soc* 51: 387–92.

Tan, J., Balci, N., Sepici, V. and Gener, F. A. (1995). Isokinetic and isometric strength in osteoarthrosis of the knee. A comparative study with healthy women. *Am J Phys Med Rehabil* 74: 364–369.

Thomas, K. S., Muir, K. R., Doherty, M., Jones, A., O'Reilly, S. C. and Bassey, E. J. (2002). Home based exercise programme for knee pain and knee osteoarthritis: randomised controlled trial. *BMJ* 325: 752–7.

Thorstensson, C. A., Roos, E. M., Petersson, I. F. and Ekdahl, C. (2005). Six-week high-intensity exercise program for middle-aged patients withknee osteoarthritis: a randomized controlled trial. *BMC Musculoskeletal Disorders* 6: 27.

Topp, R., Woolley, S., Hornyak, J., Khuder, S. and Kahaleh, B. (2002). The effect of dynamic versus isometric resistance training on pain and functioning among adults with osteoarthritis of the knee. *Arch Phys Med Rehabil* 83: 1187–95.

Tugwell, P. and Shea, B. (2004). *Evidence-based Rheumatology*. London, BMJ Books.

van Baar, M. E., Dekker, J., Lemmens, J. A., Oostendorp, R. A. and Bijlsma, J. W. (1998). Pain and disability in patients with osteoarthritis of hip or knee: the relationship with articular, kinesiological, and psychological characteristics. *J Rheumatol* 25: 125–33.

van Baar, M. E., Dekker, J., Oostendorp, R. A., Bijl, D., Voorn, T. B., Lemmens, J. A. and Bijlsma, J. W. (1998). The effectiveness of exercise therapy in patients with osteoarthritis of the hip or knee: a randomized clinical trial. *J Rheumatol* 25: 2432–9.

Wang, T.-J., Belza, B., Thompson, F. E., Whitney, J. D. and Bennett, K. (2007). Effects of aquatic exercise on flexibility, strength and aerobic fitness in adults with osteoarthritis of the hip or knee. *J Adv Nursing* 57: 141–52.

Wessel, J. (1996). Isometric strength measurements of knee extensors in women with osteoarthritis of the knee. *J Rheumatol* 23: 328–31.

Zhang, W., Moskowitz, R.W., Nuki, G., Abramson, S., Altman, R.D., Arden, N., Bierma-Zeinstra, S., Brandt, K. D., Croft, P., Doherty, M., Dougados, M., Hochberg, M., Hunter, D. J., Kwoh, K., Lohmander, L. S. and Tugwell, P. (2008). OARSI recommendtions for the management of hip and knee osteoarthritis, Part II: OARSI evidence-based, expert consensus guidelines. *Osteoarthritis Cart* 16: 137–62.

9

OSTEOPOROSIS

J. Y. Tsauo

Introduction

Osteoporosis is a serious public health issue in today's ageing societies and is recognised as one of the four major musculoskeletal conditions (osteoporosis, low back pain, osteoarthritis, rheumatoid arthritis) by the United Nations and World Health Organization (WHO) (Woolf and Pfleger 2003). Hence, osteoporosis and related health sequelae present considerable burden on individuals and health and social care systems.

What is osteoporosis?

Osteoporosis was defined by a Consensus Development Conference (1993) as 'a systemic skeletal disorder characterized by low bone mass, microarchitectural deterioration of bone tissue, with consequent increase in bone fragility and susceptibility to fracture'. Classification by aetiology was suggested by Riggs *et al.* (1982) as follows: Type I osteoporosis represents loss of trabecular bone after the menopause and Type II osteoporosis means loss of trabecular or cortical bone as a result of ageing. Therefore, the former is linked to a lack of oestrogen and the latter results from multiple factors associated with the ageing process.

Bone mineral density (BMD) accounts for 75–90 per cent of the variance in bone strength (Lauritzen *et al.*, 1996), and can be measured by dual X-ray absorptiometry (DXA). According to World Health Organization recommendations (WHO, 1994), bone mass is categorised into: 'normal' (BMD not more than 1 standard deviation (SD) below the mean value of young adults), 'osteopenia' (BMD between 1 and 2.5 SD below the mean value of young adults), 'osteoporosis' (BMD more than 2.5 SD below the mean value of young adults), and 'severe osteoporosis' (osteoporosis and presence of one or more fractures).

Osteoporosis is linked to an increased risk of bone fracture and subsequent dysfunction (or even death) and the risk of fracture rises as BMD declines (Marshall *et al.*, 1996; Johnell *et al.*, 2005). Klotzbuecher *et al.* (2000) showed that every 10 per cent loss of bone mass in the spinal vertebra doubles the risk of fracture and a 10 per cent loss of bone mass in the hip is associated with a 2.5 times greater risk of hip fracture. Additionally, as shown, in the European Prospective Osteoporosis Study (2002), the risk of vertebral fracture increases 1.5 times per 0.1 g.cm^2 decrease in spinal BMD.

Risk factors for osteoporosis and the role of exercise

The National Osteoporosis Foundation (NOF) in the USA recommend five steps to bone health and osteoporosis prevention: (i) getting daily recommended amounts of calcium and vitamin D, (ii) engaging in regular weight-bearing exercise, (iii) avoiding smoking and excessive alcohol, (iv) talking to a healthcare provider about bone health and (v) having a bone density test/taking medication when appropriate. Epidemiological studies demonstrate that genetic factors, medical conditions and medications, lifestyles, and levels of hormones and vitamins all affect bone health (Amin *et al.*, 2006). Potentially modifiable lifestyle factors include smoking (Burger *et al.*, 1998; Kanis *et al.*, 2005), alcohol (Felson *et al.*, 1995) and caffeine (Harris and Dawson-Hughes, 1994) consumption, calcium and vitamin D intake (Zhu *et al.*, 2008) and physical activity (Bonaiuti *et al.*, 2002). Peak bone mass is generally attained by the end of the third decade and this is the most important basis for prevention of osteoporosis in later life. There is evidence that aerobic exercise in combination with strength training can maintain whole body BMD in middle-aged men (Stewart *et al.*, 2005) and that high impact weight-bearing exercise can increase BMD in the lumbar spine and upper femur of premenopausal women (Vainionpää *et al.*, 2005). Resistance exercise also increases regional BMD in premenopausal women (Lohman *et al.*, 1995; Stewart *et al.*, 2005). Maddalozzo and Snow (2000) compared the effects of moderate- and high-intensity resistance exercise training in men and women aged 50–60 years. Both genders showed gains in strength and muscle mass, regardless of the exercise training intensity. Interestingly, high intensity exercise evoked a significant improvement in spine BMD in the male but not female participants. Increased BMD at the greater trochanter was observed after both high and moderate intensity exercise training in the men but not the women. The different results between the male and female participants might be explained by the effect of menopausal status on BMD.

Exercise for individuals with low bone mass

In individuals with low bone mass there has been considerable interest in the role that habitual exercise participation could have in retarding further bone loss, preventing falls and fall-related injuries. A literature review was undertaken with the aim of finding randomised controlled trials (RCTs) and clinical controlled trials

(CCTs) that had investigated the effect of exercise on physical outcomes related to reduced risk of falls, disease-specific outcomes and health-related quality of life for people (especially women) with low bone mass. Because of differences in the exercise training programmes and outcome measures across studies, meta-analyses were restricted to a limited number of outcomes. In the management of osteoporosis and related impairments, functional fitness, strength and cardiorespiratory fitness, balance and pain are important outcomes that have been frequently investigated and reported in the literature. As strength and balance are correlated with the risk of falls, these outcomes have received most attention.

Functional fitness

In the reviewed articles, measures such as the Oswestry Disability Index (ODI: used to assess how back or leg pain is affecting ability to undertake activities of daily living), the timed up and go test (TUG test: a composite performance index of balance and strength) and tests of normal walking speed have been commonly used to assess function. Two RCTs used the ODI to measure patients' function after a programme of exercise training (Liu-Ambrose *et al.*, 2005; Chien *et al.*, 2005). In the study of Liu-Ambrose *et al.* (2005), three types of group-based exercise (resistance training, agility training and general stretching) were randomly prescribed to older women with low bone mass for 25 weeks. In the study of Chien *et al.* (2005), the effect of a 12-week home-based trunk strengthening programme was studied in postmenopausal women with a diagnosis of osteoporosis or osteopenia. Although these trials reported significant improvements within the exercising groups, no differences between different exercising groups or between exercise and control groups were observed.

Four studies used the TUG test as one of their outcomes. Madureira *et al.* (2007) prescribed a balance training programme to osteoporotic women and reported a significant improvement in the intervention group compared to controls. Another study showed a positive but minimal effect on the TUG test following a workstation-based exercise programme in osteopenic women (Hourigan *et al.*, 2008). No between group difference was observed. Additionally, there was no significant difference in TUG test change scores (between the intervention and control group) in a study that investigated the effect of a 6-month home-based exercise programme of stretching, strength training and aerobics (walking) in postmenopausal women with at least one vertebral fracture (Papaioannou *et al.*, 2003). However, a significantly greater improvement on a walking speed test was observed (versus controls) following a combined programme of strength, aerobic, balance and co-ordination exercises in older women (Englund *et al.*, 2005).

Study or subgroup	Experimental			Control			Weight	Mean difference	Mean difference
	Mean	SD	Total	Mean	SD	Total		IV, fixed, 95% CI	IV, fixed, 95% CI

9.1.1 Body mass index

Study or subgroup	Mean	SD	Total	Mean	SD	Total	Weight	IV, fixed, 95% CI	
Bocalini 2009	−3	17.53	15	1	20.62	10	0.2%	−4.00 [−19.56, 11.56]	
Englund 2005	0.3	2.7	21	0.3	3.3	19	17.0%	0.00 [−1.88, 1.88]	
Swaneburg 2007	−0.1	3	10	−0.1	2.96	10	8.8%	0.00 [−2.61, 2.61]	
Subtotal (95% CI)			46			39	26.1%	−0.04 [−1.56, 1.48]	

Heterogeneity: Chi^2 = 0.25, df = 2 (P = 0.88); I^2 = 0%
Test for overall effect: Z = 0.05 (P = 0.96)

9.1.2 Body fat percentage

Study or subgroup	Mean	SD	Total	Mean	SD	Total	Weight	IV, fixed, 95% CI	
Bocalini 2009	−4	17.53	15	1	15	10	0.4%	−5.00 [−17.85, 7.85]	
Chien 2000	−0.29	10.65	22	3.65	12.3	21	1.3%	−3.94 [−10.83, 2.95]	
Engelke 2006	0.3	5.12	48	−0.1	6.66	30	7.7%	0.40 [−2.39, 3.19]	
Korpelainen 2006	1.4	2.98	84	2.2	4.18	76	46.7%	−0.80 [−1.94, 0.34]	
Subtotal (95% CI)			169			137	56.0%	−0.73 [−1.77, 0.30]	

Heterogeneity: Chi^2 = 1.90, df = 3 (P = 0.59); I^2 = 0%
Test for overall effect: Z = 1.39 (P = 0.17)

9.1.3 Lean body mass

Chien 2000	−0.01	7.11	22	1.52	5.17	21	4.4%	−1.53 [−5.23, 2.17]
Englund 2005	1.4	3.46	21	1.2	3.35	19	13.5%	0.20 [−1.91, 2.31]
Subtotal (95% CI)			43			40	17.9%	−0.22 [−2.06, 1.61]
Heterogeneity: Chi² = 0.63, df = 1 (P = 0.43); I² = 0%								
Test for overall effect: Z = 0.24 (P = 0.81)								
Total (95% CI)			258			216	100.0%	−0.46 [−1.24, 0.32]
Heterogeneity: Chi² = 3.41, df = 8 (P = 0.91); I² = 0%								
Test for overall effect: Z = 1.16 (P = 0.24)								
Test for subgroup differences: Chi² = 0.63, df = 2 (P = 0.73); I² = 0%								

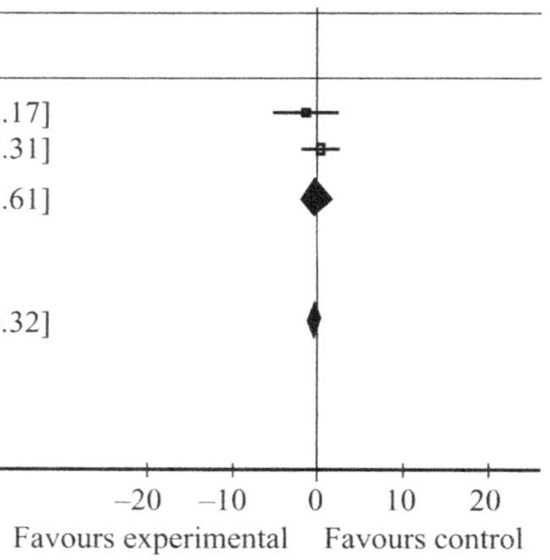

−20 −10 0 10 20

Favours experimental   Favours control

FIGURE 9.1 Forest plot: the impact of exercise training on measures of body composition.

Strength

Improvements in strength have been reported after widely differing exercise programmes. In a study by Hourigan *et al.* (2008), osteopenic women who attended a one-hour workstation-based balance training and weight-bearing exercise class twice weekly for 20 weeks showed improved strength of the hip, quadriceps and trunk extensor muscles. In another study undertaken by Bergström *et al.* (2008), 112 postmenopausal women with low BMD were randomised to physical training or a control group. The physical training included three fast 30-minute walks and 2×1 hour exercise training sessions (resistance, aerobic and flexibility exercises) per week for one year. A 'timed stand test' (time in seconds taken to stand up ten times from a standard chair) was used as an indicator of leg muscle performance and the exercise group demonstrated improved performance on this measure compared to controls. Young *et al.* (2007) used line dancing as an intervention in sedentary postmenopausal women, added home-based squats for a second group and squats with foot stamps for a third group. The number of squats to fatigue was used as a measure of low extremity strength. After 12 months, the number of squats increased in all groups but the third group achieved significantly more squats than the others. Swanenburg *et al.* (2007) investigated the effect of a combined programme of strength, balance, coordination and aerobic exercise training in older people with low BMD. An improvement in knee extensor strength between the intervention and control groups was observed after three months. Other programmes, such as the 20-week Osteofit community-based exercise programme for people with osteoporosis (resistance, stretching and posture exercises) and a 24-week aerobic exercise programme for osteopenic postmenopausal women (graded treadmill walking and stepping exercise) have also reported positive effects for lower-limb strength (Carter *et al.*, 2002; Chien *et al.*, 2000). However, a combined programme of strengthening, aerobic, balance and coordination exercises for older women did not evoke any changes in knee extensor strength and only an improvement in grip strength was reported (Englund *et al.*, 2005).

Evidence suggest that resistance exercise programmes are well tolerated in older women who are either receiving or not receiving hormone therapy and can evoke improvements in strength and functional fitness outcomes (Judge *et al.*, 2005; Bocalini *et al.*, 2009). In a study by Judge *et al.* (2005), participants on hormone therapy were grouped into a lower body intervention group and an upper body intervention group for resistance training, except that torso exercises, stretching and walking were performed by both groups. Between-group differences in one-repetition maximum (1RM) strength for the seated leg press and 6-minute walking distance were reported but there was no interaction effect between groups in time to complete five chair rises. Bocalini *et al.* (2009) studied the effect of a 24-week strength training programme in postmenopausal women not receiving hormone therapy. The strength training group demonstrated an improvement of 39 per cent in lower limb 1 RM strength, with no observed change in the controls.

Cardiorespiratory fitness, body composition and flexibility

A controlled trial (Chien *et al.*, 2000) investigated the effect of a 24-week programme of graded treadmill walking and stepping exercise (versus non-exercising controls) on maximum oxygen uptake in osteopenic postmenopausal women. Although participants in the exercise group experienced significant improvement after the exercise intervention, no between-group difference was observed. Many authors (Chien *et al.*, 2000; Englund *et al.*, 2005; Engelke *et al.*, 2006; Korpelainen *et al.*, 2006; Swanenburg *et al.*, 2007; Bocalini *et al.*, 2009) have investigated the impact of exercise training on body composition. A meta-analysis was undertaken to show the pooled results (Figure 9.1) and this shows that no between-group differences were detected in the body composition dimensions of body mass index, body fat percentage or lean body mass. Two studies measured trunk flexibility in osteopenic/osteoporotic women before and after programmes of back/trunk strengthening exercises (Chien *et al.*, 2005; Hongo *et al.*, 2007). Although no differences were reported between the intervention groups and controls, in the study of Chien *et al.* (2005), spinal range of motion of the exercise group in the sagittal plane (flextion/extension) and frontal plane (side bending) was improved from baseline after the 12-week exercise training programme.

Balance

Nine studies investigated balance performance after programmes of exercise training. Three RCTs used the Berg Balance Scale (BBS) as the outcome (Englund *et al.*, 2005; Swanenburg *et al.*, 2007; Madureira *et al.*, 2007). Englund *et al.* (2005) prescribed a one-year combined weight-bearing exercise training programme to older women, Swanenburg *et al.* (2007) investigated the effect of a combined exercise programme with calcium and vitamin D supplementation in elderly women with osteopenia and osteoporosis and Madureira *et al.* (2007) studied the impact of a balance training programme in osteoporotic women. Contrary to individual results of the two of these trials (Swanenburg *et al.*, 2007; Madureira *et al.*, 2007), the result of a meta-analysis using all three trials revealed no significant difference between the improvements in the intervention participants versus controls (Figure 9.2). This might be because of the large variance in effect sizes in these three studies.

Young *et al.* (2007) investigated the effects of three exercise programmes on one-leg standing balance. One group engaged in line dancing, a second group added home-based squats and a third group squats with foot stamps. All groups showed an improvement after the exercise programme but there was no difference between the groups. Englund *et al.* (2005) studied the effect of a one-year combined weight-bearing exercise training programme on standing leg balance. In this study, participants in the intervention group showed a 76 per cent improvement on the one leg standing test at one year of follow-up but there was no significant difference between the two groups.

Study or subgroup	Experimental			Control			Weight	Mean difference IV, random, 95% CI	Mean difference IV, random, 95% CI
	Mean	SD	Total	Mean	SD	Total			
Englund 2005	−0.19	1.51	21	0.21	2.32	19	36.2%	−0.40 [−1.63, 0.83]	
Madureira 2007	−5.5	4.95	30	0.5	5.13	30	32.6%	−6.00 [−8.55, −3.45]	
Swanenburg 2007	−3.9	3.22	10	1.3	3.5	10	31.2%	−5.20 [−8.15, −2.25]	
Total (95% CI)			61			59	100.0%	−3.72 [−7.78, 0.33]	

Heterogeneity: Tau^2 = 11.44; Chi^2 = 20.48, df = 2 (P < 0.0001); I^2 = 90%
Test for overall effect: Z = 1.80 (P = 0.07)

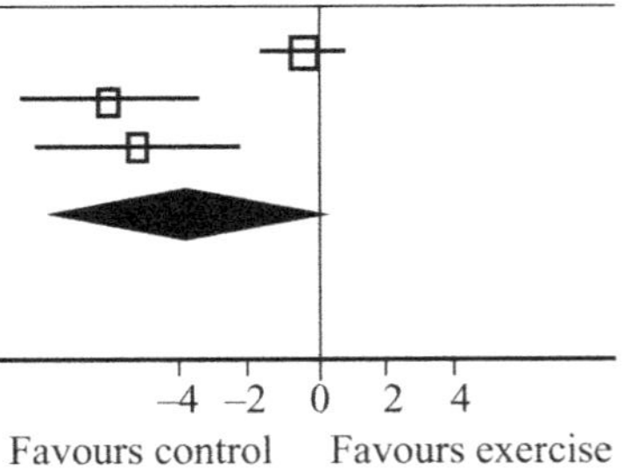

Favours control   Favours exercise

FIGURE 9.2 Forest plot: the impact of exercise training on Berg Balance Scale score.

Madureira *et al.* (2007) and Hourigan *et al.* (2008) used the Clinical Test of Sensory Interaction for Balance (CTSIB) to assess the balance function. Madureira *et al.* (2007) prescribed a 12-month balance training programme in women with osteoporosis and observed improvements in two aspects of the CTSIB compared to controls. Hourigan *et al.* (2008) investigated the effect of a workstation-based balance training and weight-bearing exercise programme in osteopenic women and reported significantly better performances in certain aspects of balance (unilateral and bilateral stance sway measures, lateral reach) versus controls.

Maciaszek *et al.* (2007) investigated the effect of a programme of Tai Chi for men with low bone mass. A computer posturographic system was used to evaluate balance. Although the Tai Chi group achieved an improvement after the 18-week exercise intervention, there was no significant difference between the exercise group and controls.

Two studies (Papaioannou *et al.*, 2003; Swanenburg *et al.*, 2007;) used force plates to assess balance. Papaioannou *et al.* (2003) investigated the effect of a 6-month home-based exercise programme comparing stretching, strength training and aerobic exercise (walking) in postmenopausal women with osteoporosis who had at least one vertebral fracture and Swanenburg *et al.* (2007) studied the effect of a 3-month exercise programme consisting of strength, coordination, balance and endurance training in elderly females aged 65 years and older with osteopenia or osteoporosis. No differences were found in the range or velocity of weight shifting after either exercise training programme.

Carter *et al.* (2002) tested static balance with a composite equilibrium score and dynamic balance with a standard 10 metre figure-of-eight course. They found no significant difference between controls and an intervention group that underwent a 20-week twice-weekly community-based exercise programme.

Disease-specific outcomes

Although researchers in the osteoporosis field have mainly focused their interests on the impact of exercise interventions on BMD, pain is a common symptom in osteoporotic patients and falls and related fractures incur medical costs and considerable social burden. Hence, these are all important outcomes to consider when assessing the effect of exercise in the management of osteoporosis.

Pain

One RCT (Gold *et al.*, 2004) and one CCT (Engelke *et al.*, 2006) assessed pain status. In the first phase (6 months) of the study of Gold *et al.* (2004), participants (older women with vertebral fractures) in the intervention group participated in three exercise classes and two coping classes each week, with control participants engaging in a weekly class on health issues for older women. Pain during activities was measured using the pain subscale of the Functional Status Index

(Jette, 1980). The change in pain score in the intervention group was not significantly different from that of the control group. Participants in the study of Engelke *et al.* (2006) participated in the intervention or control group according to their preference. The osteopenia women in the intervention group participated in low-volume high-resistance strength training and high-impact aerobic exercise for 14 months. The frequency and intensity of spinal pain decreased significantly in the intervention group, while exacerbating in the control group at three years of follow-up. However, no statistical between-group difference was observed and no difference was detected in the pain status of the main joints, within-group or between-group.

BMD

Many RCTs (Iwamoto *et al.*, 2001; Milliken *et al.*, 2003; Chan *et al.*, 2004; Englund *et al.*, 2005; Korpelainen *et al.*, 2006; Maciaszek *et al.*, 2007; Swanenburg *et al.*, 2007; Young *et al.*, 2007; Bergström *et al.*, 2008; Hourigan *et al.*, 2008; Bocalini *et al.*, 2009) and CCTs (Chien *et al.*, 2000; Judge *et al.*, 2005; Engelke *et al.*, 2006) have investigated the effect of exercise training on BMD and have reported improvements at various sites. Moreover, there are many systematic reviews and meta-analyses for this issue.

A meta-analysis by Bonaiuti *et al.* (2002) selected 18 RCTs that examined the effectiveness of exercise for preventing bone loss. This review included trials published between 1966 and 1999. It concluded that all types of exercise (aerobic, weight bearing and resistance exercises) were effective in slowing bone loss (at one year of follow-up) on spine BMD. Walking was also effective at the hip. Schmitt *et al.* (2009) then reviewed exercise trails published between January 2000 and October 2008. This review concluded from two prospective cohort studies (Feskanich *et al.*, 2002; Robbins *et al.*, 2007) that an inverse dose-response relationship existed between physical activity and the decline in bone density.

A systematic review on the impact of resistance exercise training by Zehnacker and Bemis-Dougherty (2007) provided supportive evidence for postmenopausal women. The authors emphasised the importance of high training load and programmes of long duration (over one year). Another meta-analysis by Martyn-St James and Carroll (2006) showed an increase in lumbar spine BMD of 0.006 g.cm^2 following high-intensity resistance exercise training. However, BMD at the femoral neck and total hip BMD were not significantly different between the intervention and control group.

Walking as a type of weight-bearing exercises is recommended for the elderly because of its feasibility and effect on bone mass. A meta-analysis by Bérard *et al.* (1997), investigating the impact of walking exercise in combination with other types of exercise training, reported a significant effect on bone mass only at the spine. Palombaro (2005) came to the same conclusion following a meta-analysis of walking exercise only. This was in contrast to a more recent meta-analysis, which showed that walking was effective for preserving BMD at the femoral neck but not at the spine (Martyn-St James and Carroll, 2008). A meta-analysis published in 2002 however, concluded that walking exercise was effective for slowing bone loss at both the spine and hip (Bonaiuti *et al.*, 2002).

Falls

Falls and falls prevention have mainly been investigated in relation to frailty and age-ing, rather than being the focus of studies in people with low bone mass. Moreover, the long follow-up time needed to assess falls might explain why only two RCTs have included this outcome measure. One study reported an improvement in bal-ance and strength of the knee extensors following a 3-month exercise programme consisting of muscular strength, co-ordination, balance and endurance exercises in elderly females with osteopenia or osteoporosis (Swanenburg *et al.*, 2007). Two participants in the intervention group showed a significant improvement in the Berg Balance test. These two participants sustained five falls in the three months leading up to the study but only one of them had suffered a fall by the end of the study follow-up period (12 months). In the other study, Madureira *et al.* (2007) prescribed 40 sessions of balance training (once a week) to women with osteoporo-sis. Falls per patient were calculated for the year preceding the study. The change in falls ratio between the intervention group (-0.77 ± 1.76) and controls ($+0.03 \pm 0.96$) was significant. Using a different approach, Moayyeri (2008) conducted a meta-analysis of 13 prospective cohort studies using hip fracture as the end-point to investigate the association between physical activity and risk of falls. This suggested that regular physical activity incurred a general decrease in falls risk, but both the most inactive and the most active people may be at a higher risk. Prevention of falls needs a multi-factorial approach to accompany any exercise/physical activity intervention.

Osteoporosis-related fracture

Only one RCT has reported osteoporosis-related fractures (Korpelainen *et al.*, 2006). One hundred and sixty elderly women with low BMD participated in this study and were randomised to a supervised and home-based high-impact exercise training group (n=84) or a 'no intervention' control group (n=76). The programme lasted for 30 months and comprised a warm-up, jumping and balance exercises. Six falls resulted in fractures in the exercise group compared to 16 in the control group (p=0.019) over the period of the study. In the aforementioned Moayyeri (2008) meta-analysis, the association between physical activity and osteoporotic frac-tures was also investigated. It concluded that moderate to vigorous physical activity was associated with a 45 per cent reduction in hip fracture in men and a 38 per cent reduction in women. Associations between physical activity and risk reduction at other fracture sites were mainly non-significant.

Quality of life

Six studies measured the effect of exercise on quality of life (QoL) using questionnaires (Carter *et al.*, 2002; Papaioannou *et al.*, 2003; Chien *et al.*, 2005; Devereux *et al.*, 2005; Liu-Ambrose *et al.*, 2005; Hongo *et al.*, 2007). Four of them were selected for a meta-analysis published in 2009 (Li *et al.*, 2009). According to the meta-analysis (Li, 2009), the exercise groups achieved better improvements in the domains of physical function, pain, role physical and vitality. Physical function and pain were both measured in the Quality of Life Questionnaire of the European Foundation for Osteoporosis (QUALEFFO) and Short Form 36 (SF-36), and role physical and vitality in the SF-36.

The two studies not included in the meta-analysis were those of Papaioannou *et al.* (2003) and Hongo *et al.* (2007). Papaioannou *et al.* (2003) investigated the effect of a 6-month home-based combined exercise programme in elderly women with osteoporosis-related vertebral fractures using the Osteoporosis Quality of Life Questionnaire (OQLQ). The exercising group experienced improvements in symptoms, emotion and leisure/social domains. In the study of Hongo *et al.* (2007), low-intensity back exercise was prescribed and QoL was measured using the Japanese Osteoporosis Quality of Life Questionnaire (JOQLQ). The JOQLQ contains 38 items in 6 domains and after the 4-month home exercise programme, the mean total score of participants in the exercise group was significantly greater than that of the control group. The improvement was significantly greater in the domains of 'activities of daily living', 'sense for posture and figure and falls' and 'psychological factors'.

Exercise programming for people with osteoporosis/low bone mass

Introduction

Structured exercise and non-structured physical activity is beneficial for bone health and related physical functioning across the age spectrum. High loading exercise augments bone density and improves bone quality in childhood and adolescence (Kohrt *et al.*, 2004; Guadalupe-Grau *et al.*, 2009). During adulthood, habitual exercise/physical activity appears to maintain the bone mass gained in earlier life (Kohrt *et al.*, 2004; Schwab and Klein, 2008). Moreover, promotion of balance, muscular strength and prevention of functional decline (Karinkanta *et al.*, 2007) can all result from participation in a physically active lifestyle. These factors can help to prevent the development of osteoporosis and reduce the risk of falls and/or injurious falls in older age.

However well designed an exercise programme is, its effectiveness depends on a willingness to participate and adherence to the programme. Cress *et al.* (2006) offered advice for practitioners when promoting physical activity programmes for the elderly, which include (1) emphasis on a multi-dimensional programme to match individual physiological needs and psychological interests, (2) the inclusion of behaviour management to maximise recruitment and participation and to minimise attrition and (3) attention to injury and risk management.

Multidimensional exercise programming

A well-planned exercise programme for elderly people with low bone mass should include aerobic activities, muscle-strengthening, balance and flexibility exercises (Nelson *et al.* 2007; Table 9.1). Weight-bearing or high impact exercise is used to preserve bone mass, with strengthening and balance activities also helping to reduce the risk of falls/injurious falls. Following the occurrence of vertebral fracture and/or kyphosis, trunk stabilisation and extension exercise should be emphasised (Schwab *et al.*, 2008). For all individuals, a comprehensive physical assessment to highlight weaknesses and functional deficits is needed to tailor exercise programmes to individual needs.

Knowledge of the importance and effectiveness of exercise/physical activity is insufficient for motivating people to initiate or sustain participation. Hence, strategies should be employed to facilitate adherence (Cress *et al.*, 2006). These include ensuring safety of the programme, enhancing self-efficacy by providing choices and signing a health contract, reinforcing the importance of attendance and feeding back improvements in physical status, building social support structures involving peer group and professionals.

TABLE 9.1 Recommended exercise programme for people with osteoporosis/low bone mass

Exercise modality	• Weight-bearing aerobic activities, such as brisk walking, tennis, jogging, and stair climbing • Resistance exercise (e.g. free weights, therabands, etc.) • Balance and flexibility exercises • Some structured activity, such as Tai Chi (Shen *et al.* 2007; Wayne *et al.* 2007), Yoga or dance classes (Young *et al.* 2007) maybe of interest to elderly individuals to help promote compliance
Exercise intensity	• Moderate to high, but starting from low intensity in initially sedentary individuals
Exercise frequency	• 3–5 times per week for weight-bearing aerobic activities • 2–3 times per week for resistance exercise training, including trunk, upper- and lower-limb exercises • 2–7 times per week for balance and flexibility exercises
Exercise duration	• 30–60 min per day, starting from 10 min per day in initially sedentary individuals

Injury and risk management

Individuals with severe or multiple chronic conditions should get permission from their family physician before commencing an exercise programme. Starting from a low intensity exercise programme and progression within the individual's capabilities is also important. Individualised programmes to suit different initial fitness levels work best. To avoid injuries, appropriate equipment (such as correct footwear) and a safe environment is necessary. In addition, a proper warm-up and cool-down should be built in to each exercise session. Inclusion of a variety of different types of activity will reduce the potential for overuse injuries (Holtgrefe and Glenn, 2007).

Summary and conclusions

There is evidence that exercise can increase BMD, muscle strength, walking speed and QoL in older men and women with low bone density. More limited evidence suggests that habitual exercise participation might be linked to a decrease in the frequency of falls and related fractures in older people. Improvements in balance and motor function have also been reported. On the basis of the evidence presented in this chapter, we recommend a progressive, multi-dimensional exercise programme for osteoporotic individuals and those at high risk of developing the condition. It is an important mission for health professionals to educate people about the benefits of exercise for bone health and to motivate people to participate in appropriate exercise.

References

Amin, S., Eastell, R. and Clowes, J. A. (2006) Risk factors for osteoporosis and fractures in men and women. In: Cyrus, C. and Anthony, D. W. (eds) *Osteoporosis: Best Practice and Research Compendium*. New York: Elsevier: pp. 63–78.

Bérard, A., Bravo, G. and Gauthier, P. (1997) Meta-analysis of the effectiveness of physical activity for the prevention and bone loss in postmenopausal women. *Osteoporos Int*; 7: 331–7.

Bocalini, D. S., Serra, A. J., Santos, L., Murad, N. and Levy, R. F. (2009) Strength training preserves the bone mineral density of postmenopausal women without hormone replacement therapy. *J Aging Health*; 21: 519–27.

Bonaiuti, D., Shea, B., Iovine, R., Negrini, S., Welch, V., Kemper, H. H. C. G., Wells, G. A., Tugwell, P. and Cranney, A. (2002) Exercise for preventing and treating osteoporosis in postmenopausal women. *Cochrane Database Syst Rev*, Issue 2. Art. No.: CD000333.

Bergström, I., Landgren, B. M. and Brinck, J. (2008) Physical training preserves bone mineral density in postmenopausal women with forearm fractures and low bone mineral density. *Osteoporos Int*; 19: 177–83.

Burger, H., de Laet, C. E., van Daele, P. L., Weel, A. E., Witteman, J. C., Hofman, A. and Pols, H. A. (1998) Risk factors for increased bone loss in an elderly population: the Rotterdam Study. *Am J Epidemiol*; 147: 871–9.

Carter, N. D., Khan, K. M., McKay, H. A., Petit, M. A., Waterman, C., Heinonen, A., Janssen, P. A., Donaldson, M. G., Mallinson, A., Riddell, L., Kruse, K., Prior, J. C. and Flicker, L. (2002) Community-based exercise program reduces risk factors for falls in 65- to 75-year-old women with osteoporosis: randomized controlled trial. *CMAJ*; 167: 997–1004.

Chan, K., Lau, M., Woo, J., Au, S., Choy, W., Lee, K. and Lee, S. (2004) A randomized, prospective study of the effects of Tai Chi Chun exercise on bone mineral density in postmenopausal women. *Arch Phys Med Rehabil*; 85: 717–22.

Chien, M. Y., Wu, Y. T., Hsu, A. T., Yang, R. S. and Lai, J. S. (2000) Efficacy of a 24-week aerobic exercise program for osteopenic postmenopausal women. *Calcif Tissue Int*; 67: 443–8.

Chien, M. Y., Yang, R. S. and Tsauo, J. Y. (2005) Home-based trunk-strengthening exercise for osteoporotic and osteopenic postmenopausal women without fracture – a pilot study. *Clin Rehabil*; 19: 28–36.

Consensus Development Conference. (1993) Diagnosis, prophylaxis and treatment of osteoporosis. *Am J Med* ; 94: 646–50.

Cress, M. E., Buchner, D. M., Prohaska, T., Rimmer, J., Brown, M., Macera, C., DePietro, L. and Zajko, W. C. (2006) Best practices for physical activity programs and behavior counseling in older adult populations. *Eur Rev Aging Phys Act*; 3: 34–42.

Devereux, K., Robertson, D. and Briffa, N. K. (2005) Effects of a water-based program on women 65 years and over: a randomised controlled trial. *Aust J Physiother.*; 51: 102–8.

Engelke, K., Kemmler, D., Lauber, D., Beeskow, C., Pintag, R. and Kalender, W. A. (2006) Exercise maintains bone density at spine and hip EFOPS: a 3-year longitudinal study in early postmenopausal women. *Osteoporos Int*; 17: 133–42.

Englund, U., Littbrand, H., Sondell, A., Pettersson, U. and Bucht, G. (2005) A 1-year combined weight-bearing training program is beneficial for bone mineral density and neuromuscular function in older women. *Osteoporos Int*; 16: 1117–23.

European Prospective Osteoporosis Study (EPOS) Group. (2002) The relationship between bone density and incident vertebral fracture in men and women. *J Bone Miner Res*; 17: 2214–21.

Feskanich, D., Willett, W. and Golditz, G. (2002) Walking and leisure-time activity and risk of hip fracture in postmenopausal women. *JAMA*; 288: 2300–6.

Gold, D. T., Shipp, K. M., Piper, C. F., Duncan, P. W., Martinez, S. and Lyles, K. W. (2004) Group treatment improves trunk strength and psychological status in older women with vertebral fractures: results of a randomized, clinical trial. *J Am Geriatr Soc*; 52: 1471–8.

Guadalupe-Grau, A., Fuentes, T., Guerra, B. and Calbet, J. A. L. (2009) Exercise and bone mass in adults. *Sports Med*; 39: 439–68.

Harris, S. S. and Dawson-Hughes, B. (1994) Caffeine and bone loss in healthy postmenopausal women. *Am J Clin Nutr*; 60: 573–8.

Holtgrefe, K. and Glenn, T. M. (2007) Principle of aerobic exercise. In: Kisner, C. and Colby, L. A. *Therapeuic Exercise Foundations and Techniques*. 5th edn. Philadelphia: F. A. Davis company: pp. 231–48.

Hongo, M, Itoi, E. and Sinaki, M. (2007) Effect of low-intensity back exercise on quality of life and back extensor strength in patients with osteoporosis: a randomized controlled trial. *Osteoporos Int*; 18: 1389–95.

Hourigan, S. R., Nitz, J. C., Brauer, S. G., O'Neill, S., Wong, J. and Richardson, C. A. (2008) Positive effects of exercise on falls and fracture risk in osteopenic women. *Osteoporos Int*; 19: 1077–86.

Iwamoto, J., Takeda, T. and Ichimura, S. (2001) Effect of exercise training and detraining on bone mineral density in postmenopausal women with osteoporosis. *J Orthop Sci*; 6: 128–32.

Jette, A. M. (1980) Functional status index: reliability of a chronic disease evaluation instrument. *Arch Phys Med Rehabil*; 61: 395–401.

Johnell, O., Kanis, J. A., Oden, A., Johansson, H., De Laet, C., Delmas, P., Eisman, J. A., Fujiwara, S., Kroger, H., Mellstrom, D., Meunier, P. J., Melton, L. J. 3rd, O'Neill, T., Pols, H., Reeve, J., Silman, A. and Tenenhouse, A. (2005) Predictive value of BMD for hip and other fractures. *J Bone Miner Res*; 20: 1185–94.

Judge, J. O., Kleppinger, A., Kenny, A., Smith, J. A., Biskup, B. and Marcella, G. (2005) Home-based resistance training improves femoral bone mineral density in women on hormone therapy. *Osteoporos Int*; 16: 1096–108.

Karinkanta, S., Heinonen, A., Sievänen, H., Uusi-Rasi, K., Pasanen, M., Ojala, K., Fogelholm, M. and Kannus, P. (2007) A multi-component exercise regimen to prevent functional decline and bone fragility in home-dwelling elderly women: randomized, controlled trial. *Osteoporos Int*; 18: 453–62.

Kanis, J. A., Johnell, O., Oden, A., Johansson, H., De Laet, C., Eisman, J. A., Fujiwara, S., Kroger, H., McCloskey, E. V., Mellstrom, D., Melton, L. J., Pols, H., Reeve, J., Silman, A. and Tenenhouse, A. (2005) Smoking and fracture risk: a meta-analysis. *Osteoporosis Int*; 16: 155–62.

Klotzbuecher, C. M., Ross, P. D., Landsman, P. B., Abbott, T. A. 3rd and Berger, M. (2000) Patients with prior fractures have an increased risk of future fractures: a summary of the literature and statistical synthesis. *J Bone Miner Res*; 15: 721–39.

Kohrt, W. M., Bloomfield, S. A., Little, K. D., Nelson, M. E. and Yingling, V. R. (2004) American College of Sport Medicine position stand on physical activity and bone health. *Med Sci Sports Exer*; 36: 1985–96.

Korpelainen, R., Keinäenei-Kiukaammiemi, S., Heikkinen, J., Väänänen, K. and Korpelainen, J. (2006) Effect of impact exercise on bone mineral density in elderly women with low BMD: a population-based randomized controlled 30-month intervention. *Osteoporos Int*; 17: 109–18.

Lauritzen, J. B. (1996) Hip fracture: incidence, risk factors, energy absorption and prevention. *Bone*; 18: S65–75.

Li, W. C., Chen, Y. C., Yang, R. S. and Tsauo, J. Y. (2009) Effect of exercise programmes on quality of life in osteoporotic and osteopenic postmenopausal women: a systematic review and meta-analysis. *Clin Rehabil*; 23: 888–96.

Liu-Ambrose, T. Y. L., Khan, K. M., Eng, J. J., Lord, S. R., Lentle, B. and McKay, H. A. (2005) Both resistance and agility training reduce back pain and improve health-related quality of life in older women with low bone mass. *Osteoporos Int*; 16: 1321–9.

Lohman, T., Going, S., Pamenter, R., Hall, M., Boyden, T., Houtkooper, L., Ritenbaugh, C., Bare, L., Hill, A. and Aickin, M. (1995) Effects of resistance training on regional and total bone mineral density in premenopausal women: a randomized prospective study. *J Bone Miner Res*; 10: 1015–24.

Maciaszek, J., Osiński, W., Szeklicki, R. and Stemplewski, R. (2007) Effect of Tai Chi on body balance: randomized controlled trial in men with osteopenia or osteoporosis. *Am J Chin Med*; 35: 1–9.

Maddalozzo, G. F. and Snow, C. M. (2000) High intensity resistance training: effects on bone in older men and women. *Calcif Tissue Int*; 66: 399–404.

Madureia, M. M., Takayama, L., Gallinaro, A. L., Caparbo, V. F., Costa, R. A., Pereira, R. M. (2007) Balance training program is highly effective in improving functional status and reducing the risk of falls in elderly women with osteoporosis: a randomized controlled trial. *Osteoporos Int*; 18: 419–25.

Marshall, D., Johnell, O. and Wedel, H. (1996) Meta-analysis of how well measures of bone mineral density predict occurrence of osteoporotic fractures. *BMJ*; 312: 1254–9.

Martyn-St James, M. and Carroll, S. (2006) High-intensity resistance training and postmenopausal bone loss: a meta-analysis *Osteoporos Int.*; 17: 1225–40.

Martyn-St James, M. and Carroll, S. (2008) Meta-analysis of walking for preservation of bone mineral density in post menopausal women. *Bone*; 43: 521–31.

Milliken, L. A., Going, S. B., Houtkooper, L. B., Flint-Wagner, H. G., Figueroa, A., Metcalfe, L. L., Blew, R. M., Sharp, S. C. and Lohman, T. G. (2003) Effects of exercise training on bone remodeling, insulin-like growth factors, and bone mineral density in postmenopausal women with and without hormone replacement therapy. *Calcif Tissue Int*; 72: 478–84.

Moayyeri, A. (2008) The association between physical activity and osteoporotic fractures: a review of the evidence and implications for future research. *Physical Activity and Osteoporosis*; 18: 827–35.

Nelson, M. E., Rejeski, W. J., Blair, A. N., Duncan, P. W., Judge, J. O., King, A. C., Macera, C. A. and Castaneda-Sceppa, C. (2007) Physical activity and public health in older adult: recommendation from the American College of Sports Medicine and the American Heart Association. *Med Sci Sports Exerc*; 39: 1435–45.

Palombaro, K. M. (2005) Effect of walking-only intervention on bone mineral density at various skeletal sites: a meta-analysis. *J Geriat Physic Ther*; 28: 1027–107.

Papaioannou, A., Adachi, J. D., Winegard, K., Ferko, N., Parkinson, W., Cook, R. J., Webber, C. and McCartney, N. (2003) Efficacy of home-based exercise for improving quality of life among elderly women with symptomatic osteoporosis-related vertebral fractures. *Osteoporos Int*; 14: 677–82.

Riggs, B. L., Wahner, H. W., Seeman, E., Offord, K. P., Dunn, W. L., Mazess, R. B., Johnson, K. A. and Melton, L. J. 3rd (1982) Change in bone mineral density of the proximal femur and spine with aging. Difference between the postmenopausal and senile osteoporosis syndromes. *J Clin Invest*; 70: 716–23.

Robbins, J., Aragaki, A. K., Kooperberg, C., Watts, N., Wactawski-Wende, J., Jackson, R. D., LeBoff, M. S., Lewis, C. E., Chen, Z., Stefanick, M. L. and Cauley, J. (2007) Factor associated with 5-year risk of hip fracture in postmenopausal women. *JAMA*; 298: 2389–98.

Schmitt, N.M., Schmitt, J. and Dören, M. (2009) The role of physical activity in the prevention of osteoporosis in postmenopausal women – an update. *Maturitas*; 63: 34–8.

Schwab, P. and Klein, R. F. (2008) Nonpharmacological approaches to improve bone health and reduce osteoporosis. *Curr Opin Rheumatol*; 20: 213–17.

Shen, C. L., Williams, J. S. and Chyu, M. C. (2007) Comparison of the effects of Tai Chi and resistance training on bone metabolism in the elderly: a feasibility study. *Am J Chin Med*; 35: 369–81.

Stewart, K. J., Bacher, A. C., Hees, P. S., Tayback, M., Ouyang, P. and Jan de Beur, S. (2005) Exercise effects on bone mineral density relationship to changes in fitness and fatness. *Am J Prev Med*; 28: 453–60.

Swanenburg, J., de Bruin, E. D., Stauffacher, M., Mulder, T. and Uebelhart, D. (2007) Effects of exercise and nutrition on postural balance and risk of falling in elderly people with decreased bone mineral density: randomized controlled trial pilot study. *Clin Rehabil*; 21: 523–34.

Vainionpää, A., Korpelainen, R., Leppäluoto, J. and Jämsä, T. (2005) Effects of high-impact exercise on bone mineral density: a randomized controlled trial in premenopausal women. *Osteoporos Int*; 16: 191–7.

Wayne, P. M., Kiel, D. P., Krebs, D. E., Davis, R. B., Savetsky-German, J., Connelly, M. and Buring, J. E. (2007) The effects of Tai Chi on bone mineral density in postmenopausal women: A systematic review. *Arch Phys Med Rehabil*; 88: 673–80.

Woolf, A. D. and Pfleger B. (2003) Burden of major musculoskeletal conditions. *Bulletin of the World Health Organization*; 81:646–56.

World Health Organization. (1994) Assessment of fracture risk and its application to screening for postmenopausal women. *WHO Technical Report Series* 843. Geneva: WHO.

Young, C. M., Week, B. K. and Beck, B. R. (2007) Simple, novel physical activity maintains proximal femur bone mineral density, and improves muscle strength and balance in sedentary, postmenopausal Caucasian women. *Osteoporos Int*; 18: 1379–87.

Zehnaker, C. H. and Bemis-Dougherty A. (2007) Effect of weighted exercises on bone mineral density in post menopausal women. A systematic review. *J Geriatr Phys Ther*; 30: 79–88.

Zhu, K., Devine, A., Dick, I. M., Wilson, S. G. and Prince, R. L. (2008) Effects of calcium and vitamin D supplementation on hip bone mineral density and calcium-related analytes in elderly ambulatory Australian women: a five-year randomized controlled trial. *J Clin Endocrinol Metab.*; 93: 743–9.

10

RHEUMATOID ARTHRITIS

C. H. M. van den Ende

Introduction

Rheumatoid arthritis (RA) is a chronic inflammatory, multisystem disorder of unknown aetiology. The disease is characterised by symmetric arthritis and destructive synovitis and affects primarily cartilage and bone of small and middle-sized joints. In addition, larger joints and several organs such as lungs, vessels and the hematopoietic system may be involved. Locally, inflammatory cells invade the synovium, leading to hyperplasia and formation of pannus-tissue, which causes destruction of cartilage, erosion of the adjacent bone and ultimately loss of function of the affected joint. Systemic inflammation, in parallel, has long-term impact on various organs, considerably increasing the risk for atherosclerosis and lymphoma development (Kvien *et al.*, 2009).

A patient is said to have RA if s/he satisfies at least 4 out of the 7 criteria of the American College of Rheumatology (ACR): (1) morning stiffness, (2) arthritis of three or more joints, (3) arthritis of the hand joints, (4) symmetric arthritis, (5) rheumatoid nodules, (6) serum rheumatoid factor, or (7) radiologic changes (Arnett *et al.*, 1988).

The disease predominantly affects the joints of the hands and feet. Joints with inflammation are painful, tender and the patient perceives stiffness on movement. The patients may also observe that the joints are swollen. A general feeling of morning stiffness is common and typical. Other frequently occurring general symptoms include fatigue and loss of energy. For reasons largely unknown, the individual presentation of disease ranges from mild cases with non-erosive, even sometimes spontaneously remitting disease, to severe, rapidly progressive and destructive RA. Also, the course of the disease is highly variable, with periods of remission alternating with periods of flare. A flare is any worsening of disease activity that would, if persistent, in most cases lead to initiation or change of therapy (Bingham *et al.*, 2009). A flare is usually accompanied by pain, swollen joints and fatigue.

In established disease, joint involvement is often dominated by deformities as a consequence of longstanding inflammation and radiographic damage. Any joint may be involved in the disease process but the most common sites are the joints of the hands, feet and knees. Common deformities of the hand joints are Boutonierre deformity (flexion of the proximal interphalangeal (PIP) joint and hyperextension of the distal interphalangeal (DIP) joint resulting from lack of ligament support) and Swan-Neck deformity of the finger describing the combination of hyperextension of the PIP joint and flexion of the DIP joint. Deformities of the metacarpophalangeal (MCP) joints include volar subluxation which may be seen as ulnar drift (often in combination with radial deviation of the wrist joint) and flexion deformities. Within the foot the subtalar and mid-tarsal joints are more frequently involved than the ankle joint. Forefoot deformity starts with synovitis of the MTP joints and the involvement of flexor tendons which is often followed by clawing of the toes and dorsal dislocation of the MTP joints. Reduction of knee extension might be result of inflammation of the joint and/or the presence of a so-called Baker's cyst: a cyst of the popliteal region. Destruction of the knee may lead to instability as a result of laxity of the collateral and cruciate ligaments (Kvien *et al.*, 2009).

RA affects approximately 0.5–1 per cent of European and North-American adults, with considerable regional differences. Annual incidence rates are estimated to be 16.5 cases (per 10,000) in Southern Europe, 29 cases in Northern Europe and 38 cases in North America (Alamanos *et al.*, 2006). The prevalence is almost a 2:1 ratio for women to men.

Consequences of RA on body functions and activities

The World Health Organization International Classification of Functioning, Disability and Health (ICF) provides a framework for classifying the consequences of a disease (World Health Organization, 2002). According to the ICF, the consequences of a disease may concern 'Body (anatomical) Structures and (physiological) Functions' and 'Activities and Participation'. Disease consequences are modified by 'Contextual Factors', including both environmental and personal factors. Non-problematic aspects of health are summarised under the umbrella term 'functioning', whereas 'disability' serves as an umbrella term for impairment of body functions or body structures, activity limitations or participation restrictions.

The ICF Core Set for RA defines the areas that are relevant to functioning in RA patients and contains goals for treatment. Exercise therapy aims to improve body functions, the performance of activities and, ultimately, participation. Table 10.1 depicts the categories of body functions, activities and participation of the ICF brief core for RA that are considered important by a majority of experts (Stucki *et al.*, 2004). This table shows that RA has an impact on body structures, body functions, activities and environmental factors. The impact of RA on body functions and activities, the main focus for exercise, are discussed briefly next.

TABLE 10.1 Categories of body functions, activities and participation of the ICF brief core for RA that are considered important by a majority of experts (Stucki *et al.*, 2004)

Body functions	Sensation of pain
	Mobility of joint functions
	Muscle power functions
	Exercise tolerance functions
	Sensations related to muscles and movement functions
Body structures	Structure of lower extremity
	Structure of upper extremity
	Structure of head and neck region
	Structure of shoulder region
Activities and participation	Walking
	Remunerative employment
	Fine hand use
	Changing basic body position
	Hand and arm use
	Carrying out daily routine
Environmental factors	Immediate family
	Health services, systems and policies
	Health professionals
	Products and technology for personal use in daily living
	Social security services, systems and policies

TABLE 10.2 Requirements for the successful design, implementation and maintenance of an exercise routine (Vliet Vlieland *et al.*, 2009; Westby, 2001)

- Establish reasonable goals on the basis of discussion with the patients.
- Choose a mode of delivery that matches the patient's preferences and circumstances.
- Adapt the programme to individual preferences, possibilities and disabilities.
- Avoid activities and exercises that induce pain and discomfort.
- Identify possible barriers for exercising.
- Monitor effectiveness and feasibility: both the patient and the health care provider need to monitor programme success.

Body functions

Pain is the leading symptom in patients with RA and one of the key domains for treatment. Pain in RA is typically present in the different body parts of the loco-motor system and may specifically involve the joints. Loss of joint mobility may result from (a) pain, (b) capsular distension from increased amounts of synovial fluid or synovial tissue, (c) contraction of the capsule, periarticular ligaments or tendons, or (d) degenerative processes such as loss of articular cartilage, bone loss and deformities (Ytterberg *et al.*, 1994). Information about the extent of loss of joint mobility in early and later stages of the disease is sparse. Half of the patients show limited mobility of the hand joints already at first presentation. In later years, loss of joint motion is present in about 25–35 per cent of the ankle, knee, hip, elbow or shoulder joints (Eberhardt and Fex, 1995).

While pain and loss of mobility of the joints are the main impairments of RA, they are closely followed by skeletal muscle weakness. There are multiple reasons for muscular weakness in RA. Several histological investigations showed alterations in muscle biopsies, suggesting the influence of inflammatory processes on muscle fibres (Brooke and Kaplan, 1972; Edstrom and Nordemar, 1974; Haslock *et al.*, 1970). Even in the absence of pain, joint pathology can inhibit muscle activity and so cause both weakness and wasting. Joint inflammation affects muscle function as a result of afferent impulses from mechanoreceptors and joint nocioreceptors – the so-called arthrogeneous reflex muscle inhibition (Stokes and Young, 1984). This theory is based on observations that muscle weakness is more pronounced in injured joints (Haggmark *et al.*, 1986; Rutherford *et al.*, 1990; Young *et al.*, 1982). Apart from the disease process on muscle function, physical inactivity and medication, in particular the use of corticosteroids, may further contribute to muscle weakness.

In mildly disabled patients, strength of knee and hip muscle groups is reduced to 50–75 per cent (Bearne *et al.*, 2002; Ekblom *et al.*, 1974; Ekdahl and Broman, 1992; Hsieh *et al.*, 1987) and muscle endurance to 45 per cent (Ekdahl and Broman, 1992) when compared to age-matched healthy persons. The reduction of muscle strength is more pronounced in patients using corticosteroids (Danneskiold-Samsoe and Grimby, 1986a; Danneskiold-Samsoe and Grimby, 1986b). The maximal and explosive muscle strength has also been reported to be reduced in female RA patients, able to maintain their aerobic fitness at the same level as age-matched healthy people by using various physical exercises on a regular basis (Hakkinen *et al.*, 2002).

In addition to muscle weakness, poor cardiorespiratory function has been reported in patients with RA. The reduction in aerobic capacity ($\dot{V}O_{2max}$) by submaximal or maximal ergometer testing varies between 20 and 30 per cent (Ekblom *et al.*, 1974; Ekdahl and Bromen, 1992; Minor *et al.*, 1988). This may be due to the observation that patients with RA spend less time per week on physical activity (van den Berg *et al.*, 2007a).

Postural balance is markedly reduced in patients with RA compared to healthy persons and an association has been found with gender, age, body mass index and functional ability but not with disease activity (Aydog *et al.*, 2006). Patients with RA have an increased risk of falls (Smulders *et al.*, 2009b) which might be associated with a reduced ability to avoid obstacles (Smulders *et al.*, 2009a).

Finally, fatigue and a general feeling of unwellness have been identified as an important outcome of disease (Carr *et al.*, 2003; Hewlett *et al.*, 2005). Severe fatigue is experienced by as many as 50 per cent of RA patients (Repping-Wuts *et al.*, 2007).

Activities of daily living

Activities of daily living (ADLs) can be limited by impairments in body structures related to the rheumatoid disease (tissue inflammation and structural damage) and restrictions of body functions such as range of movement, skeletal muscle strength, balance, global pain and morning stiffness. Joint tenderness and pain are the most important factors for limitations in activities (Plant *et al.*, 2005; Rupp *et al.*, 2006; van den Ende *et al.*, 1997).

The most commonly used outcome measure to describe limitations in ADLs is the Health Assessment Questionnaire (HAQ) (Fries *et al.*, 1980). This questionnaire incorporates a range of ADLs, such as dressing and grooming, reaching for objects, dexterity and mobility. The HAQ is questioned for its insensitivity for change in exercise trials (van den Ende *et al.*, 1997); for that reason patient-oriented questionnaires like the McMaster Toronto Arthritis (MACTAR) questionnaire (Tugwell *et al.*, 1987) are preferred which assesses change in those activities that are important for each individual patient.

RA is associated with a >7-fold risk of disability compared with that in a general population of adults in the same community. In 30–79-year-old patients with RA, 17–45 per cent of women and 7–32 per cent of men reported HAQ scores greater than the adjusted reference values. The impact of disability due to RA appears to be greater in younger and middle-age people than in elderly patients (Sokka *et al.*, 2003). Many patients with RA experience limitations in ADLs, such as personal care, house keeping and transport. Limitations in upper extremity activities, particularly with regard to personal hygiene, are associated with impaired strength of the internal shoulder rotator muscles (Bostrom, 2000) and reduced joint mobility (Badley *et al.*, 1984; van den Ende *et al.*, 1997). Mild walking disability is present in the majority of patients at initial presentation (van der Leeden *et al.*, 2008), which might be explained by impairments (pain and swelling) of the joints of the forefoot (van der Leeden *et al.*, 2008) and limited range of motion of the MTP joints (Laroche *et al.*, 2006).

Management of RA

Pharmacological and non-pharmacological treatments

The management of RA includes a variety of pharmacological and non-pharmacological treatment options. The pharmacological treatment is directed towards suppressing pain, disease activity and the reduction of risk factors of cardiovascular disease (Peters *et al.*, 2009). Disease-modifying anti-rheumatic drugs (DMARDs) constitute the backbone of RA pharmacological treatment and comprise those drugs that have positive impact on radiological outcome of joint damage (erosions and joint space narrowing). DMARDs include a heterogeneous group of drugs including the most commonly used drugs such as methotrexate, suflfasalazine and glucocorticosteroids as well as recently introduced biological agents (McInnes *et al.*, 2009). Modern insights legitimate early and aggressive pharmacological treatment to achieve remission, or at least a low disease activity state in order to prevent joint damage in the long term (Sokka and Makinen, 2009). Indicators of disease activity are, among others, erythrocyte sedimentation rate (ESR) and the number of tender and swollen joints.

In addition to pharmacological treatment, health professionals like occupational therapists and physiotherapists offer treatment modalities aimed at improving and maintaining physical, psychological and social functioning. Regular participation in exercise therapy is considered to be an important cornerstone in the management of RA (American College of Rheumatology subcommittee on rheumatoid arthritis guidelines, 2002). Exercise therapy aims to reduce the consequences of the disease on body functions and the performance of activities.

In patients who have unacceptable levels of pain, loss of range of motion or limitation of function because of structural joint damage, surgical procedures are being considered. Surgical procedures for RA include carpal tunnel release, synovectomy, resection of the metatarsal heads, total joint arthroplasty and joint fusion (American College of Rheumatology subcommittee on rheumatoid arthritis guidelines, 2002).

Possible benefits and adverse effects of exercise therapy for patients with RA

Specific goals of exercise therapy in RA are to increase and maintain joint flexibility, muscle function, cardiorespiratory function and the performance of activities. Secondary goals of exercise in RA are to improve well-being, to improve social interactions and to prevent comorbidity such as osteoporosis and cardiovascular disease, as patients with RA are as a consequence of their disease, its treatment (glucocorticosteroids) and physical inactivity more at risk of osteoporosis or osteoporotic fractures (Gough et al., 1994; Huusko et al., 2001) and cardiovascular disease (Avina-Zubieta et al., 2008; Metsios et al., 2009). Traditionally, patients with RA have been cautioned against vigorous exercise. In particular, dynamic exercises against resistance were considered to enhance pain and disease activity (Hazes and van den Ende, 1996). Low intensity isometric exercises and range of motion exercises, on the other hand, were thought to be safe. As a result, besides establishing the effectiveness of exercise therapy, an important focus of research in this field should be the safety of exercises for patients with this condition.

Evidence on the effectiveness of exercise in RA

Dynamic exercise therapy

The available literature on exercise therapy for RA focuses mainly on dynamic exercise, i.e. rhythmic exercise with large skeletal muscle groups of sufficient intensity, duration and frequency to improve aerobic capacity and/or skeletal muscle strength. Conclusions of systematic reviews on the effectiveness of dynamic exercise therapy differ slightly due to differences in applied methods (e.g. eligibility criteria for studies to be included) and consequently, conclusions being drawn from different numbers of studies. In general, systematic reviews conclude that dynamic exercise has small to moderate effects on aerobic capacity and skeletal muscle strength (Baslund *et al.*, 1993; Cairns and McVeigh, 2009; Gaudin *et al.*, 2008; Hurkmans *et al.*, 2009; Stenstrom and Minor, 2003). Results on the effectiveness of dynamic exercise on functional ability are unclear but the majority of the studied interventions did not report improvements in daily functioning.

In a recently updated Cochrane review, applying pertinent eligibility criteria regarding the intensity of the exercise intervention, a distinction was made between land-based and water-based exercise therapy (Hurkmans *et al.*, 2009). In this review, eight studies were included (Baslund *et al.*, 1993; de Jong *et al.*, 2003; Hansen *et al.*, 1993; Harkcom *et al.*, 1985; Lyngberg *et al.*, 1994; Minor *et al.*, 1989; Sanford-Smit *et al.*, 1998; van den Ende *et al.*, 1996); four of which were deemed to be of methodological high quality (Baslund *et al.*, 1993; Hansen *et al.*, 1993; Lyngberg *et al.*, 1994; Sanford-Smit *et al.*, 1998). It was concluded that short-term land-based dynamic exercise programmes (lasting three months or less) have a positive effect on aerobic capacity and skeletal muscle strength immediately after the intervention, but not after a follow-up period. There is evidence that short-term water-based dynamic exercise therapy has a positive effect on functional ability, but is unknown whether these effects are maintained over longer follow-up periods (Hurkmans *et al.*, 2009). Long-term, land-based dynamic exercise programmes (lasting two years) have a positive effect on functional ability, aerobic capacity and skeletal muscle strength immediately after the intervention. This latter conclusion is based on the results of one trial with high methodological quality. Patients enrolled on a 2-year high-intensity exercise programme showed improvements in functional ability, as measured by the MACTAR questionnaire but not by the HAQ, compared to controls (de Jong *et al.*, 2003). After 18 months of follow-up, the original gains in functional ability were sustained, irrespective of continuation of exercises. The majority of the RA patients who participated in a 2-year high-intensity exercise programme continued, in a 'real-life' situation, exercising at a similar level of intensity but at a lower frequency (de Jong *et al.*, 2009).

Resistance exercise training to improve muscular strength

A systematic review on the effectiveness of different types of resistance exercise (strength) training concluded that increases in strength were highest in the studies that included high intensity training compared to lower intensity mixed strength and/or aerobic exercise training programmes (de Jong *et al.*, 2003; Hakkinen 2004). One study reported a 5.5 per cent increase in the cross-sectional area of the quadriceps femoris muscle after a programme of resistance exercise training in patients with RA (Hakkinen *et al.*, 1994).

Tai Chi

Tai Chi combines deep diaphragmatic breathing and relaxation, with slow and gentle movements, both isometric and isotonic, while maintaining good postures. Isometric exercises allow the patient to exercise specific muscle groups while avoiding joint motion. Isotonic exercises contract muscles in a way that causes joint movement. Tai Chi involves stepping with full weight-bearing on both lower extremities, but has a gentler heel-strike than walking because of slow and deliberate foot placement (Han *et al.*, 2004). There is fairly strong evidence that Tai Chi improves the range of motion of the ankle, hip and knee in people with RA (Han *et al.*, 2004).

Dance exercise

The effects of dance exercise have been investigated in many non-randomised trials and the weight of evidence suggests that improvements in aerobic capacity, walking ability, muscular strength and psychological parameters such as anxiety and depression can be attained (Metsios *et al.*, 2009).

Hand exercises

In a systematic review on the effectiveness of hand exercises in RA, nine randomised controlled trials with relatively small number of patients were included. Although hand exercises are advocated for RA, it was concluded that there is little evidence to support or refute hand exercise as an intervention. Limited evidence that hand exercises performed against a resistance over a long enough time period of time results in an increase in hand-grip strength (Wessel, 2004).

Interventions to increase physical activity

In a meta-analysis the effectiveness of a variety of interventions for patients with arthritis (both rheumatoid arthritis and osteoarthritis) on the amount of physical activity was summarised. The content of interventions of studies included in this meta-analysis ranged from (combinations of) supervised exercise to interventions to increase self-management skills such as goal setting, problem solving, self-monitoring and decision making (Conn *et al.*, 2008). A positive effect on physical activity was found; authors concluded that exercise and/or interventions promoting physical activity are successful to incorporate physical activity into their lifestyles for individuals with arthritis.

Safety of exercise in RA

Pain and disease activity

In none of the trials included in systematic reviews of the effectiveness of exercise therapy in RA has an increase in pain levels or measures of disease activity been observed (Cairns *et al.*, 2009; Gaudin *et al.*, 2008; Hakkinen, 2004; Hurkmans *et al.*, 2009; Metsios *et al.*, 2008; Stenstrom and Minor, 2003). However, it should be noted that these reviews generally included patients with well-controlled disease. One study, which included patients hospitalised because of active disease, showed that isokinetic exercise and cycling to improve aerobic capacity (during the period of hospitalisation) resulted in an improvement of disease activity compared to a conservative exercise regimen consisting of isometric exercise and active-assisted exercise to improve joint mobility (van den Ende *et al.*, 2000). Hence, there is currently no evidence that either high or low intensity exercise therapy has any detrimental effect on pain or disease activity.

Joint damage

Data on the effect of intensive exercise on joint damage, as measured by radiography, in patients with rheumatoid arthritis are scarce. Furthermore, only one trial (de Jong *et al.*, 2003) included a sufficient number of patients to draw grounded conclusions. From the available evidence, it can be concluded that high intensive exercise does not affect the rate of damage of the small joints of the hand and feet (de Jong and Vliet Vlieland, 2005).

However, there is some evidence that prolonged high intensity might affect the rate of damage of the large joints (shoulders, elbows, hips, knees and ankles). In a trial comparing the effectiveness of 2-year high intensity exercise and usual care a non-significant trend toward a greater increase in joint damage of the large joints in the exercise group was observed. Compared to the control group more patients in the exercise group showed a relevant progression in damage of the large joints (Munneke *et al.*, 2005). The authors concluded that in the absence of sufficient data on exercise and radiologic progression of the large joints, RA patients with significant radiologic damage of the large joints should not be encouraged to participate in high intensity exercise unless individually curved protective measures are taken for the specific damaged joints (de Jong and Vliet Vlieland, 2005; Munneke *et al.*, 2005).

Structuring an exercise programme for people with RA

The first step in the design of an exercise programme is to establish mutually agreed goals on the basis of discussion with patients (Table 10.2). Exercise programmes of reasonable length, frequency, intensity and complexity, designed to reduce impairments and improve activities important to the individual patient will be most likely to be maintained.

Patients' preferences and circumstances should be taken into account in the choice for the optimum mode of delivery. Studies on planned and structured exercises as described in this chapter have been performed mainly in clinical environments with physical therapists supervising their patients. However, there is little evidence on the superiority of supervised exercising above other modes of care delivery. Communication with the patient can range from face-to-face contact, contact by telephone, contact by the internet (e-mail and/or web-based interactions) and written communication (written instructions, leaflets). Also, the intensity of communication can vary considerably ranging from a single contact to frequent contacts over a long period of time. In many programmes interaction with other patients is stimulated by organising sessions in groups, but there is no knowledge about the added value of group sessions above individualised sessions in chronic diseases (Newman *et al.*, 2004).

Exercise forms should be adapted to individual preferences, possibilities and disabilities. Individual preferences about forms of exercising (e.g. bicycling, swimming or recreational activities) should be identified and discussed. Many patients prefer to wear their everyday special footwear (extra depth shoes, custom-made foot orthosis) or functional wrist splints while exercising. Soft exercise materials (e.g. the use of a foam ball for game activities) or adapted materials (e.g. rackets with a broadened handle) may be considered.

Positions and activities that are stressful for joints and cause pain and discomfort should be avoided. It may be helpful to offer alternative body positions in periods of increased pain and disease activity. Patients with existing large joint damage should be discouraged to participate in sports and activities involving twisting and rapid joint loading or unloading (Cairns and McVeigh, 2009).

It is important to discuss with the patient possible barriers for exercising. Many patients with RA have the belief that exercise will contribute to joint damage and provoke inflammation (van den Berg *et al.*, 2007b). A clear policy with regard to pain and fatigue during and after exercising might help overcome barriers for exercising.

RA is a progressive disease that runs a variable course. Therefore, it is important to monitor effectiveness and feasibility of a planned exercise regimen to adjust goals and content when necessary. How and how often to evaluate are important considerations that should be based on clear goals and a determination when changes can be expected.

Summary and conclusions

Patients with RA are, as a consequence of their disease and its treatment, at risk for decreased physical capacity and functional ability and at increased risk for cardiovascular morbidity and mortality compared with their healthy counterparts. It has been consistently demonstrated that in patients with RA dynamic exercises, supervised and/or home-based are effective with respect to improvement of aerobic capacity and muscle strength, with no detrimental effects on disease activity, pain or radiological damage. It is important to underline that, contrary to a rather common belief, exercising inflamed joints does not have any deleterious effects. However, pain during and after exercising should be avoided to ensure compliance. Also, non-weight bearing exercises should be considered for patients with damage of the large joints.

Given the potential health benefits, it is generally acknowledged that RA patients should be advised to achieve and/or maintain an amount of physical activity that at least equals public health recommendations. Coaching or supervision might be necessary to overcome barriers for exercising such as local disease activity or joint damage, co-morbidity or movement anxiety, Furthermore, (temporal) limitations in specific movement patterns or daily activities need to be addressed in an individualised structured exercise programme.

References

Alamanos, Y., Voulgari, P. V., and Drosos, A. A. (2006), Incidence and prevalence of rheumatoid arthritis, based on the 1987 American College of Rheumatology criteria: a systematic review, *Semin Arthritis Rheum*, 36(3), 182–188.

American College of Rheumatology subcommittee on rheumatoid arthritis guidelines (2002) Guidelines for the management of rheumatoid arthritis. 2002 update, *Arthritis Rheum*, 46(2), 328–346.

Arnett, F. C., Edworthy, S. M., Bloch, D. A., McShane, D. J., Fries, J. F., Cooper, N. S., Healey, L. A., Kaplan, S. R., Liang, M. H., Luthra, H. S., Medsger, T. A. Jr., Mitchell, D. M., Neustadt, D. H., Pinals, R. S., Schaller, J. G., Sharp, J. T., Wilder, R. L. and Hunder, G. G. (1988), The American Rheumatism Association 1987 revised criteria for the classification of rheumatoid arthritis, *Arthritis Rheum*, 31(3), 315–324.

Avina-Zubieta, J. A., Choi, H. K., Sadatsafavi, M., Etminan, M., Esdaile, J. M., and Lacaille, D. (2008) Risk of cardiovascular mortality in patients with rheumatoid arthritis: a meta-analysis of observational studies, *Arthritis Rheum*, 59(12), 1690–1697.

Aydog, E., Bal, A., Aydog, S. T., and Cakci, A. (2006) Evaluation of dynamic postural balance using the Biodex Stability System in rheumatoid arthritis patients, *Clin Rheumatol*, 25(4), 462–467.

Badley, E. M., Wagstaff, S., and Wood, P. H. (1984) Measures of functional ability (disability) in arthritis in relation to impairment of range of joint movement, *Ann Rheum Dis*, 43(4), 563–569.

Baslund, B., Lyngberg, K., Andersen, V., Halkjaer, K. J., Hansen, M., Klokker, M., and Pedersen, B. K. (1993) Effect of 8 wk of bicycle training on the immune system of patients with rheumatoid arthritis, *J Appl Physiol*, 75(4), 1691–1695.

Bearne, L. M., Scott, D. L., and Hurley, M. V. (2002) Exercise can reverse quadriceps sensorimotor dysfunction that is associated with rheumatoid arthritis without exacerbating disease activity, *Rheumatology (Oxford)*, 41(2), 157–166.

Bingham, C. O. 3rd, Pohl, C., Woodworth, T. G., Hewlett, S. E., May, J. E., Rahman, M. U., Witter, J. P., Furst, D. E., Strand, C. V., Boers, M., and Alten, R. E. 2009, Developing a standardized definition for disease 'flare' in rheumatoid arthritis (OMERACT 9 Special Interest Group), *J Rheumatol*, 36(10), 2335–2341.

Bostrom, C. (2000) Shoulder rotational strength, movement, pain and joint tenderness as indicators of upper-extremity activity limitation in moderate rheumatoid arthritis, *Scand J Rehabil Med*, 32(3), 134–139.

Brooke, M. H. and Kaplan, H. (1972) Muscle pathology in rheumatoid arthritis, polymyalgia rheumatica, and polymyositis: a histochemical study, *Arch Pathol*, 94(2), 101–118.

Cairns, A. P. and McVeigh, J. G. (2009) A systematic review of the effects of dynamic exercise in rheumatoid arthritis, *Rheumatol Int*, 30(2) 147–158.

Carr, A., Hewlett, S., Hughes, R., Mitchell, H., Ryan, S., Carr, M., and Kirwan, J. (2003) Rheumatology outcomes: the patient's perspective, *J Rheumatol*, 30(4), 880–883.

Conn, V. S., Hafdahl, A. R., Minor, M. A., and Nielsen, P. J. (2008) Physical activity interventions among adults with arthritis: meta-analysis of outcomes, *Semin Arthritis Rheum*, 37(5), 307–316.

Danneskiold-Samsoe, B. and Grimby, G. (1986a) Isokinetic and isometric muscle strength in patients with rheumatoid arthritis. The relationship to clinical parameters and the influence of corticosteroid, *Clin Rheumatol*, 5(4), 459–467.

Danneskiold-Samsoe, B. and Grimby, G. (1986b) The relationship between the leg muscle strength and physical capacity in patients with rheumatoid arthritis, with reference to the influence of corticosteroids, *Clin Rheumatol*, 5(4), 468–474.

de Jong Z., Munneke, M., Zwinderman, A. H., Kroon, H. M., Jansen, A., Ronday, K. H., Van Schaardenburg D., Dijkmans, B. A., van den Ende, C. H., Breedveld, F. C., Vliet Vlieland, T. P., and Hazes, J. M. (2003) Is a long-term high-intensity exercise program effective and safe in patients with rheumatoid arthritis? Results of a randomized controlled trial, *Arthritis Rheum*, 48(9), 2415–2424.

de Jong, Z., Munneke, M., Kroon, H. M., van, Schaardenburg, D., Dijkmans, B. A., Hazes, J. M., and Vliet Vlieland, T. P. (2009) Long-term follow-up of a high-intensity exercise program in patients with rheumatoid arthritis, *Clin Rheumatol*, 28(6), 663–671.

de Jong, Z. and Vliet Vlieland, T. P. (2005) Safety of exercise in patients with rheumatoid arthritis, *Curr Opin Rheumatol*, 17(2), 177–182.

Eberhardt, K. B. and Fex, E. (1995) Functional impairment and disability in early rheumatoid arthritis – development over 5 years, *J Rheumatol*, 22(6), 1037–1042.

Edstrom, L. and Nordemar, R. (1974) Differential changes in type I and type II muscle fibres in rheumatoid arthritis. A biopsy study, *Scand J Rheumatol*, 3(3), 155–160.

Ekblom, B., Lovgren, O., Alderin, M., Fridstrom, M., and Satterstrom, G. (1974) Physical performance in patients with rheumatoid arthritis, *Scand J Rheumatol*, 3(3), 121–125.

Ekdahl, C. and Broman, G. (1992) Muscle strength, endurance, and aerobic capacity in rheumatoid arthritis: a comparative study with healthy subjects, *Ann Rheum Dis*, 51(1), 35–40.

Fries, J. F., Spitz, P., Kraines, R. G., and Holman, H. R. (1980) Measurement of patient outcome in arthritis, *Arthritis Rheum*, 23(2), 137–145.

Gaudin, P., Leguen-Guegan, S., Allenet, B., Baillet, A., Grange, L., and Juvin, R. (2008) Is dynamic exercise beneficial in patients with rheumatoid arthritis?, *Joint Bone Spine*, 75(1), 11–17.

Gough, A. K., Lilley, J., Eyre, S., Holder, R. L., and Emery, P. (1994) Generalised bone loss in patients with early rheumatoid arthritis, *Lancet*, 344(8914), 23–27.

Haggmark, T., Eriksson, E., and Jansson, E. (1986) Muscle fiber type changes in human skeletal muscle after injuries and immobilization, *Orthopedics*, 9(2), 181–185.

Hakkinen, A. (2004) Effectiveness and safety of strength training in rheumatoid arthritis, *Curr Opin Rheumatol*, 16(2), 132–137.

Hakkinen, A., Haanonan, P., Nyman, K., and Hakkinen, K. (2002) Aerobic and neuromuscular performance capacity of physically active females with early or long-term rheumatoid arthritis compared to matched healthy women, *Scand J Rheumatol*, 31(6), 345–350.

Hakkinen, A., Hakkinen, K., and Hannonen, P. (1994) Effects of strength training on neuromuscular function and disease activity in patients with recent-onset inflammatory arthritis, *Scand J Rheumatol*, 23(5), 237–242.

Han, A., Robinson, V., Judd, M., Taixiang, W., Wells, G., and Tugwell, P. (2004) Tai chi for treating rheumatoid arthritis, *Cochrane Database Syst Rev* no. 3, p. CD004849.

Hansen, T. M., Hansen, G., Langgaard, A. M., and Rasmussen, J. O. (1993) Longterm physical training in rheumatoid arthritis. A randomized trial with different training programs and blinded observers, *Scand J Rheumatol*, 22(3), 107–112.

Harkcom, T. M., Lampman, R. M., Banwell, B. F., and Castor, C. W. (1985) Therapeutic value of graded aerobic exercise training in rheumatoid arthritis, *Arthritis Rheum*, 28(1), 32–39.

Haslock, D. I., Harriman, D. F., and Wright, V. (1970) Neuromuscular disorders associated with rheumatoid arthritis, *Ann Rheum Dis*, 29(2), 197.

Hazes, J. M. and van den Ende, C. H. (1996) How vigorously should we exercise our rheumatoid arthritis patients?, *Ann Rheum Dis*, 55(12), 861–862.

Hewlett, S., Cockshott, Z., Byron, M., Kitchen, K., Tipler, S., Pope, D., and Hehir, M. (2005) Patients' perceptions of fatigue in rheumatoid arthritis: overwhelming, uncontrollable, ignored, *Arthritis Rheum*, 53(5), 697–702.

Hsieh, L. F., Didenko, B., Schumacher, H. R. Jr., and Torg, J. S. 1987, Isokinetic and isometric testing of knee musculature in patients with rheumatoid arthritis with mild knee involvement, *Arch Phys Med Rehabil*, 68(5) Pt 1, 294–297.

Hurkmans, E., van der Giesen, F. J., Vliet Vlieland, T. P., Schoones, J., and Van den Ende, E. C. (2009) Dynamic exercise programs (aerobic capacity and/or muscle strength training) in patients with rheumatoid arthritis, *Cochrane Database Syst Rev* no. 4, p. CD006853.

Huusko, T. M., Korpela, M., Karppi, P., Avikainen, V., Kautiainen, H., and Sulkava, R. (2001) Threefold increased risk of hip fractures with rheumatoid arthritis in Central Finland, *Ann Rheum Dis*, 60(5), 521–522.

Kvien, T. K., Scherer, H., and Burmester, G. R. (2009) 'Rheumatoid Arthritis,' in Bijlsma, J. W., Burmester, G. R., Da Silva, J. A., Faarvang, K. L., Hachulla, E. and Mariette, X. (eds) *Eular Compendium on Rheumatic Diseases*, BMJ Publishing Group Ltd, 61–80.

Laroche, D., Pozzo, T., Ornetti, P., Tavernier, C., and Maillefert, J. F. (2006) Effects of loss of metatarsophalangeal joint mobility on gait in rheumatoid arthritis patients, *Rheumatology (Oxford)*, 45(4), 435–440.

Lyngberg, K. K., Harreby, M., Bentzen, H., Frost, B., and Danneskiold-Samsøe, B. (1994) Elderly rheumatoid arthritis patients on steroid treatment tolerate physical training without an increase in disease activity, *Arch Phys Med Rehabil*, 75(11), 1189–1195.

McInnes, I., Jacobs, J. W., Woodburn, J., and Van Laar, J. (2009) 'Treatment of rheumatoid arthritis,' in Bijlsma, J. W., Burmester, G. R., Da Silva, J. A., Faarvang, K. L., Hachulla, E. and Mariette, X. (eds), *Eular Compendium on Rheumatic Diseases*, 1st edn, BMJ Publishing Group Ltd, London, pp. 81–91.

Metsios, G. S., Stavropoulos-Kalinoglou, A., Panoulas, V. F., Wilson, M., Nevill, A. M., Koutedakis, Y., and Kitas, G. D. (2009) Association of physical inactivity with increased cardiovascular risk in patients with rheumatoid arthritis, *Eur J Cardiovasc Prev Rehabil*, 16(2), 188–194.

Metsios, G. S., Stavropoulos-Kalinoglou, A., Veldhuijzen van Zanten, J. J., Treharne, G. J., Panoulas, V. F., Douglas, K. M., Koutedakis, Y., and Kitas, G. D. (2008) Rheumatoid arthritis, cardiovascular disease and physical exercise: a systematic review, *Rheumatology (Oxford)*, 47(3), 239–248.

Minor, M. A., Hewett, J. E., Webel, R. R., Anderson, S. K., and Kay, D. R. (1989) Efficacy of physical conditioning exercise in patients with rheumatoid arthritis and osteoarthritis, *Arthritis Rheum*, 32(11), 1396–1405.

Minor, M. A., Hewett, J. E., Webel, R. R., Dreisinger, T. E., and Kay, D. R. (1988) Exercise tolerance and disease related measures in patients with rheumatoid arthritis and osteoarthritis, *J Rheumatol*, 15(6), 905–911.

Munneke, M., de Jong, Z., Zwinderman, A. H., Ronday, H. K., van, Schaardenburg, D., Dijkmans, B. A., Kroon, H. M., Vliet Vlieland, T. P., and Hazes, J. M. (2005) Effect of a high-intensity weight-bearing exercise program on radiologic damage progression of the large joints in subgroups of patients with rheumatoid arthritis, *Arthritis Rheum*, 53(3), 410–417.

Newman, S., Steed, L., and Mulligan, K. (2004) Self-management interventions for chronic illness, *Lancet*, 364(9444), 1523–1537.

Peters, M. J., Symmons, D. P., McCarey, D., Dijkmans, B. A., Nicola, P., Kvien, T. K., McInnes, I. B., Haentzschel, H., Gonzalez-Gay, M. A., Provan, S., Semb, A. G., Sidiropoulos, P., Kitas, G., Smulders, Y. M., Soubrier, M. J., Szekanecz, Z., Sattar, N. G., and Nurmohamed, M. T. (2009) EULAR evidence-based recommendations for cardiovascular risk management in patients with rheumatoid arthritis and other forms of inflammatory arthritis, *Ann Rheum Dis*, 69(2), 325–31.

Plant, M. J., O'Sullivan, M. M., Lewis, P. A., Camilleri, J. P., Coles, E. C., and Jessop, J. D. (2005) What factors influence functional ability in patients with rheumatoid arthritis. Do they alter over time?, *Rheumatology (Oxford)*, 44(9), 1181–1185.

Repping-Wuts, H., Fransen, J., van Achterberg, T., Bleijenberg, G., and van Riel, P. (2007) Persistent severe fatigue in patients with rheumatoid arthritis, *J Clin Nurs*, 16(11C), 377–383.

Rupp, I., Boshuizen, H. C., Dinant, H. J., Jacobi, C. E., and van den Bos, G. A. (2006) Disability and health-related quality of life among patients with rheumatoid arthritis: association with radiographic joint damage, disease activity, pain, and depressive symptoms, *Scand J Rheumatol*, 35(3), 175–181.

Rutherford, O. M., Jones, D. A., and Round, J. M. (1990) Long-lasting unilateral muscle wasting and weakness following injury and immobilisation, *Scand J Rehabil Med*, 22(1), 33–37.

Sanford-Smit, S., MacKay-Lyons, M., and Nunes-Clement, S. (1998) Therapeutic beneift of aquarobics for individuals with rheumatoid arthritis, *Physiother Can* (Winter), 40–46.

Smulders, E., Schreven, C., van, L. W., Duysens, J., and Weerdesteyn, V. (2009a) Obstacle avoidance in persons with rheumatoid arthritis walking on a treadmill, *Clin Exp Rheumatol*, 27(5), 779–785.

Smulders, E., Schreven, C., Weerdesteyn, V., van den Hoogen, F. H., Laan, R., and van, L. W. (2009b) Fall incidence and fall risk factors in people with rheumatoid arthritis, *Ann Rheum Dis*, 68(11), 1795–1796.

Sokka, T., Krishnan, E., Hakkinen, A., and Hannonen, P. (2003) Functional disability in rheumatoid arthritis patients compared with a community population in Finland, *Arthritis Rheum*, 48(1), 59–63.

Sokka, T. and Makinen, H. (2009) Drug management of early rheumatoid arthritis – 2008, *Best Pract Res Clin Rheumatol*, 23(1), 93–102.

Stenstrom, C. H. and Minor, M. A. (2003) Evidence for the benefit of aerobic and strengthening exercise in rheumatoid arthritis, *Arthritis Rheum*, 49(3), 428–434.

Stokes, M. and Young, A. (1984) The contribution of reflex inhibition to arthrogenous muscle weakness, *Clin Sci (Lond)*, 67(1), 7–14.

Stucki, G., Cieza, A., Geyh, S., Battistella, L., Lloyd, J., Symmons, D., Kostanjsek, N., and Schouten, J. (2004) ICF Core Sets for rheumatoid arthritis, *J Rehabil Med* 44 (Suppl), 87–93.

Tugwell, P., Bombardier, C., Buchanan, W. W., Goldsmith, C. H., Grace, E., and Hanna, B. (1987) The MACTAR Patient Preference Disability Questionnaire – an individualized functional priority approach for assessing improvement in physical disability in clinical trials in rheumatoid arthritis, *J Rheumatol*, 14(3), 446–451.

van den Berg, M. H., de, Boer, I., le Cessie, S., Breedveld, F. C., and Vliet Vlieland, T. P. (2007a) Are patients with rheumatoid arthritis less physically active than the general population?, *J Clin Rheumatol*, 13(4), 181–186.

van den Berg, M. H., de Boer, I., le Cessie, S., Breedveld, F. C., and Vliet Vlieland, T. P. (2007b) Most people with rheumatoid arthritis undertake leisure-time physical activity in the Netherlands: an observational study, *Aust J Physiother*, 53(2), 113–118.

van den Ende, C. H., Breedveld, F. C., Dijkmans, B. A., and Hazes, J. M. (1997) The limited value of the Health Assessment Questionnaire as an outcome measure in short term exercise trials, *J Rheumatol*, 24(10), 1972–1977.

van den Ende, C. H., Breedveld, F. C., le Cessie, S., Dijkmans, B. A., de Mug, A. W. and Hazes, J. M. (2000) Effect of intensive exercise on patients with active rheumatoid arthritis: a randomised clinical trial, *Ann Rheum Dis*, 59(8), 615–621.

van den Ende, C. H., Hazes, J. M., Le Cessie S., Mulder, W. J., Belfor, D. G., Breedveld, F. C., and Dijkmans, B. A. (1996) Comparison of high and low intensity training in well controlled rheumatoid arthritis. Results of a randomised clinical trial, *Ann Rheum Dis*, 55(11), 798–805.

van der Leeden, M., Steultjens, M. P., Ursum, J., Dahmen, R., Roorda, L. D., Schaardenburg, D. V., and Dekker, J. (2008) Prevalence and course of forefoot impairments and walking disability in the first eight years of rheumatoid arthritis, *Arthritis Rheum*, 59(11), 1596–1602.

Vliet Vlieland, T. P., van den Ende, C. H., and Pinheiro, J. 2009, 'Principles of rehabilitation of rheumatic diseases,' in Bijlsma, J. W., Burmester, G. R., Da Silva, J. A., Faarvang, K. L., Hachulla, E. and Mariette, X. (eds), *Eular Compendium on Rheumatic Diseases*, 1st edn, BMJ Publising Group Ltd, pp. 590–600.

Wessel, J. (2004) The effectiveness of hand exercises for persons with rheumatoid arthritis: a systematic review, *J Hand Ther*, 17(2), 174–180.

Westby, M. D. (2001) A health professional's guide to exercise prescription for people with arthritis: a review of aerobic fitness activities, *Arthritis Rheum*, 45(6), 501–511.

World Health Organization. (2002) The International Classification of Functioning, Disability and Health – ICF. Geneva, World Health Organization.

Young, A., Hughes, I., Round, J. M., and Edwards, R. H. (1982) The effect of knee injury on the number of muscle fibres in the human quadriceps femoris, *Clin Sci (Lond)*, 62(2), 227–234.

Ytterberg, S. R., Mahowald, M. L., and Krug, H. E. (1994), Exercise for arthritis, *Baillieres Clin Rheumatol*, 8(1), 161–189.

11

ANKYLOSING SPONDYLITIS

Hanne Dagfinrud, Silje Halvorsen and Nina K. Vøllestad

Introduction

Epidemiology and etiology of ankylosing spondylitis

Ankylosing spondylitis (AS) is a common inflammatory rheumatic disease affecting mainly the spinal column and sacroiliac joints, causing characteristic inflammatory back pain. AS can lead to structural and functional impairments and may also be associated with extraspinal manifestations, involving peripheral joints, eye, bowel and heart (Braun and Sieper, 2007). AS is found worldwide, but more often in Caucasians than in other races. Overall, the prevalence is between 0.1 per cent and 1.4 per cent (Braun and Sieper, 2007). The disease onset is most commonly between the ages of 20 and 30 years. About 80 per cent of patients develop the first symptoms at an age younger than 30 years, and less than 5 per cent of patients present at older than 45 years. Men are more often affected than women, with a ratio of roughly 2:1 (Braun and Sieper., 2007; Feldtkeller *et al.*, 2003).

Despite advances in research, the etiology of AS is still unclear. A strong inherited component is evident, and about a third of this effect is explained by the Human Leukocyte Antigen B27 (HLA B27). Approximately 90–95 per cent of patients with AS are positive for HLA B27 and the risk of this disease developing is as high as about 5 per cent in HLA B27-positive individuals, and substantially higher in HLA B27-positive relatives of patients. However, most HLA B27-positive individuals remain healthy (Sieper, 2009).

Clinical features and skeletal manifestations

The main clinical features of AS are inflammatory back pain caused by inflammation in the axial skeleton (especially sacroiliitis), enthesitis and anterior uveitis (Braun and Sieper, 2007). Peripheral joint involvement is reported in about 30 per cent of patients with AS, most often hip, shoulder and knee joints. Sacroiliac joint involvement is regarded as the hallmark of the disease, and the presence of radiographic sacroiliitis is considered obligatory for classification of AS according to the modified New York criteria (van der Linden *et al.*, 1984).

The most characteristic symptom of AS is loss of spinal mobility, a consequence of spinal inflammation and structural damage. Most often AS starts with inflammation at the bone/cartilage interface in the sacroiliac joint, and syndesmophytes and ankylosis are the most characteristic features (Braun and Sieper, 2007). The initial lesions of the spine consist of inflammatory granulation tissue at inter-vertebral discs and margin of vertebral bone, later on resulting in syndesmophytes and 'squaring' of vertebrae (the characteristic 'bamboo spine' observed radiographically) (Braun and Sieper, 2007). The structural changes are mainly caused by osteoproliferation rather than osteodestruction, and can result in complete or incomplete ankylosis of the spine (including the facet joints and the sacroiliac joints) (Sieper, 2009). The spinal inflammation can arise as spondylitis, spondylodiscitis or spondylarthritis. Inflammation of the spinal ligaments, intervertebrae and spinal facet joints and the secondary fibrosis and calcification of the spinal elastic structures lead to varying degrees of pain, stiffness and limitations of spinal mobility.

The association between inflammation and new bone formation in AS is, however, not clear. Although inflammation is assumed to trigger new bone formation, there is no close correlation between inflammation and osteoproliferation. In rheumatoid arthritis, structural damage has been shown to be a direct consequence of inflammation, but the link between inflammation and new bone formation is less clear in AS. This topic is further complicated because exaggerated local bone formation in the spine exists, together with bone loss of the whole spine. AS patients have an increased risk only of vertebral fractures, but not of non-vertebral fractures, probably indicating osteoporosis preferentially of the spine in AS (Vosse *et al.*, 2008).

Consequences of AS

A study comparing the self-reported general health of patients with AS with the general population revealed that AS patients report significant worse health for all actual health dimensions (including pain, vitality, mental health, physical and social functioning). However, the differences from the general population were largest for the physical dimensions, underlining that AS mainly influence patients' physical health, i.e. physical function, vitality and bodily pain (Dagfinrud *et al.*, 2004).

Among the main consequences of AS are reduced spinal mobility and loss of flexibility of the thoracic cage. The pathological processes of the spinal column may lead to loss of important dynamic functions, resulting in problems with daily activities, such as car driving, housekeeping, social interaction and work in those who are most affected (Dagfinrud *et al.*, 2004 ; Dagfinrud *et al.*, 2005a).

Due to these typical clinical features, a main focus in the management of AS has traditionally been on improvement or maintenance of the mobility of the spinal column, the thoracic cage and the hip joints.

Recent evidence also suggests that metabolic syndrome might be more prevalent in patients with AS. Metabolic syndrome has been shown to promote mortality from cardiovascular disease and some studies pointed out an association between metabolic syndrome and inflammation (Heeneman and Daemen, 2007; Malesci *et al.*, 2007). Patients with AS have an increased mortality risk compared to the general population, explained in part by the excess mortality from cardiovascular disease (Lehtinen, 1993). Furthermore, some studies suggest that systemic inflammation in patients with AS is directly related to vascular damage and the development of aortic insufficiency, accompanied by conduction disturbances similar to other rheumatic diseases such as rheumatoid arthritis (Divecha *et al.*, 2005). Additional risk factors for cardiovascular disease in patients with AS may be chronic steroid use, decreased physical activity and, related to decreased physical activity and steroids, the development of obesity and hypercholesterolemia.

Physical activity and ankylosing spondylitis

Patients with chronic musculoskeletal diseases such as rheumatoid arthritis are shown to have a lower physical activity level than the general population (Hootman *et al.*, 2003). Furthermore, a study by Carter *et al.* reported that patients with AS have significantly reduced physical capacity compared to age-matched healthy individuals (Carter *et al.*, 1999). The reduced physical activity may be a consequence of disease activity and reduced spinal mobility. Specifically, inflammation-induced pain may lead to a typical deconditioning process: pain or fear of pain may reduce physical activity level, which in the short term decreases spinal mobility and muscle strength and in the long term aerobic capacity and exercise tolerance are reduced. Patients with AS also suffer from fatigue (Dagfinrud *et al.*, 2005b), which might contribute to reduced physical activity levels.

Physical activity is strongly recommended for health promotion in healthy populations (Haskell *et al.*, 2007; Warburton *et al.*, 2006). Current treatment guidelines for AS recommend exercises as a cornerstone of the management programme (Zochling *et al.*, 2006) and recommendations for physical activity for persons with rheumatoid arthritis is 30 minutes 4 to 7 times per week with an intensity of 50–70 per cent of age predicted maximum heart rate (Stenstrom and Minor, 2003). However, studies of exercise habits in patients with AS show that only 24 per cent are physically active more than three times per week and that more than 40 per cent are physically active less than once a week (Santos *et al.*, 1998; Sundstrom *et al.*, 2002).

Exercise responses in patients with AS

There is a limited number of studies investigating the physiological changes with exercise or physical activity in AS patients. In a case-control study, Carter and co-workers examined cardiovascular and muscular factors in relation to exercise. The purpose of the study was to investigate factors possibly responsible for limiting aerobic capacity in patients with AS, and the results of a cardiopulmonary exercise test were compared to age and gender matched healthy controls. Variables that might influence exercise tolerance, including pulmonary function tests, respiratory muscle strength and endurance, AS severity assessment including chest expansion, thoracolumber movement, wall tragus distance and peripheral muscle strength, hand grip strength and lean body mass were measured in the patients with AS. The study concluded that peripheral muscle strength was the most important determinant of exercise intolerance in AS patients, suggesting that deconditioning is the main factor in the production of the reduced aerobic capacity (Carter *et al.*, 1999).

In another study, Carbon and co-workers examined the responses to 30 minutes of cycling exercise in patients with AS (Carbon *et al.*, 1996). They showed increased circulating levels of neutrophils, leukocytes and lymphocytes which normalized quickly after exercise. The responses were similar to those observed in healthy controls. Interestingly, they also showed a small improvement in spinal flexibility immediately after exercise which normalized over the subsequent 3–5 hours (Carbon *et al.*, 1996).

Over the last decade, a number of studies have documented marked changes in cytokines, especially interleukin-6 (IL-6), during acute bouts of exercise in healthy individuals. It is well established that IL-6 is released from contracting muscle to the blood and the serum levels may increase 100-fold during exercise (Pedersen and Febbraio, 2008). It seems that the response is substantial, quite similar in different kinds of exercise and closely related to duration of exercise. Following the rise in IL-6, other cytokines also rise, including the anti-inflammatory cytokine IL-10. However, tumor necrosis factor alpha (TNF-α) seems to be unaffected by exercise. Hence, the cytokine cascade during exercise differs from that seen in infections, which are characterized by an increase in TNF-α (preceding the rise in IL-6) (Pedersen and Febbraio, 2008). The increasing interest in inflammatory response systems, as studied by for instance IL-6 and TNF-α, should be of particular focus in future research of patients with inflammatory diseases such as AS. The fact that the inflammation response system seems to operate differently in exercise and infection raises interesting questions regarding how they interact in exercise.

Current guidelines for management of AS

Current treatment guidelines for AS recommend appropriate medication (mainly nonsteroidal anti-inflammatory drugs (NSAIDs) and in severe cases tumor necrosis factor-alpha inhibitors (TNF-α), and mobility exercise as the corner-stones of treatment (Zochling *et al.*, 2006). Development of the TNF-α inhibitors has revolutionized the treatment of AS, but the combination of NSAIDs and physical therapy is still the first step in the management of AS (Elyan and Khan, 2008; Zochling *et al.*, 2006). Physiotherapy and exercises for AS patients are first of all considered important to maintain or improve spinal mobility and to reduce pain. The patients are routinely encouraged to exercise and to spend a lot of effort trying to limit the negative consequences of their lifelong disease. It is therefore important that they receive accurate information and relevant advice for optimal management of their disease.

Exercise for ankylosing spondylitis: systematic review of the evidence

Description of the studies

The following review is based on a systematic literature search in relevant data-bases (Pubmed, Embase, Cinahl, PEDro) up to August 2009. The literature synthesis includes data from a total of 16 randomized controlled trials (RCTs) and uncontrolled studies. Six of the studies compared different types of exer-cise programmes with no intervention (Durmus *et al.*, 2009b; Ince *et al.*, 2006; Kraag *et al.*, 1990; Lee *et al.*, 2008; Lim *et al.*, 2005; Sweeney *et al.*, 2002) and five studies compared supervised exercise programmes with non-supervised (Altan *et al.*, 2006; Analay *et al.*, 2003; Cagliyan *et al.*, 2007; Hidding *et al.*, 1993; Karapolat *et al.*, 2008), individualized programmes, including home exercise programmes. Four studies compared two or three different exercise programmes (Durmus *et al.*, 2009b; Fernandez-de-las-Penas *et al.*, 2005; Helliwell *et al.*, 1996; van Tubergen *et al.*, 2001) and the last had a non-comparison study (before-after) design (Ortancil *et al.*, 2009). For a description of interventions, see Table 11.1.

TABLE 11.1 Main results, comparisons and study quality (PEDro points) of the reviewed studies

Study	n	Design and quality	Comparison	Main results – spinal mobility and BASMI	Main results – BASFI, BASDAI, BAS-G	Main results – cardiorespiratory fitness
Kraag et al. 1990 Canada	53	RCT 7/10	1	FFD: ES=0.72 Schober: neg. effect effect	Function score: ES=1.12 Pain: neg. effect	
Hidding et al. 1993 The Netherlands	144	RCT 5/10	2	Sig. more improvement on spinal mobility in the SV-group compared to the IV-group (p<0.05)	Sig. more improvement on global health assessment in the SV-group compared to the IV-group (p<0.05) No difference in pain improvement between the groups	Sig. More improvement on physical fitness in the SV-group compared to the IV-group (p<0.05)
Helliwell et al. 1996 United Kingdom	44	RCT 4/10	4	No difference between groups	SV-groups reported more subjective improvement in pain (p=0.001)	Not measured
Van Tubergen et al. 2001 The Netherlands	120	RCT 5/10	4	Not measured	SV: BASFI: ES=0.67 BASDAI: ES=0.56 well-being ES=0.60 SV: BASFI: ES=0.4 BASDAI: ES=0.60 well-being ES=0.83 IV: BASFI: no effect BASDAI: ES=0.15 well-being ES=0.12	Not measured
Sweeney et al. 2002 United Kingdom	200	RCT 4/10	1	Not measured	BASFI ES=0.18 BASDAI: ES=0.17 BAS-G: ES=0.08	Not measured
Analay et al. 2003 TurkeyCotni	51	RCT 7/10	2	SV: FFD: ES=0.38 Shober ES=0.31 IV: FFD: ES=0/05 Shober: ES=0.24	SV: BASFI ES=0.32 Pain: ES=0.15 OV: BASFI: ES=0.02 Pain: ES=0.02	SV: $\dot{V}O_{2max}$ ES: 0.09 IV: neg. effect

Continued

TABLE 11.1 *continued*

Study	n	Design and quality	Comparison	Main results – spinal mobility and BASMI	Main results – BASFI, BASDAI, BAS-G	Main results – cardiorespiratory fitness
Lim *et al.* 2005 Korea	58	RCT 6/10	1	Sig. more improvement on FFD in the EG group compared to CG (p<0.001)	Sig. more improvement on BASI and pain in the EG group compared o CG (p<0.0001)	Not measured
Fernandez-de-las-Penas *et al.* 2005 Spain	45	RCT 5/10	3	Program 1: Schober: ES=0.15 Program 2: Schober: ES=0.46	Program 1: BASFI ES=0.03 BASDAI: ES=0.223 Program 2: NASFO ES=0.29 BASDI: ES=0.18	Not measured
Altan *et al.* 2006 Turkey	60	RCT 5/10	2	SV: Schober: ES=0.30 IV: Schober: ES=0.14	SV: BASFI: ES=0.68 BASDAI: ES=1.47 global assessment of disease activity: ES=1.11 IV: BASFI ES=0.40 BASDAI: ES=0.8 global assessment of disease activity: ES=0.56	Not measured
Ince *et al.* 2006 Turkey	30	RCT 6/10	1	FFD: ES=0.21 Schober: ES=0.11	Not measured	W/kg: ES=2.19
Cagliyan *et al.* 2007 Turkey	46	RCT 4/10	2	SV: FFD: ES=0.67 Schober ES=0.39 IV: 0.03	SV: BASFI: ES=0.94 BASDAI: ES=1 IV: Neg. effect	Not measured
Lee *et al.* 2008 South Korea	40	Clinical trial 1 n/r		FFD: ES=0.33	BASDAI: ES=0.65	Not measured

Study	n	Design and quality	Comparison	Main results – spinal mobility and BASMI	Main results – BASFI, BASDAI, BAS-G	Main results – cardiorespiratory fitness
Karapolat et al. 2005 Turkey	41	Clinical trial n/r	2	SV: BASMI: ES=0.27 IV: BASMI: ES=0.05	SV: BASFI: ES=0.27 BASDI: ES=0.36 IV: BASFI: no effect BASDAI: ES=0.46	Not measured
Durmus et al. 2009 (a) Turkey	56	Clinical trial n/r	3	Not measured	Program 1: BASFI: ES=0.67 BASDAI: ES=1.20 Program 2: BASFI: ES0.55 BASDAI: ES=1.07	Not measured
Durmas et al. 2009 (b) Turkey	43	Clinical trial n/r	1	Not measured	BASFI: ES=0.63 BASDAI:0.94	Not measured
Ortaneil et al. 2009 Turkey	22	Pre/post test		Schober: ES=0.06	BASFI: ES=0.1	Not measured

N = participants included in the trial.

n/r = no randomization.

SV = supervised.

IV = individualized.

CG = control group.

EG = exercise group.

Comparisons:

1: Exercise program vs no intervention.

2: Supervised vs individualized (incl home based) programs.

3: Two different programs.

4: Three different programs.

BAS = Bath Ankylosing Spondylitis; BASMI = Metrology Index; BASFI = Function Index; BASDAI = Disease Activity Index; BAS-G = global assessment of well-being; FFD = fingertip-to-floor distance.

Assessment of the methodological quality of the studies

The studies included 22 to 200 patients with AS, with most of them having 40 to 60 participants. The Physiotherapy Evidence Database (PEDro) quality scoring method was used for the assessment of the methodological quality of the studies. According to this method, quality is rated on the basis of ten methodological criteria: random allocation, concealed allocation, comparability, blinded subjects, blinded therapists, blinded assessors, adequate follow-up, intention-to-treat analysis, between group comparisons and point estimates/variability for outcome measures (de Morton, 2009). Two of the RCTs met 7 out of 10 criteria (Analay *et al.*, 2003; Hidding *et al.*, 1993), 2 studies met 6 (Fernandez-de-las-Penas *et al.*, 2005; Lim *et al.*, 2005), 4 studies met 5 and 3 studies met 4 out of 10 PEDro points (see Table 11.2).

TABLE 11.2 Description of the exercise interventions performed in the reviewed studies

Study	Intervention
Comparison 1: exercise programs vs no intervention	
Kraag *et al.* 1990 Canada	G1: Daily home exercises + physiotherapy 8–16 times
	G2: Daily home exercises + physiotherapy as needed
	Objectives: disease education, pain control, posture and function
Sweeney *et al.* 2002 United Kingdom	G1: Exercise/educational video
	G2: Control group
Lim *et al.* 2005 Korea	G1: 16 exercises for relaxation, flexibility, muscular strength, breathing and posture. Twenty minutes per day for eight weeks
	G2: No intervention
Ince *et al.* 2006 Turkey	G1: aerobic (30 minutes low intensity), stretching and pulmonary exercises. Fifty × three time a week for three months
	G2: No intervention
Durmus *et al.* 2009b Turkey	G1: Home based. Twenty exercises per day for 12 weeks Relaxation, flexibility, strength, breathing and posture
	G2: No intervention
Lee *et al.* 2008 South Korea	G1: Group tai-chi for 45 minutes × twice a week, + daily home exercises
	G2: No intervention

Study	Intervention
Comparison 2: supervised vs non-supervised exercise programs	
Hidding *et al.* 1993 The Netherlands	G1: unsupervised daily mobility exercises 30 minutes G2: unsupervised daily mobility exercises + weekly group physical therapy (one hour physical training (strengthening/flexibility), one hour sports activity, one hour hydrotherapy)
Analay *et al.* 2003 Turkey	G1: Supervised exercise program (50 minutes × three times a week) G2: Home-based exercise program Exercise program: stretching, mobilization, strengthening, bicycling (15–30 minutes), posture, respiration Duration: six weeks
Altan *et al.* 2006 Turkey	G1: Balneotherapy 30 minutes per day + home-based exercise program 30 minutes per day for three weeks G2: Home-based exercise program 30 minutes per day for three weeks Exercise program: respiration/posture. Dorsal/lumbal
Cagliyan *et al.* 2007 Turkey	G1: Group exercises, two hours per week for three months G2: Home exercise (dose not specified) Range of motion flexibility, stretching, strengthening, respiration and posture exercises
Karapolat *et al.* 2008 Turkey	G1: Group-based exercise program G2: Home-based exercise program Exercise program: walking, mobility, flexibility, strength, respitation Fourty-five minutes three time per week for six weeks
Comparison 3 and 4: comparing two or three different exercise programs or not control group	
Helliwell *et al.* 1996 United Kingdom	G1: intensive in patients physiotherapy. Five hour group exercise + three hour hydrotherapy per week for three weeks G2: Out-patient hydrotherapy × two hours per week + home exercises for six weeks G3: Home exercises twice a day for six weeks All patients = flexibility and breathing exercises
Van Tubergen *et al.* 2001 The Netherlands	G1: one hour spa therapy + one hour group exercises + 30 minutes walking × five times a week for three weeks G2: one hour spa therapy + one hour group exercises + 30 minutes walking × five times per week for three weeks G3: Home exercises + one hour exercises, one hour sports, one hour hydrotherapy per week for three weeks All = walking and flexibility exercises

Continued

TABLE 11.2 *continued*

Study	Intervention
Fernandez-de-las-Penas *et al.* 2005 Spain	G1: 20 exercises of motion and flexibility G2: Global Posture Relearning (GPR): strengthening and flexibility exercises for shortened muscles, one hour per week for four months
Durmus *et al.* 2009a Turkey	G1: 20 motion and flexibility exercises daily for 12 weeks G2 GPR: specific strengthening and flexibility exercises daily for 12 weeks G3: No intervention
Ortancil *et al.* 2009 Turkey	G1: Breathing exercises, upper-extremity exercises three time per week for six weeks No control group

Presentation of results

Effect sizes were calculated where possible, based on the difference score (between baseline and post-treatment score) for the different outcome measures for each intervention group, divided by the standard deviation of the baseline score. The effect sizes were interpreted according to Cohen's effect size index, in which 0.2 refers to a small difference, 0.5 refers to a moderate difference and 0.8 or above refers to a large difference (Cohen, 1988). Such effect sizes are unit less and have the advantage of allowing comparisons across different studies and scales.

Content of exercise programmes

There are no studies available showing that physical activity reduces the risk of comorbidity or mortality in patients with AS. However, it is reasonable to assume that general exercise recommendations for promoting health benefits in healthy individuals also are suitable for patients with AS. Thus, it is important that exercise programmes prescribed for patients with AS comply with recommendations for improving cardiorespiratory fitness, muscle strength and mobility/flexibility in healthy individuals. Physiological responses to exercise are determined by the mode, frequency, intensity and duration of exercise and the effects of exercise programmes are therefore dependent on the way the interventions are administered. Moreover, a dose-response relationship for exercises exists, as it does for drugs, and the effect of exercise is therefore dependent on adherence to the prescribed programme.

In the following sections, the exercise interventions applied in the reviewed papers are evaluated in relation to general recommendations for improving cardiorespiratory fitness, muscle strength and mobility/flexibility (ACSM, 1998; Kohrt *et al.*, 2004).

Cardiorespiratory fitness

For developing cardiorespiratory fitness, training 3–5 days a week at an intensity of 55–90 per cent of maximum heart rate and duration between 20 and 60 minutes is recommended. Duration is dependent on the intensity of the activity; lower activities should be conducted over a longer period of time (30 minutes or more). The American College of Sports Medicine (ACSM) recommend that the length of the exercise period should be between 12 and 15 weeks (ACSM, 1998).

The intervention of Hidding *et al.* (1993) included an aerobic endurance exercise component (volleyball and badminton), but the intensity was not controlled, and even though the duration was one hour, the intensity should be over 50 per cent of maximal heart rate to have an effect on cardiorespiratory fitness (ACSM, 1998). In Analay *et al.* (2003) the participants exercised on a cycle ergometer and again, intensity was not controlled. Thus, the aerobic components of these programmes did not comply with current recommendations. A low intensity group aerobic programme was performed in the study of Ince *et al.* (2006) and the intensity was controlled by participants measuring their heart rate during the session. This study was the only one meeting the ACSM's recommendations for duration and frequency and the impact on cardiorespiratory fitness in this study was large (ES 2.19) (Ince *et al.*, 2006) (see Table 11.1).

In summary, very few studies have focused on improving cardiorespiratory fitness, and even if the programmes include an aerobic exercise component, current recommendations for intensity, duration and frequency were not met. The only study meeting the recommendations for duration and frequency showed a large cardiorespiratory improvement (Ince *et al.*, 2006).

Muscular strength

The ACSM recommends a minimum of 8–10 exercises involving the major skeletal muscle groups in the body with a minimum of one set of 8–12 repetitions of each exercise performed 2–3 days a week to develop muscular strength. The exercise period should be at least 15–20 weeks. Eight of the included studies had muscular strength training as a part of the intervention, but none of them used muscular strength as an outcome measure.

Karapolat *et al.* (2008) was the only study that used free weights as resistance. None of the other studies used external resistance in their strengthening programme and the majority of the trials have a poor description of muscle strength intervention. Karapolat *et al.* had an intervention consisting of strengthening exercises for the whole body, whereas the other studies focused on strengthening exercises for the back. The majority of trials described the strengthening exercises more like exercises for developing core stability. In three studies, strengthening exercises were performed daily (Durmus *et al.*, 2009a; Durmus *et al.*, 2009b; Lim *et al.*, 2005), and in two studies, strengthening exercises were performed only once a week (Fernandez-de-las-Penas *et al.*, 2005; Hidding *et al.*, 1993).

Although strength was not included as an outcome, these studies show that controlled strength training can be prescribed in patients with AS with minimum risk of adverse events.

Flexibility/mobility exercises

The ACSM recommends that at least four repetitions per muscle group should be performed a minimum of 2–3 days a week to develop flexibility. The flexibility programme should include the major muscle groups in the body. Stretching should include appropriate static and/or dynamic techniques. Static stretches should be held for 10–30 seconds, whereas dynamic techniques should include a 6-second active contraction followed by a 10–30 second stretch (ACSM, 1998).

Five studies included dynamic mobility exercises (Helliwell *et al.*, 1996; Hidding *et al.*, 1993; Lim *et al.*, 2005; Cagliyan *et al.*, 2007; Lee *et al.*, 2008), and six studies included both dynamic movements and stretching (Analay *et al.*, 2003; Durmus *et al.*, 2009a; Durmus *et al.*, 2009b; Fernandez-de-las-Penas *et al.*, 2005; Ince *et al.*, 2006; Karapolat *et al.*, 2008). The majority of the studies focused mainly on flexibility exercises for the back, but some also included exercises for the whole body.

The dose of flexibility exercises was described in only one study, in which the dynamic movements were repeated 3–5 times (Helliwell *et al.*, 1996). Stretching exercises formed part of the intervention in six studies but none of them described the techniques used, holding time or number of repetitions (Analay *et al.*, 2003; Durmus *et al.*, 2009a; Durmus *et al.*, 2009b; Fernandez-de-las-Penas *et al.*, 2005; Ince *et al.*, 2006; Karapolat *et al.*, 2008). In most of these studies, flexibility exercises were performed daily on several days a week and there was no evidence of adverse events.

Summary of the results

The ASessment in Ankylosing Spondylitis (ASAS) working group defined a core set of domains and instruments for assessing the most important aspects of disease assessments in AS, including pain, spinal mobility, physical function and patient global assessment of disease (van der Heijde *et al.*, 1999). Measures of aerobic capacity or physical fitness are not included in the core set, reflecting the main treatment goal of improving or maintaining spinal mobility and reducing pain. Accordingly, the outcome measures selected in this review were the Bath Ankylosing Spondylitis (BAS) Metrology Index (BASMI) (Jenkinson *et al.*, 1994) or a separate spinal mobility measure (Schober test or fingertip-to-floor distance, FFD), BAS Functioning Index (BASFI) (Calin *et al.*, 1994), BAS Disease Activity Index (BASDAI) (Garrett *et al.*, 1994) or a single pain scale and global assessment of well-being (BAS-G) (Jones *et al.*, 1996). Additionally, three studies had cardiorespiratory fitness as an outcome measure.

BASMI and spinal mobility

Exercise programmes versus no intervention

Four studies (Ince *et al.*, 2006; Kraag *et al.*, 1990; Lim *et al.*, 2005; Lee *et al.*, 2008) that compared exercise programmes with no intervention used spinal mobility as an outcome measure. All studies reported more improvement in the exercise group than in the control group. The effect sizes varied between the studies and were generally small to moderate (from 0.11 to 0.72) (see Table 11.1). Two of the RCTs were rated with six PEDro points and one with seven PEDro points, indicating moderate evidence for effect of exercise on spinal flexion when compared to no intervention.

Supervised vs non-supervised exercise programmes

Five studies compared supervised exercise or physical therapy programmes with individualized, home-based programmes (Analay *et al.*, 2003; Hidding *et al.*, 1993; Karapolat *et al.*, 2008; Cagliyan *et al.*, 2007; Karapolat *et al.*, 2008). All studies reported significantly more improvement in spinal mobility or BASMI after the supervised exercise programmes. The effect sizes for the supervised groups were small to moderate (between 0.11 and 0.67) whereas the non-supervised groups showed generally small effect sizes (0.03–0.24). Two of these RCTs were rated with five PEDro points, one with seven and one with four points (Table 11.1). Thus, patients with AS seem to benefit more from supervised exercise programmes than non-supervised programmes and the effect of supervised exercise programmes on spinal mobility is moderate.

Comparing two or three different exercise programmes

Four studies (Durmus *et al.*, 2009b; Fernandez-de-las-Penas *et al.*, 2005; Helliwell *et al.*, 1996; van Tubergen *et al.*, 2001) investigated the efficacy of two or three different exercise programmes. These studies reported similar results for spinal mobility in the intervention groups. Effect sizes were only calculated for one study (0.46 for the experimental exercise programme) (Fernandez-de-las-Penas *et al.*, 2005). These trials were judged to have four or five PEDro points (Table 11.1).

Patient reported measures

Exercise programmes versus no intervention

Four studies (Kraag *et al.*, 1990; Lee *et al.*, 2008; Lim *et al.*, 2005; Sweeney *et al.*, 2002) comparing exercise programmes with no-intervention control groups included patient reported measures. These generally reported significantly more effect on patient function, disease activity and global assessment

(BAS-G) for the exercise groups. The within-group effects were small to moderate (0.17 to 0.65) for these trials, which were judged to have 4–7 PEDro points (Table 11.1).

Supervised versus non-supervised exercise programmes

Five trials (Altan *et al.*, 2006; Analay *et al.*, 2003; Cagliyan *et al.*, 2007; Hidding *et al.*, 1993; Karapolat *et al.*, 2008) compared supervised with non-supervised exercise. Effect sizes for the supervised groups were generally higher for all the patient reported outcome measures. For the supervised groups, the mean effect size changes for BASDAI/pain, BASFI and global assessment (BAS-G) were 0.75, 0.60 and 1.1 respectively, in comparison to 0.43, 0.21 and 0.56, respectively, for the non-supervised groups. Two of the trials were judged to have five PEDro points, one with four and one with seven PEDro points (Table 11.1), indicating that there is moderate evidence for large effect of supervised exercise programmes on patient reported outcome measures.

Comparing two or three different exercise programmes

The efficacy of different exercise programmes on patient reported outcomes were studied in four trials (Fernandez-de-las-Penas *et al.*, 2005; Helliwell *et al.*, 1996; van Tubergen 2001; Durmus *et al.*, 2009b). Between group differences were rarely observed and within-group effect sizes for the exercise programmes were generally moderate (Table 11.1). These trials were judged to have 4 or 5 PEDro points (Table 11.1).

Cardiorespiratory fitness

Exercise programmes versus no intervention

Three studies had cardiorespiratory fitness as an outcome measure (Analay *et al.*, 2003; Hidding *et al.*,1993; Ince *et al.*, 2006). One RCT that compared an exercise intervention with no intervention reported a large effect size change in cardiorespiratory fitness (2.19), which improved significantly more than in the control group (Ince *et al.*, 2006).

Supervised versus non-supervised exercise programmes

Two studies compared supervised exercise with an individualized, home-based programme and both studies reported significantly more improvement in the supervised versus the control group (Analay *et al.*, 2003; Hidding *et al.*, 1993). The effect size was small (0.09) in one study (Analay *et al.*, 2003), and the other (Hidding *et al.*, 1993) did not report effect size changes.

Compliance to exercise

Only three of the 16 included studies in this review reported compliance to the exercise programmes. Hidding *et al.* (1993) monitored compliance using exercise diaries and by an instructor recording attendance at group sessions. The mean attendance at group sessions was 73.5 per cent, and the participants exercised at home 1.4–1.9 hours per week, when according to the protocol, they should have exercised for 3.5 hours per week. Lee *et al.* (2008) also monitored compliance to home-based exercise with exercise diaries and reported a mean compliance of 93.3 per cent, whereas van Tubergen *et al.* (2001) reported a mean attendance of 99 per cent in supervised groups.

Summary and conclusions

Patients with AS experience health benefits from exercise participation, such as reduced levels of pain and improved spinal mobility, self-reported physical functioning and global assessment of well-being. A systematic literature review of exercise studies reached this conclusion, but the reviewed studies had a number of methodological weaknesses (Dagfinrud *et al.*, 2008). A frequent weakness in studies of complex health interventions is incomplete description of the exercise programme (Glasziou *et al.*, 2008). Lack of thorough descriptions of the interventions used makes it difficult to reproduce the programme and to utilize possible positive findings. Recent research has shown that the implementation of positive findings is slow, and that a barrier for implementation may be clinicians' ability to carry out the treatment on the basis of the information provided in published reports (Dopson *et al.*, 2001; Glasziou *et al.*, 2008). Furthermore, when descriptions are missing, it is difficult to ensure that the exercise programmes have sufficient dose, intensity and frequency to achieve specific physiological responses. Currently, physical activity and exercise rehabilitation are increasingly being considered as part of the treatment programme for several musculoskeletal diseases such as AS. As a dose-response relationship for exercise exists (as it does for pharmacological treatments), it is important that the prescription and monitoring of exercise as part of disease management is as specific and accurate as possible.

The reported effect size changes in key health outcomes were generally moderate, but the results were consistent across studies. Overall, greater benefits were observed after supervised exercise programmes than after individualized, home-based programmes. This may be due to better compliance with the exercise programme, but also due to better quality in terms of control of exercise intensity and duration. Adherence to prescribed exercise programmes was described in only a few studies and the longer-term benefits of exercise are unknown. Nevertheless, supervised exercise programmes should be recommended where possible, to ensure maximal efficacy.

The reported studies were mainly focused on spinal mobility, pain and physical function as outcome measures, and only three of the studies included measure of cardiorespiratory fitness as an end-point. Furthermore, many of the exercise programmes delivered in the reviewed studies did not comply with current physical activity recommendations, but where they did, effect size changes were generally greater. Hence, it is important that exercise programmes are planned in accordance with recommendations for developing physical fitness and that relevant outcome measures are included. Additionally, to ensure implementation of positive findings, the description must provide enough information for facilitating reproduction of the exercise programmes.

The treatment options for patients with AS have been dramatically improved with the introduction of biological medication (anti-TNF-α drugs) and promising results have been reported, in terms of reduced pain and disease activity for many patients. So far, no studies have compared treatment with TNF inhibitors in combination with exercise therapy versus TNF inhibitors alone (Elyan and Khan, 2008). However, a study from the UK reported that patients who benefit from such medication become more motivated for physiotherapy/exercise therapy and show a higher degree of adherence to exercise programmes (Dubey *et al.*, 2008). These drugs have positive effects on disease symptoms, but do not contribute to improved muscle strength, mobility and physical fitness (Braun *et al.*, 2006), thus, exercises remains an essential part of the management plan (Elyan and Khan, 2008). Such pharmacological treatments might augment the beneficial effects of exercise, but more research is needed.

References

ACSM (1998) 'American College of Sports Medicine position stand. The recommended quantity and quality of exercise for developing and maintaining cardiorespiratory and muscular fitness in healthy adults', *Med Sci Sports Exerc*, 22(2), 265–274.

Altan, L., Bingol, U., Aslan, M. and Yurtkuran, M. (2006) 'The effect of balneotherapy on patients with ankylosing spondylitis', *Scand J Rheumatol*, 35(4), 283–289.

Analay, Y., Ozcan, E., Karan, A., Diracoglu, D. and Aydin, R. (2003), 'The effectiveness of intensive group exercise on patients with ankylosing spondylitis', *Clin Rehabil*, 17(6), 631–636.

Braun, J., Davis, J., Dougados, M., Sieper, J., van der Linden, S., van der Heijde, D. and for the ASAS Working Group (2006) 'First update of the international ASAS consensus statement for the use of anti-TNF agents in patients with ankylosing spondylitis', *Annals of the Rheumatic Diseases*, 65(3), 316–320.

Braun, J. and Sieper, J. (2007) 'Ankylosing spondylitis', *Lancet*, 369(9570), 1379–1390.

Cagliyan, A., Kotevoglu, N., Onal, T., Tekkus, B. and Kuran, B. (2007) 'Does group exercise program add anything more to patients with ankylosing spondylitis', *Jounal of Back and Muskuloskeletal Rehabilitation*, 20, 79–85.

Calin, A., Garrett, S., Whitelock, H., Kennedy, L. G., O'Hea, J., Mallorie, P. and Jenkinson, T. (1994) 'A new approach to defining functional ability in ankylosing spondylitis: the development of the Bath Ankylosing Spondylitis Functional Index', *J Rheumatol*, 21(12), 2281–2285.

Carbon, R. J., Macey, M. G., McCarthy, D. A., Pereira, F. P., Perry, J. D., and Wade, A. J. (1996), 'The effect of 30 min cycle ergometry on ankylosing spondylitis', *Br J Rheumatol.*, 35(2), 167–177.

Carter, R., Riantawan, P., Banham, S. W. and Sturrock, R. D. (1999) 'An investigation of factors limiting aerobic capacity in patients with ankylosing spondylitis', *Respir Med*, 93(10), 700–708.

Cohen, J. (1988) *Statistical Power Analysis for the Behavioral Sciences – The Effect Size*, 2nd edn, Lawrence Erlbaum Associates, Inc., Hillsdale, N.J.

Dagfinrud, H., Kjeken, I., Mowinckel, P., Hagen, K. B. and Kvien, T. K. (2005a) 'Impact of functional impairment in ankylosing spondylitis: impairment, activity limitation, and participation restrictions', *J Rheumatol*, 32(3), 516–523.

Dagfinrud, H., Kvien, T. K. and Hagen, K. B. (2008) 'Physiotherapy interventions for ankylosing spondylitis', *Cochrane Database Syst Rev*, no. 1, p. CD002822.

Dagfinrud, H., Mengshoel AM, Hagen, K. B., Loge, J. H. and Kvien, T. K. (2004) 'Health status in patients with ankylosing spondylitis: a comparison with the general population'. *Ann Rheum Dis*, 63, 1605–1610.

Dagfinrud, H., Vollestad, N. K., Loge, J. H., Kvien, T. K. and Mengshoel, A. M. (2005b) 'Fatigue in patients with ankylosing spondylitis: A comparison with the general population and associations with clinical and self-reported measures', *Arthritis Rheum*, 53(1), 5–11.

de Morton, N. A. (2009) 'The PEDro scale is a valid measure of the methodological quality of clinical trials: a demographic study', *Aust J Physiother*, 55(2), 129–133.

Divecha, H., Sattar, N., Rumley, A., Cherry, L., Lowe, G. D. and Sturrock, R. (2005) 'Cardiovascular risk parameters in men with ankylosing spondylitis in comparison with non-inflammatory control subjects: relevance of systemic inflammation', *Clin Sci (Lond)*, 109(2), 171–176.

Dopson, S., Locock, L., Chambers, D. and Gabbay, J. (2001) 'Implementation of evidence-based medicine: evaluation of the Promoting Action on Clinical Effectiveness programme', *J Health Serv Res Policy*, 6(1), 23–31.

Dubey, S. G., Leeder, J. and Gaffney, K. (2008) 'Physical therapy in anti-TNF treated patients with ankylosing spondylitis', *Rheumatology (Oxford)*, 47(7), 1100–1101.

Durmus, D., Alayli, G., Cil, E. and Canturk, F. (2009a) 'Effects of a home-based exercise program on quality of life, fatigue, and depression in patients with ankylosing spondylitis', *Rheumatol Int*, 29(6), 673–677.

Durmus, D., Alayli, G., Uzun, O., Tander, B., Canturk, F., Bek, Y. and Erkan, L. (2009b) 'Effects of two exercise interventions on pulmonary functions in the patients with ankylosing spondylitis', *Joint Bone Spine*, 76(2), 150–155.

Elyan, M. and Khan, M. A. 2008, 'Does physical therapy still have a place in the treatment of ankylosing spondylitis?', *Curr Opin Rheumatol*, 20(3), 282–286.

Feldtkeller, E., Khan, M. A., van der Heijde, D., van der Linden, S. and Braun, J. (2003) 'Age at disease onset and diagnosis delay in HLA-B27 negative vs. positive patients with ankylosing spondylitis', *Rheumatol Int*, 23(2), 61–66.

Fernandez-de-las-Penas, C., Alonso-Blanco, C., Morales-Cabezas, M. and Miangolarra-Page, J. C. (2005) 'Two exercise interventions for the management of patients with ankylosing spondylitis: a randomized controlled trial', *Am J Phys Med Rehabil*, 84(6), 407–419.

Garrett, S., Jenkinson, T., Kennedy, L. G., Whitelock, H., Gaisford, P. and Calin, A. (1994) 'A new approach to defining disease status in ankylosing spondylitis: the Bath Ankylosing Spondylitis Disease Activity Index', *J Rheumatol*, 21(12), 2286–2291.

Glasziou, P., Meats, E., Heneghan, C. and Shepperd, S. (2008) 'What is missing from descriptions of treatment in trials and reviews?', *BMJ*, 336(7659), 1472–1474.

Haskell, W. L., Lee, I. M., Pate, R. R., Powell, K. E., Blair, S. N., Franklin, B. A., Macera, C. A., Heath, G. W., Thompson, P. D. and Bauman, A. (2007) 'Physical activity and public health: updated recommendation for adults from the American College of Sports Medicine and the American Heart Association', *Med Sci Sports Exerc*, 39(8), 1423–1434.

Heeneman, S. and Daemen, M. J. (2007) 'Cardiovascular risks in spondyloarthritides', *Curr Opin Rheumatol*, 19(4), 358–362.

Helliwell, P., Abbott, C. A. and Chamberlain, M. A. (1996) 'A randomised trial of three different physiotherapy regimes in ankylosing spondylitis', *Physiotherapy*, 82(2), 85–90.

Hidding, A., van der Linden, S., Boers, M., Gielen, X., de Witte, L., Kester, A., Dijkmans, B. and Moolenburgh, D. (1993) 'Is group physical therapy superior to individualized therapy in ankylosing spondylitis? A randomized controlled trial', *Arthritis Care Res*, 6(3), 117–125.

Hootman, J. M., Macera, C. A., Ham, S. A., Helmick, C. G. and Sniezek, J. E. (2003) 'Physical activity levels among the general US adult population and in adults with and without arthritis', *Arthritis Rheum*, 49(1), 129–135.

Ince, G., Sarpel, T., Durgun, B. and Erdogan, S. (2006) 'Effects of a multimodal exercise program for people with ankylosing spondylitis', *Phys Ther*, 86(7), 924–935.

Jenkinson, T. R., Mallorie, P. A., Whitelock, H. C., Kennedy, L. G., Garrett, S. L. and Calin, A. (1994), 'Defining spinal mobility in ankylosing spondylitis (AS). The Bath AS Metrology Index', *J Rheumatol*, 21(9), 1694–1698.

Jones, S. D., Steiner, A., Garrett, S. L. and Calin, A. 1996, 'The Bath Ankylosing Spondylitis Patient Global Score (BAS-G)', *Br J Rheumatol*, 35(1), 66–71.

Karapolat, H., Akkoc, Y., Sari, I., Eyigor, S., Akar, S., Kirazli, Y. and Akkoc, N. (2008) 'Comparison of group-based exercise versus home-based exercise in patients with ankylosing spondylitis: effects on Bath Ankylosing Spondylitis Indices, quality of life and depression', *Clin Rheumatol*, 27(6), 695–700.

Kohrt, W. M., Bloomfield, S. A., Little, K. D., Nelson, M. E. and Yingling, V. R. (2004) 'American College of Sports Medicine Position Stand: physical activity and bone health', *Med Sci Sports Exerc*, 36(11), 1985–1996.

Kraag, G., Stokes, B., Groh, J., Helewa, A. and Goldsmith, C. (1990) 'The effects of comprehensive home physiotherapy and supervision on patients with ankylosing spondylitis – a randomized controlled trial', *J Rheumatol*, 17(2), 228–233.

Lee, E. N., Kim, Y. H., Chung, W. T. and Lee, M. S. (2008) 'Tai chi for disease activity and flexibility in patients with ankylosing spondylitis – a controlled clinical trial', *Evid Based Complement Alternat Med*, 5(4), 457–462.

Lehtinen, K. (1993) 'Mortality and causes of death in 398 patients admitted to hospital with ankylosing spondylitis', *Ann Rheum Dis*, 52(3), 174–176.

Lim, H. J., Moon, Y. I. and Lee, M. S. (2005) 'Effects of home-based daily exercise therapy on joint mobility, daily activity, pain, and depression in patients with ankylosing spondylitis', *Rheumatol Int*, 25(3), 225–229.

Malesci, D., Niglio, A., Mennillo, G. A., Buono, R., Valentini, G. and La, M. G. (2007) 'High prevalence of metabolic syndrome in patients with ankylosing spondylitis', *Clin Rheumatol.*, 26(5), 710–714.

Ortancil, O., Sarikaya, S., Sapmaz, P., Basaran, A. and Ozdolap, S. (2009) 'The effect(s) of a six-week home-based exercise program on the respiratory muscle and functional status in ankylosing spondylitis', *J Clin Rheumatol*, 15(2), 68–70.

Pedersen, B. K. and Febbraio, M. A. (2008) 'Muscle as an endocrine organ: focus on muscle-derived interleukin-6', *Physiol Rev*, 88(4), 1379–1406.

Santos, H., Brophy, S. and Calin, A. (1998) 'Exercise in ankylosing spondylitis: how much is optimum?', *J Rheumatol*, 25(11), 2156–2160.

Sieper, J. (2009) 'Can structural damage be prevented in ankylosing spondylitis?', *Curr. Opin.Rheumatol.*, 21(4), 335–339.

Stenstrom, C. H. and Minor, M. A. (2003) 'Evidence for the benefit of aerobic and strengthening exercise in rheumatoid arthritis', *Arthritis Rheum*, 49(3), 428–434.

Sundstrom, B., Ekergard, H., and Sundelin, G. (2002) 'Exercise habits among patients with ankylosing spondylitis. A questionnaire based survey in the County of Vasterbotten, Sweden.PG -', *Scand J Rheumatol*, 31(3).

Sweeney, S., Taylor, G. and Calin, A. (2002) 'The effect of a home based exercise intervention package on outcome in ankylosing spondylitis: a randomized controlled trial', *J Rheumatol*, 29(4), 763–766.

van der Heijde, D., Calin, A., Dougados, M., Khan, M. A., van der Linden, S. and Bellamy, N. (1999), 'Selection of instruments in the core set for DC-ART, SMARD, physical therapy, and clinical record keeping in ankylosing spondylitis. Progress report of the ASAS Working Group. Assessments in Ankylosing Spondylitis', *J Rheumatol*, 26(4), 951–954.

van der Linden, S., Valkenburg, H. A. and Cats, A. (1984), 'Evaluation of diagnostic criteria for ankylosing spondylitis. A proposal for modification of the New York criteria', *Arthritis Rheum*, 27(40, 361–368.

Van Tubergen, A., Landewe, R., van der Heijde, D., Hidding, A., Wolter, N., Asscher, M., Falkenbach, A., Genth, E., The, H. G., and van der Linden, S. (2001) 'Combined spa-exercise therapy is effective in patients with ankylosing spondylitis: a randomized controlled trial', *Arthritis Rheum*, 45(5), 430–438.

Vosse, D., Landewe, R., van der Heijde, D., van der Linden, S., van Staa, T. P. and Geusens, P. (2008), 'Ankylosing spondylitis and the risk of fracture: results from a large primary care-based nested case control study', *Ann Rheum Dis*, 68(12), 1839–1842.

Warburton, D. E., Nicol, C. W. and Bredin, S. S. (2006) 'Prescribing exercise as preventive therapy', *CMAJ*, 174(7), 961–974.

Zochling, J., van der Heijde, D., Burgos-Vargas, R., Collantes, E., Davis, J. C., Jr., Dijkmans, B., Dougados, M., Geher, P., Inman, R. D., Khan, M. A., Kvien, T. K., Leirisalo-Repo, M., Olivieri, I., Pavelka, K., Sieper, J., Stucki, G., Sturrock, R. D., van der Linden, S., Wendling, D., Bohm, H., Van Royen, B. J. and Braun, J. (2006) 'ASAS/EULAR recommendations for the management of ankylosing spondylitis', *Annals of the Rheumatic Diseases*, 65(4), 442–452.

12

MULTIPLE SCLEROSIS

Ulrik Dalgas

Introduction

Multiple sclerosis

Multiple sclerosis (MS) is a clinically and pathologically complex and heterogeneous disease of unknown etiology (Kantarci, 2008). The generally accepted view is, that primarily, MS is an autoimmune disease of the CNS that is precipitated by environmental factors in a genetically predisposed host (Kurtzke, 2005). MS is the most common neurological disease affecting young adults in Western countries (Pilz *et al.*, 2008), with most patients being diagnosed between 20 to 40 years of age (Liguori *et al.*, 2000). In 28 European countries with a total population of 466 million people, it is estimated that 380,000 individuals are affected by MS (Sobocki *et al.*, 2007). More females than males have MS and in Denmark the female to male ratio has increased from 1.31 in 1950 to 2.02 in 2005 (Bentzen *et al.*, 2010).

Strong evidence exists that both genetic and environmental factors affects susceptibility to MS. Studies have shown a MS risk of approximately 0.3 per cent in the general population, 3–5 per cent in first-degree relatives and a 25–30 per cent risk in monozygotic twins, where one is affected by the disease (Kantarci, 2008). Furthermore, migration studies have clearly demonstrated that changes to early environment, by moving from one region to another, can affect susceptibility to MS (Ebers, 2008). Consequently, several environmental candidates have been investigated, including viral agents (e.g. Epstein-Barr virus), latitude, hours of sunlight, vitamin D and smoking (Ebers, 2008) among which virus infection has gained most attention. Diagnosis of MS is based on internationally accepted consensus criteria (McDonald *et al.*, 2001). The disorder is progressive but more than 80 per cent of all MS patients live with the disease for more than 35 years (Koch-Henriksen *et al.*, 1998) and 5–10 years of life are lost to the disease (Bronnum-Hansen *et al.*, 2004).

Pathology, clinical course and treatment

The pathology of MS is defined as an inflammatory process leading to focal lesions with primary demyelination in the white matter of the brain and spinal cord. Inflammation is dominated by T cells and activated macrophages or microglia. In active lesions, this inflammatory process is accompanied by degradation of the blood brain barrier and profound disturbances of the local expression of proinflammatory cytokines and chemokines, as well as of their cognate receptors. Complete demyelination is accompanied by a varying degree of acute axonal injury and loss. Occasionally, remyelination occurs leading to remission (for references see Lassmann *et. al.*, 2007).

The clinical course of MS is characterized by heterogeneity. However, five basic clinical courses of MS are recognized, namely relapsing-remitting MS (RRMS), primary progressive MS (PPMS), secondary progressive MS (SPMS), progressive-relapsing MS (PRMS) and benign MS (Table 12.1). Depending on the type of MS, individuals demonstrate neurological and functional decline ranging from very slow progression to rapid deterioration. In a cross-sectional study from a Hungarian county of 400,000 inhabitants, it was reported that 54 per cent had RRMS, 20 per cent had SPMS, 15 per cent had the benign form of MS and 11 per cent had PPMS (Bencsik *et al.*, 2001).

TABLE 12.1 Definitions of subgroups of multiple sclerosis according to clinical course (Lublin and Reingold, 1996)

Relapsing-remitting multiple sclerosis
Clearly defined disease relapses with full recovery or with residual deficit upon recovery; periods between disease relapses characterized by a lack of disease progression.

Benign multiple sclerosis
Disease course in which the patient remains fully functional in all neurologic systems 15 years after disease onset.

Primary-progressive multiple sclerosis
Disease progression from onset with occasional plateaus, temporary minor improvements being allowed.

Secondary-progressive multiple sclerosis
Initial relapsing-remitting disease course followed by progression with or without occasional relapses, minor remissions, and plateaus.

Progressive-relapsing multiple sclerosis
Progressive disease from onset, with clear acute relapses, with or without full recovery; periods between relapses characterized by continuing progression.

After disease onset, the majority of people with MS (~85 per cent) develop a RRMS course, characterized by exacerbations, after which symptoms persist or partially remit leading to cumulative disability over time (Rovaris *et al.*, 2006).

A significant sub-group of MS patients (approximately 30 per cent) have little disease progression and minimal or no disability after many years of the disease which is referred to as benign. The definitions of benign MS have varied in terms of the disability and duration of disease (5–15 years) (Pittock and Rodriguez, 2008). Most authors consider benign MS as a disease course in which the patient remains fully functional in all neurologic systems 15 years after disease onset (Lublin and Reingold, 1996). Approximately 40–65 per cent of the patients with RRMS will eventually experience slow progression (SPMS) (Coyle, 1996). However, in MS surveys, the longer duration of the follow-up, the higher the proportion of cases with a RRMS onset who will have converted to SPMS. An estimate of the median time from RRMS onset to SPMS is about 19 years (Rovaris *et al.*, 2006). About 10–15 per cent of patients with MS present with gradually increasing neurological disability, a clinical course known as PPMS. Compared with RRMS, people with PPMS are older at onset, with a higher proportion being men (Miller and Leary, 2007). The classification, PRMS, refers to a small proportion of patients (probably less than 5–10 per cent) who begin as PPMS but eventually experience one or more acute relapses (Coyle, 1996).

Awareness of the different courses of MS is important because there is increasing evidence that they are pathologically different. Clinical and MRI data suggest that inflammation and the formation of new white matter lesions are common characteristics of RRMS, while in PPMS new inflammatory demyelinating lesions are rare and diffuse atrophy of grey and white matter and changes of the normal-appearing white matter become prominent (Lassmann *et al.*, 2007). Disease progression is assessed using the Expanded Disability Status Score (EDSS), which is a scale from 0–10 with 0 denoting no impairments caused by the disease and 10 denoting dead caused by the disease.

Physiological and functional impairments in MS

Patients having MS are characterized by both reduced aerobic capacity (Mostert and Kesselring, 2002; Tantucci *et al.*, 1996) and muscle strength (Armstrong *et al.*, 1983; Carroll *et al.*, 2005; Chen *et al.*, 1987; de Haan *et al.*, 2000; Garner and Widrick, 2003; Kent-Braun *et al.*, 1994; Kent-Braun *et al.*, 1997; Lambert *et al.*, 2001; Ng *et al.*, 2004; Ponichtera *et al.*, 1992; Rice *et al.*, 1992; Schwid *et al.*, 1999; Sharma *et al.*, 1995). The impaired muscle strength may be due to reduced neural activation (de Haan *et al.*, 2000; Ng *et al.*, 2004; Rice *et al.*, 1992) or reduced skeletal muscle mass (Formica *et al.*, 1997; Garner and Widrick 2003; Kent-Braun *et al.*, 1997). In conjunction with other common symptoms like spasticity, fatigue, bowel and bladder problems, balance problems and visual problems, these physiological deficits translate into reduced functional capacity (Morris *et al.*, 2002; Savci *et al.*, 2005; Thoumie and Mevellec 2002). Furthermore, MS patients have increased risk of developing depression (Arnett *et al.*, 2008). Consequently, health-related quality of life (QoL) is often impaired in MS patients (Miller and Dishon, 2006).

Exercise rehabilitation for MS

For many years the general advice given to individuals with MS was not to participate in physical exercise. This advice was given because participation in physical exercise was reported to lead to deterioration of symptoms or fatigue (Sutherland and Andersen, 2001). During the last decade, it has been more common to recommend exercise for MS patients, because of the emerging evidence for its beneficial effects (Petajan and White, 1999; Ponichtera-Mulcare, 1993; Sutherland and Andersen, 2001). Subsequently, a number of reviews (Brown and Kraft, 2005; Heesen *et al.*, 2006; Karpatkin, 2006; Petajan and White, 1999; Ponichtera-Mulcare, 1993; Poser and Ronthal, 1991; Sutherland and Andersen, 2001; White and Dressendorfer, 2004) and meta-analyses (Baker and Tickle-Degnen, 2001; Rietberg *et al.*, 2005) have been published regarding different aspects of exercise and MS. Furthermore, it has recently been shown that a worsening of the number and/or intensity of sensory symptoms, which is experienced by more than 40 per cent of all MS patients after exercise, is temporal, and will be normalized within half an hour after exercise cessation in most (85 per cent) patients (Smith *et al.*, 2006). Today, exercise is, therefore, generally recommended for MS patients (Dalgas *et al.*, 2008; White and Dressendorfer, 2004).

Before the mid-1990s, there were only a few studies on exercise in MS but during the last 10–15 years several studies have emerged. While there are many reports of exercise-induced benefits, only half of all studies are randomized controlled trials (RCTs). Additionally, it should be mentioned that almost all studies have included MS patients able to walk independently for 20 metres or more, making it impossible to draw conclusions regarding the effects of exercise in the most severely impaired patients. Furthermore, most studies have evaluated exercise in the form of either resistance exercise training (i.e. a few skeletal muscle contractions against heavy loads) or aerobic exercise training (i.e. multiple skeletal muscle contractions against relatively lighter loads). This chapter, therefore, focuses on the effects of these training modalities conducted separately or in combination.

Exercise, functional capacity, fatigue and quality of life

Resistance exercise training and functional capacity

Functional capacity has been shown to be reduced in MS patients. Several studies have reported reduced gait speed at both comfortable and maximal gait velocity (Morris *et al.*, 2002; Schwid *et al.*, 1999; Thoumie and Mevellec 2002). In accordance with these results, it has also been demonstrated that MS patients walked significantly shorter than healthy individuals during a 6-minute walk test (Goldman *et al.*, 2008; Savci *et al*, 2005). Studies evaluating the effects of resistance exercise training in MS patients have, in general, shown mixed results on functional capacity. Harvey *et al.* (1999) reported a 23 per cent increase in 'chair transfer', whereas no change was observed in gait speed after eight weeks of daily weighted leg raises. De Souza-Teixeira *et al.* (2009) reported improvements (8 per cent) of the timed up and go test after eight weeks of bi-weekly resistance exercise training for the lower extremity. This finding is supported by a preliminary report, where Kraft *et al.* (1996) showed an increase in gait speed, stair climbing and 'timed up and go' after 12 weeks of resistance exercise training, three times a week. An improvement in timed up and go could, however, not be demonstrated in a RCT by DeBolt and McCubbin (2004), where the participants underwent eight weeks of home-based resistance exercise training three times a week. Taylor *et al.* (2006) reported an improvement (6 per cent) in maximal gait velocity in a 10 m walk-test after 10 weeks of bi-weekly resistance exercise training, but found no change in a 2-minute walk-test or in stair climbing performance. White and Dressendorfer (2004) reported improved performance during a step-test, but found no improvements in gait. Finally, a recent study found significant improvements in maximal gait speed (12 per cent), walking distance during a six-minute walk test (6MWT) (12 per cent), stair climbing (15 per cent) and chair rise performance (28 per cent) in a RCT, where the participants underwent intense bi-weekly resistance exercise training for the lower extremity for a 12-week period (Dalgas *et al.*, 2009). Although not consistent, the majority of studies show improvements in various functional tasks, thought to reflect important activities of daily living (ADLs) following resistance exercise training. This conclusion is in concordance with a recent meta-analysis showing that exercise in general (effect size: 0.19) and resistance exercise training in particular (effect size: 0.34), improve gait in MS patients (Snook and Motl, 2008).

Aerobic exercise training and functional capacity

The reported effects of aerobic exercise training on functional capacity are inconsistent. Most studies evaluating the effects of cycle ergometry exercise training (Rasova *et al.*, 2006; Schapiro *et al.*, 1988) or arm-leg ergometry exercise training (Petajan *et al.*, 1996) have reported improvements in endurance exercise performance during maximal testing on the ergometer used for exercise training. Furthermore, six studies (Mostert and Kesselring 2002; Petajan *et al.*, 1996; Ponichtera-Mulcare *et al.*, 1997; Rampello *et al.*, 2007; Rasova *et al.*, 2006; Schulz *et al.*, 2004) have evaluated how aerobic exercise training affects aerobic capacity. Petajan *et al.* (1996) and Ponichtera-Mulcare *et al.* (1997) found marked improvements (22 per cent and 15 per cent) in $\dot{V}O_{2max}$ after 15 and 24 weeks of arm-leg ergometry exercise, training three days a week at an intensity of 55–60 per cent of $\dot{V}O_{2max}$. Measurements during the intervention period after five and ten weeks (Petajan *et al.*, 1996) and at week 12 (Ponichtera-Mulcare *et al.*, 1997), also showed significant improvements in $\dot{V}O_{2max}$ at these time intervals (9 per cent, 19 per cent and 10 per cent, respectively). Rampello *et al.* (2007) reported an improvement of 17 per cent in $\dot{V}O_{2max}$ after eight weeks of cycle ergometry exercise performed three times a week. However, studies that evaluated the effects of cycle ergometry for four weeks (training five days a week) (Mostert and

Kesselring, 2002) or eight weeks (training two days a week) (Rasova *et al.*, 2006; Schulz *et al.*, 2004) at similar exercise intensities could not demonstrate significant improvements in $\dot{V}O_{2max}$. This suggests that aerobic exercise training for at least three days a week is necessary for improvements in $\dot{V}O_{2max}$ to occur within the first eight weeks of exercise training using a moderate (55–60 per cent of $\dot{V}O_{2max}$) exercise training intensity. This raises the question of whether training at that intensity for two days a week will provide an adequate stimulus for improving $\dot{V}O_{2max}$. It should, however, be noted that although the study by Mostert and Kesselring (2002) did not show an improvement of $\dot{V}O_{2max}$, five weeks of cycle ergometry exercise did result in a rightward shift in, what the authors called, the aerobic threshold, indicating an improvement in aerobic capacity when exercising at sub-maximal intensities.

Several studies have investigated how aerobic exercise training influences gait velocity. The findings show great diversity, as it has been reported that gait velocity is either reduced (Rodgers *et al.*, 1999), unaffected (Gehlsen *et al.*, 1986; Heesen *et al.*, 2003; O'Connell *et al.*, 2003) or improved (Kileff and Ashburn 2005; Rampello *et al.*, 2007; van den Berg *et al.*, 2006) after programmes of aerobic exercise. This suggests that aerobic exercise training, at best, results in modest improvements in this important ADL, which might be more dependent on skeletal muscle strength. This conclusion is also in accordance with a recent meta-analysis showing that aerobic exercise training has a smaller effect size than resistance exercise training (0.25 vs. 0.34) when the effect on gait is evaluated in MS patients (Snook and Motl, 2008). The one study that has evaluated the effects of combined aerobic and resistance exercise training on gait, found improvements in both a short and a long gait test after six months of exercise training, implying that combined exercise training programmes can improve functional capacity (Romberg *et al.*, 2004).

Fatigue

Fatigue is one of the most frequent symptoms reported by MS patients (Krupp *et al.*, 1988). As 55 per cent of all MS patients describe fatigue as one of the most severe symptoms (Fisk *et al.*, 1994), interventions that can reduce fatigue are of particular interest. In a non-controlled study White *et al.* (2004) reported a reduction in fatigue score evaluated with the Modified Fatigue Impact Scale (MFIS) after eight weeks of lower extremity resistance exercise training. In another non-controlled study Dodd *et al.* (2006), using a qualitative approach, reported reduced fatigue in seven out of nine patients after 10 weeks of bi-weekly resistance exercise training. A recent randomized controlled trial showed a small, but significant improvement in the Fatigue Severity Scale (FSS) score after 12 weeks of bi-weekly resistance exercise training of the lower limbs. Furthermore, changes in General Fatigue on the Mulidimensional Fatigue Inventory (MFI) scale improved significantly in the resistance exercise training group versus controls. These data, therefore, provide support that resistance exercise training has a beneficial effect on MS-induced fatigue (Dalgas *et al.*, 2010).

Aerobic exercise training also has the potential to reduce fatigue, but findings are inconsistent. Some studies show an effect (McCullagh *et al.*, 2008; Oken *et al.*, 2004; Rasova *et al.*, 2006), whereas others do not (Kileff and Ashburn, 2005; Mostert and Kesselring, 2002; Petajan *et al.*, 1996; Schulz *et al.*, 2004; van den Berg *et al.*, 2006). Interestingly, studies that reported an effect of endurance training on fatigue either used the multidimensional Modified Fatigue Impact Scale (McCullagh *et al.*, 2008; Rasova *et al.*, 2006) or the MFI (Oken *et al.*, 2004). All studies, except one (Schulz *et al.*, 2004) that were unable to demonstrate an effect of aerobic exercise training used the one-dimensional FSS. This could indicate that the FSS is not as sensitive a measure of MS-related fatigue as some of the multidimensional scales. A few studies (Fragoso *et al.*, 2008; Surakka *et al.*, 2004) have studied the effect of combined resistance and endurance training on MS fatigue. Fragoso *et al.* (2008) reported that 20 weeks of combined training 3 days a week reduced Chalder's score of fatigue, whereas no effect was found by Surakka *et al.* (2004) after 23 weeks of combined training at home. Consequently, exercise has the potential to reduce fatigue, resistance training being at least as successful as endurance training.

Exercise, depression and quality of life

One recent study evaluated the effects of resistance exercise training on mood in MS patients. Twelve weeks of bi-weekly resistance exercise resulted in a significant decrease in the Major Depression Inventory (MDI) score of the exercise group compared to the control group (Dalgas *et al.*, 2010). Mood scores were reduced from a baseline score of 10.3 ± 5.9 to 7.9 ± 4.9 after the programme of exercise training, approaching data from healthy Danish subjects aged 35–49 years having a MDI score of 7.7 (Olsen *et al.*, 2004).

A large study by Petajan *et al.* (1996) reported that 15 weeks of arm-leg ergometry three times a week improved depression scores, as measured by the Profile Of Mood States (POMS). This finding earned support from another large study evaluating the effects of eight weeks of bi-weekly cycle ergometry, where a significant improvement in the Becks Depression Inventory (BDI) was reported (Rasova *et al.*, 2006). However, two studies (Oken *et al.*, 2004; Schulz *et al.*, 2004) did not show any effect on mood or depression scores after programmes of cycle ergometry exercise training. These differences might well be explained by low exercise training frequency and intensity in the study by Oken *et al.* (2004) and by a general lack of any exercise training effects in the study by Schultz *et al.* (2004). Only one study has evaluated the effects of combined exercise training on depression score (Centre for Epidemiologic Studies Depression Scale), reporting no change after six months of mainly home-based exercise training (Romberg *et al.*, 2005). In summary, both aerobic and resistance exercise training have the potential to beneficially influence mood and depression scores in MS patients but the findings are inconsistent.

Only one study has examined the effects of resistance exercise training on quality of life (QoL) in individuals with MS. After twelve weeks of bi-weekly resistance exercise training, a significant increase was found in the physical domain of the SF-36 questionnaire and a trend was observed in the mental domain (p=0.09) (Dalgas *et al.*, 2010).

Aerobic exercise training also seems to positively influence health-related QoL, as assessed using the SF36 (Mostert and Kesselring, 2002; Oken *et al.*, 2004), Multiple Sclerosis Quality Of Life (MSQOL) (Rasova *et al.*, 2006), Hamburg Quality Of Life Questionnaire for MS (HAQUAMS) (Schulz *et al.*, 2004) and POMS scales (Petajan *et al.*, 1996; Sutherland *et al.*, 2007). Improvements have been reported for vitality (Mostert and Kesselring, 2002), social functioning (Mostert and Kesselring, 2002; Schulz *et al.*, 2004), mood (Schulz *et al.*, 2004), energy (Oken *et al.*, 2004; Sutherland *et al.*, 2007), fatigue (Oken *et al.*, 2004; Petajan *et al.*, 1996; Sutherland *et al.*, 2007), anger (Petajan *et al.*, 1996) and sexual function (Sutherland *et al.*, 2007). This interpretation is in accordance with a recent meta-analysis evaluating the effects of aerobic exercise training on quality of life in individuals with MS, showing a small but significant effect of aerobic exercise training on QoL (Motl and Gosney 2008). However, studies evaluating the effects of combined exercise training on QoL have not reported any significant effects, which could be explained by low statistical power (Bjarnadottir *et al.*, 2007) or the use of home-based exercise training programmes (Romberg *et al.*, 2005). In summary, there is evidence that different exercise modalities can influence various dimensions of health-related QoL in a positive way.

Mode, intensity, frequency and progression of exercise for individuals with MS

Resistance exercise training

Studies of resistance exercise training and MS have been conducted with supervision at a fitness facility (Dalgas *et al.*, 2009; Taylor *et al.*, 2006; White *et al.*, 2004) or without supervision at home using weighted vests (DeBolt and McCubbin, 2004; Harvey *et al.*, 1999). None of the studies on resistance exercise training reported significant problems tolerating this exercise training modality. In most studies on resistance exercise training (Aimet *et al.*, 2006; Dalgas *et al.*, 2009; DeBolt and McCubbin, 2004; Harvey *et al.*, 2004), the intervention was aimed at the lower extremities, corresponding to the clinical observation of a predominant strength deficit in the legs (Schwid *et al.*, 1999). However, notable improvements (3–29 per cent) were also present in the upper extremity (elbow extensors, elbow flexors, shoulder abductors and shoulder adductors) after resistance exercise training (Kasser and McCubbin, 1996; Kraft *et al.*, 1996; Taylor *et al.*, 2006). Not all studies have quantified exercise training intensity precisely, but those that have, report resistance exercise training intensities of 60–80 per cent of the one-repetition maximum strength (1RM) (Aimet *et al.*, 2006; Taylor *et al.*, 2006;

White *et al.*, 2004) or sets of the 8–12 RM strength (Dalgas *et al.*, 2009). A training frequency of two (Aimet *et al.*, 2006; Dalgas *et al.*, 2009; Kasser and McCubbin, 1996; Taylor *et al.*, 2006; White *et al.*, 2004) or three (DeBolt and McCubbin, 2004; Fisher *et al.*, 2000; Kraft *et al.*, 1996) days a week have been prescribed in most studies and have been shown to evoke improvements in both skeletal muscle strength and functional capacity. Three days a week would be expected to be superior to two days a week, but no studies have compared this in individuals with MS. However, some individuals with MS will need a much longer time for recovery than healthy persons, which could make a frequency of two days a week superior. Different types of progression models have also been applied. In one study, one set of each exercise was performed and the weight was increased by 2–5 per cent of the maximum voluntary contraction (MVC) force when 15 repetitions of an exercise could be performed (White *et al.*, 2004). In another study, a progression from three sets of 10 repetitions at a load of 15 RM strength to four sets of eight repetitions at a load of 8 RM strength was used (Dalgas *et al.*, 2009).

Aerobic exercise training

Aerobic exercise training modalities that have been investigated in individuals with MS include cycle ergometry (Heesen *et al.*, 2003; Kileff and Ashburn, 2005; Mostert and Kesselring, 2002; Oken *et al.*, 2004; Rampello *et al.*, 2007; Rasova *et al.*, 2006; Schapiro *et al.*, 1988; Schulz *et al.*, 2004; Sosnoff *et al.*, 2009), arm-leg ergometry (Petajan *et al.*, 1996; Ponichtera-Mulcare *et al.*, 1997; Rodgers *et al.*, 1999), arm ergometry (Marsh *et al.*, 1986), aquatic exercise (Gehlsen *et al.*, 1986; Gehlsen *et al.*, 1984; Sutherland *et al.*, 2007) and treadmill walking (Marsh *et al.*, 1986; van den Berg *et al.*, 2006). Although these studies have shown that aerobic exercise training is a highly feasible exercise modality for individuals with MS, many of the aerobic exercise regimens used were insufficiently described and the exercise training intensity poorly controlled. Nonetheless, a recent review concluded that aerobic exercise training at low to moderate intensities has proven to be well tolerated among individuals with MS (Dalgas *et al.*, 2008). Studies have generally evaluated aerobic exercise training intensities in the range of 50–70 per cent of $\dot{V}O_{2max}$ (Gehlsen *et al.*, 1984; Kileff and Ashburn, 2005; Marsh *et al.*, 1986; Mostert and Kesselring, 2002; Petajan *et al.*, 1996; Ponichtera-Mulcare *et al.*, 1997; Rampello *et al.*, 2007; Rasova *et al.*, 2006; Schapiro *et al.*, 1988; Schulz *et al.*, 2004; van den Berg *et al.*, 2006) corresponding to 60–80 per cent of the maximum heart rate. No studies have evaluated interval-type aerobic exercise training involving repeated short bouts of higher intensity exercise in individuals with MS. In most studies, one exercise training session lasted 15–30 minutes (Marsh *et al.*, 1986; Mostert and Kesselring, 2002; Ponichtera-Mulcare *et al.*, 1997; Rampello *et al.*, 2007; Rasova *et al.*, 2006; Schapiro *et al.*, 1988; Schulz *et al.*, 2004; van den Berg *et al.*, 2006), whereas in a few studies exercise sessions lasted from 40 minutes (Koudouni and Orologas, 2004; Petajan *et al.*, 1996) to one hour (Gehlsen *et al.*, 1984). Studies have applied exercise training frequencies of one

(Koudouni and Orologas 2004; Oken *et al.*, 2004), two (Heesen *et al.*, 2003; Kileff and Ashburn, 2005; Marsh *et al.*, 1986; Rasova *et al.*, 2006), three (Dettmers *et al.*, 2009; Gehlsen *et al.*, 1984; O'Connell *et al.*, 2003; Petajan *et al.*, 1996; Ponichtera-Mulcare *et al.*, 1997; Rampello *et al.*, 2007; Sosnoff *et al.*, 2009; Sutherland *et al.*, 2007; van den Berg *et al.*, 2006) and five (Mostert and Kesselring, 2002; Schapiro *et al.*, 1988) days a week, but no studies have evaluated the effects of different exercise training frequencies in individuals with MS. Long-term (>15 weeks) studies on endurance training for three days a week have consistently been shown to result in significant improvements of aerobic capacity ($\dot{V}O_{2max}$) in individuals with MS (Petajan *et al.*, 1996; Ponichtera-Mulcare *et al.*, 1997). Measurements during the intervention period at 5, 10 (Petajan *et al.*, 1996) and 12 (Ponichtera-Mulcare *et al.*, 1997) weeks, showed significant improvements in $\dot{V}O_{2max}$ of 9 per cent, 19 per cent and 10 per cent, respectively. However, studies that evaluated the effects of cycle ergometry for four weeks (five days a week)(Mostert and Kesselring, 2002) or eight weeks (two days a week) (Rasova *et al.*, 2006; Schulz *et al.*, 2004) at similar exercise training intensities could not demonstrate significant improvements of $\dot{V}O_{2max}$. This might suggest that exercise training at least three days a week is important for improvements in $\dot{V}O_{2max}$ within the first eight weeks when a moderate (60 per cent $\dot{V}O_{2max}$) training intensity is used. In most studies, the progression model consisted of maintaining the same relative exercise training intensity throughout the study period without increasing the length of the exercise session (Gehlsen *et al.*, 1984; Kileff and Ashburn, 2005; Marsh *et al.*, 1986; Mostert and Kesselring, 2002; Petajan *et al.*, 1996; Ponichtera-Mulcare *et al.*, 1997; Rampello *et al.*, 2007; Rasova *et al.*, 2006; Schapiro *et al.*, 1988; Schulz *et al.*, 2004; van den Berg *et al.*, 2006). However, no description of the exercise training progression model was reported in several studies (Koudouni and Orologas, 2004; O'Connell *et al.*, 2007). No studies to date have compared different exercise training progression models but this is an avenue that is worthy of future research.

Combined exercise training programmes

As described earlier, little is known about combined exercise training in individuals with MS. It has been shown that two weekly days of resistance exercise training and two weekly days of aerobic exercise training is well tolerated by MS patients (Romberg *et al.*, 2004). In other studies, an exercise training frequency of three days a week have been applied, where each session contains equal portions of resistance and aerobic exercise training (Bjarnadottir *et al.*, 2007; Carter and White, 2003; Fragoso *et al.*, 2008). None of the existing studies have controlled exercise training intensity, and details of the applied progression models were not reported.

Exercise and MS aetiology

MS is a chronic disease with no known cure. However, it has been suggested that exercise might have the potential to slow down the disease process

(Heesen *et al.*, 2006; Le-Page C. *et al.*, 1994). Only a few studies have addressed this important question. Because of the associated methodological difficulties in designing a study evaluating this in individuals with MS, most studies have used experimental autoimmune encephalomyelitis (EAE) rats (or mice) as the study population, which is an animal model of MS. In a study by Le Page *et al.* (1996) two groups of rats (exercise training and control) were followed after they were induced with EAE. This study showed that the onset of the disease was delayed in the group of rats that had exercised on a treadmill for 60–120 minutes each day. More recently, Rossi *et al.* (2009) explored this further and showed that EAE mice with free access to a running wheel consistently exhibited less severe neurological deficits compared to control EAE animals during a time period of 50 days after EAE induction. In humans, a more indirect approach has been taken, where the effects of exercise have been measured on mediators related to disease activity. From animal studies it is known that aerobic exercise training can increase neuroprotection through elevations of brain-derived neurotrophic factor (BDNF) secretion in the brain (Berchtold *et al.*, 2001). An increase of BDNF after aerobic exercise training in humans might have a positive effect on the disease process. In humans with MS, Castellano and White (2008) evaluated whether eight weeks of cycling three times a week, would affect serum concentrations of BDNF. After four weeks of endurance training, a significant increase in BDNF was found, but the concentration was normalized after eight weeks of exercise training. However, the authors concluded that serum BDNF concentration may be influenced by long-term exercise. Also, changes in the concentrations of certain cytokines, in particular IFN-g and TNF-a, have been associated with changes in disease status in MS, and elevated concentrations of pro-inflammatory cytokines may contribute to neurodegeneration and disability (Ozenci *et al.*, 2002). It is, therefore, notable that White *et al.* (2006) in a pilot study, reported that resting levels of IL-4, IL-10, CRP and IFN-g were reduced, while TNF-a, IL-2 and IL-6 levels remained unchanged after eight weeks of bi-weekly resistance exercise training. These results suggest that progressive resistance exercise training may have an impact on cytokine concentrations and thus, could have an impact on overall immune function and disease course in individuals with MS. However, the small number of existing studies, combined with the low number of participants, makes it necessary to confirm these findings in studies with stronger statistical power. Taken together, these data suggest that exercise in general may have an anti-inflammatory effect which could be beneficial for conditions that are mediated by inflammatory processes, such as MS.

Exercise recommendations

Exercise prescription recommendations are presented in Tables 12.2–4. After approval from a medical doctor, MS patients should consult an exercise specialist (e.g. a physiotherapist or an exercise physiologist) before embarking on an exercise programme (White and Dressendorfer 2004). It is important that the programme is designed and prescribed on an individual basis so that individual capabilities and impairments (and the potential impact of environmental conditions) can be taken into account. These recommendations are limited to MS patients that are able to walk at least 20 metres (EDSS ≤ 6.5), because at present, too little is known about the effects of exercise in more severely impaired individuals with MS. In general, the recommendations are based on the literature reviewed in this chapter; however, solid evidence-based recommendations regarding optimal resistance exercise training cannot be given solely on the basis of the existing scientific literature. Consequently, resistance exercise training recommendations are a composite of the limited literature which has investigated the impact of resistance exercise training in individuals with MS, and general resistance exercise training recommendations considered safe for individuals with MS to follow (Kraemer *et al.*, 2002; Kraemer and Ratamess 2004). The recommendations for combined exercise training programmes are based on the limited scientific evidence available.

TABLE 12.2 Resistance exercise training recommendations for individuals with MS

---

1 To secure safety, resistance training should be supervised by an expert until the patient has acquired proper skills.
2 In the initial phase of training the use of training machines should be preferred over free weights.
3 Although often less effective than machine training, home-based resistance exercise training, using elastic bands and/or exercises using body weight as load, represents an alternative approach.
4 Intensities in the range of 8–15 repetition maximum (RM) strength are recommended. Intensities of 15 RM strength are recommended during the initial training phase and should be progressively (over several months) increased toward intensities around 8–10 RM strength.
5 The number of sets should initially be in the range of 1–3, which can be increased toward 3–4 sets of every exercise after a few months. Rest periods between sets and exercises in the range of 2–4 min. are recommended.
6 A training frequency in the range of 2–3 days per week is well tolerated and results in meaningful improvements in MS patients.
7 In general, a whole body programme consisting of 4–8 exercises is recommended. Only in very special cases where the training frequency is exceeding three times a week, should a split program be considered (where different exercises are performed on different days).
8 In general, the exercise order should be planned so that large muscle group exercises are performed before small muscle group exercises, and multiple-joint exercises before single-joint exercises.
9 For individuals with MS, lower extremity exercises should have higher priority, because it has been shown that the extent of the strength deficit in the lower extremities is of greater magnitude than in the upper extremity.

Reprinted from Dalgas *et al.* (2009), Int MS J;16: 5–11, with permission from Cambridge Medical Publications.

TABLE 12.3 Aerobic exercise recommendations for individuals with MS

1 Cycle ergometry, arm-leg ergometry, arm ergometry, aquatic exercise and treadmill walking have all been shown to induce favourable improvements in MS patients, whereas running, road cycling and rowing are only suitable for well-functioning individuals.
2 A training frequency of 2–3 sessions per week using an initial training intensity of 50–70% of $\dot{V}O_{2max}$, corresponding to 60–80% of maximum heart rate is recommended.
3 An initial exercise duration of 10–40 min is recommended, depending on the disability level of the MS patient.
4 During the first 2–6 months, progression should be based on increasing the exercise training volume, by extending the duration of the sessions or by adding an extra training day. After this period, it should be determined if a higher exercise training intensity can be tolerated.

Reprinted from *Dalgas et al. 2009*, Int MS J;16: 5–11, with permission from Cambridge Medical Publications.

TABLE 12.4 Combined exercise training recommendations for individuals with MS

1 Combined exercise training, based on equal proportions of resistance- and endurance exercise, performed on alternate days is recommended.
2 Two days of resistance exercise training and two days of aerobic exercise training is recommended as the maximal initial weekly training frequency.
3 The two bouts of resistance exercise training, as well as the two bouts of aerobic exercise training, should be separated by an interval of 24–48 hours to allow adequate recovery.
4 The recommendations described earlier regarding resistance and aerobic exercise training should be followed when designing the combined programme.

Reprinted from Dalgas *et al.* 2009, Int MS J;16: 5–11, with permission from Cambridge Medical Publications.

Future research priorities

The existing studies have almost exclusively included MS patients with preserved mobility (able to walk at least 20 metres). Furthermore, most studies have included heterogeneous cohorts of patients having different disease courses. Consequently, future training studies should include participants with more severe disease and the disease course and potential co-morbidities should be standardized. Regarding optimal exercise training modalities, it is clear that there is a need for future RCT studies to evaluate the effects of combined exercise training programmes to establish more solid guidelines for individuals with MS. These studies should clearly document the relative proportions of resistance and aerobic exercise training, exercise training frequency, intensity, duration and total volume. Also, it would be of great interest to establish whether MS patients can tolerate more intense interval-type aerobic exercise training. If so, more rapid and greater exercise-induced improvements might be possible, helping to prevent a fast plateau in any improvements caused by too little overload. Finally, studies evaluating interventions which are aimed at reducing exacerbations of sensory symptoms that are observed in up to 40 per cent of all individuals with MS after exercise (Smith *et al.*, 2006) are needed. Because the worsening of symptoms after exercise might be related to increases in core temperature (White *et al.*, 2000), one approach is to use cooling before and during exercise. Another approach would be to study whether some exercise modalities result in less symptom exacerbations than other exercise modalities in this particular group of patients. Resistance exercise training is not accompanied by the same increases in core temperature as aerobic exercise training. It is therefore possible that resistance exercise training, more rarely than aerobic exercise training, will cause unpleasant experiences in thermo-sensitive patients but this is still unexplored. Also, more studies aimed at evaluating immunologically and MRI outcomes in individuals with MS who engage in exercise are warranted.

At the design level, longer intervention periods should be applied in future studies. From classical exercise physiology, it is known that an exercise training intervention lasting for 12 weeks or longer is more likely to obtain measurable cardiovascular, morphological and neural adaptations (Jones *et al.*, 1989). An exercise training intervention lasting 12 weeks or more is therefore recommended, regardless of the training modality being investigated. In future studies, it is very important that the exercise training intensity is better controlled and described.

Summary and conclusions

Physical exercise, contrary to earlier beliefs, is well tolerated and induces beneficial effects in individuals with MS. Both aerobic and resistance exercise training performed at moderate intensity are very well tolerated among moderately impaired individuals. To date, more studies have evaluated the effects of aerobic exercise training than resistance exercise training and only few studies have evaluated the efficacy of combined exercise training programmes. Aerobic exercise training and, particularly, resistance exercise training have the potential to improve functional capacity during activities of daily living. Also, aerobic and resistance exercise training appear to improve symptoms of fatigue, depression and QoL in individuals with MS. Improvements in the maximal oxygen consumption have been reported after aerobic exercise training and improvements in skeletal muscle strength have been reported after resistance exercise training in individuals with MS. It has also been suggested that exercise might positively influence the disease process but more research is needed to verify this. Future studies should evaluate longer exercise training interventions (> 12 weeks), the impact of exercise therapy in more severely impaired participants (EDSS > 6.5) and the relative benefits of different exercise training intensities. There should be more emphasis on studies of resistance exercise training and combined exercise training programmes.

Acknowledgements

Ass. Professor, MD Egon Stenager, Department of Neurology, Hospitals of Southern Denmark/Institute of Regional Research, University of Southern Denmark and Professor Johannes, Department of Neurology, Aarhus University Hospital, Denmark, are thanked for providing valuable comments to the present chapter.

References

Aimet, M., Lampichler, J. Musil, U., Spiesberger, R., Pelikan, J., Schmid, J., Haudum, G., Weisshaidinger, G., Rupp, M., Pokan, R. and Zifko U.A. (2006). 'High and moderate intensities in strength training in multiple sclerosis'. *Isokin Exerc Sci*, 14 (2): 153.

Armstrong, L.E., Winant, D.M., Swasey, P.R., Seidle, M.E., Carter, A.L. and Gehlsen, G. (1983). 'Using isokinetic dynamometry to test ambulatory patients with multiple sclerosis'. *Phys Ther*, 63 (8): 1274–1279.

Arnett, P.A., Barwick, F.H. and Beeney, J.E. (2008). 'Depression in multiple sclerosis: review and theoretical proposal'. *J Int Neuropsychol Soc*, 14 (5): 691–724.

Baker, N.A. and Tickle-Degnen, L. (2001). 'The effectiveness of physical, psychological, and functional interventions in treating clients with multiple sclerosis: a meta-analysis'. *Am J Occup Ther*, 55 (3): 324–331.

Bencsik, K., Rajda, C., Fuvesi, J., Klivenyi, P., Jardanhazy, T., Torok, M. and Vecsei, L. (2001). 'The prevalence of multiple sclerosis, distribution of clinical forms of the disease and functional status of patients in Csongrad County, Hungary'. *Eur Neurol*, 46 (4): 206–209.

Bentzen, J., Flachs, E.M., Stenager, E., Brønnum-Hansen, H. and Koch-Henriksen, N. (2010). 'Prevalence of multiple sclerosis in Denmark 1950–2005'. *Mult Scler*, 16(5): 520–525.

Berchtold, N.C., Kesslak, J.P., Pike, C.J., Adlard, P.A. and Cotman, C.W. (2001). 'Estrogen and exercise interact to regulate brain-derived neurotrophic factor mRNA and protein expression in the hippocampus'. *Eur J Neurosci*, 14 (12): 1992–2002.

Bjarnadottir, O.H., Konradsdottir, A.D., Reynisdottir, K. and Olafsson, E. (2007). 'Multiple sclerosis and brief moderate exercise. A randomised study'. *Mult Scler*, 13 (6): 776–782.

Brønnum-Hansen, H., Koch-Henriksen, N. and Stenager, E. (2004). 'Trends in survival and cause of death in Danish patients with multiple sclerosis'. *Brain*, 127 (pt 4): 844–850.

Brown, T.R. and Kraft, G.H. (2005). 'Exercise and rehabilitation for individuals with multiple sclerosis'. *Phys Med Rehabil Clin N Am*, 16 (2): 513–555.

Carroll, C.C., Gallagher, P.M., Seidle, M.E. and Trappe, S.W. (2005). 'Skeletal muscle characteristics of people with multiple sclerosis'. *Archives of Physical Medicine and Rehabilitation*, 86 (2): 224–229.

Carter, P. and White, C.M. (2003). 'The effect of general exercise training on effort of walking in patients with multiple sclerosis'. 14th International World Confederation for Physical Therapy, Barcelona RR-PL-1517.

Castellano, V. and White, L.J. (2008). 'Serum brain-derived neurotrophic factor response to aerobic exercise in multiple sclerosis'. *J Neurol Sci*, 269 (1–2): 85–91.

Chen, W.Y., Pierson, F.M. and Burnett, C.N. (1987). 'Force-time measurements of knee muscle functions of subjects with multiple sclerosis'. *Phys Ther*, 67 (6): 934–940.

Coyle, P.K. (1996). 'The neuroimmunology of multiple sclerosis'. *Adv Neuroimmunol*, 6 (2): 143–154.

Dalgas, U., Stenager, E., Jakobsen, J., Petersen, T., Hansen, H., Knudsen, C., Overgaard, K. and Ingemann-Hansen, T. (2009). 'Resistance training improves muscle strength and functional capacity in multiple sclerosis'. *Neurology*, 73 1478–1484.

Dalgas, U., Stenager, E. and Ingemann-Hansen, T. (2008). 'Multiple sclerosis and physical exercise: recommendations for the application of resistance-, endurance- and combined training'. *Mult Scler*, 14 (1): 35–53.

Dalgas, U., Stenager, E., Jakobsen, J., Petersen, T., Hansen, H., Knudsen, C., Overgaard, K. and Ingemann-Hansen, T. (2010). 'Fatigue, mood and quality of life improve in MS patients after progressive resistance training'. *Mult Scler*, 16 (4): 480–490.

de Haan, A., de Ruiter, C.J., Der Woude, L.H. and Jongen, P.J. (2000). 'Contractile properties and fatigue of quadriceps muscles in multiple sclerosis'. *Muscle Nerve*, 23 (10): 1534–1541.

DeBolt, L.S. and McCubbin, J.A. (2004). 'The effects of home-based resistance exercise on balance, power, and mobility in adults with multiple sclerosis'. *Archives of Physical Medicine and Rehabilitation*, 85 (2): 290–297.

de Souza-Teixeira, F., Costilla, S., Ayán, C., García-López, D., González-Gallego, J., de Paz, J.A. (2009). 'Effects of resistance training in multiple sclerosis'. *Int J Sports Med*, 30 (4): 245–50.

Dettmers, C., Sulzmann, M., Ruchay-Plossl, A., Gutler, R. and Vieten, M. (2009). 'Endurance exercise improves walking distance in MS patients with fatigue'. *Acta Neurol Scand*, 120 (4): 251–257.

Dodd, K.J., Taylor, N.F., Denisenko, S. and Prasad, D. (2006). 'A qualitative analysis of a progressive resistance exercise programme for people with multiple sclerosis'. *Disabil Rehabil*, 28 (18): 1127–1134.

Ebers, G.C. (2008). 'Environmental factors and multiple sclerosis'. *Lancet Neurol*, 7 (3): 268–277.

Fisher, N.M., Lenox, J., Granger, C.V., Brown-scheidle, C. and Jacobs, L. (2000). 'Effects of an anti-fatiguing exercise program on fatigue and physiological function in patients with Multiple Sclerosis'. *Neurology*, 54 (7): A338.

Fisk, J.D., Pontefract, A., Ritvo, P.G., Archibald, C.J. and Murray, T.J. (1994). 'The impact of fatigue on patients with multiple sclerosis'. *Can J Neurol Sci*, 21 (1): 9–14.

Formica, C.A., Cosman, F., Nieves, J., Herbert, J. and Lindsay, R. (1997). 'Reduced bone mass and fat-free mass in women with multiple sclerosis: effects of ambulatory status and glucocorticoid Use'. *Calcif Tissue Int*, 61 (2): 129–133.

Fragoso, Y.D., Santana, D.L. and Pinto, R.C. (2008). 'The positive effects of a physical activity program for multiple sclerosis patients with fatigue'. *Neuro Rehabilitation*, 23 (2): 153–157.

Garner, D.J. and Widrick, J.J. (2003). 'Cross-bridge mechanisms of muscle weakness in multiple sclerosis'. *Muscle Nerve*, 27 (4): 456–464.

Gehlsen, G., Beekman, K., Assmann, N., Winant, D., Seidle, M. and Carter, A. (1986). 'Gait characteristics in multiple sclerosis: progressive changes and effects of exercise on parameters'. *Archives of Physical Medicine and Rehabilitation*, 67 (8): 536–539.

Gehlsen, G.M., Grigsby, S.A. and Winant, D.M. (1984). 'Effects of an aquatic fitness program on the muscular strength and endurance of patients with multiple sclerosis'. *Phys Ther*, 64 (5): 653–657.

Goldman, M.D., Marrie, R.A. and Cohen, J.A. (2008). 'Evaluation of the six-minute walk in multiple sclerosis subjects and healthy controls'. *Mult Scler*, 14 (3): 383–390.

Harvey, L., Smith, A. and Jones, R. (1999). 'The effect of weighted leg raises on quadriceps strength, EMG parameters and funtional activities in people with multiple sclerosis'. *Physiotherapy*, 85 (3): 154–161.

Heesen, C., Gold, S.M., Hartmann, S., Mladek, M., Reer, R., Braumann, K.M., Wiedemann, K. and Schulz, K.H. (2003). 'Endocrine and cytokine responses to standardized physical stress in multiple sclerosis'. *Brain Behav Immun*, 17 (6): 473–481.

Heesen, C., Romberg, A., Gold, S. and Schulz, K.H. (2006). 'Physical exercise in multiple sclerosis: supportive care or a putative disease-modifying treatment'. *Expert Rev Neurother*, 6 (3): 347–355.

Jones, D.A., Rutherford, O.M. and Parker, D.F. (1989). 'Physiological changes in skeletal muscle as a result of strength training'. *Q J Exp Physiol*, 74 (3): 233–256.

Kantarci, O.H. (2008). 'Genetics and natural history of multiple sclerosis'. *Semin Neurol*, 28 (1): 7–16.

Kasser, S. and McCubbin, J.A. (1996). 'Effects of progressive resistance exercise on muscular strength in adults with multiple sclerosis'. *Med Sci Sports Exerc*, 28: S143.

Kent-Braun, J.A., Ng, A.V., Castro, M., Weiner, M.W., Gelinas, D., Dudley, G.A. and Miller, R.G. (1997). 'Strength, skeletal muscle composition, and enzyme activity in multiple sclerosis'. *J Appl Physiol*, 83 (6): 1998–2004.

Kent-Braun, J.A., Sharma, K.R., Weiner, M.W. and Miller, R.G. (1994). 'Effects of exercise on muscle activation and metabolism in multiple sclerosis'. *Muscle Nerve*, 17 (10): 1162–1169.

Kileff, J. and Ashburn, A. (2005). 'A pilot study of the effect of aerobic exercise on people with moderate disability multiple sclerosis'. *Clin Rehabil*, 19 (2): 165–169.

Koch-Henriksen, N., Bronnum-Hansen, H. and Stenager, E. (1998). 'Underlying cause of death in Danish patients with multiple sclerosis: results from the Danish Multiple Sclerosis Registry'. *J Neurol Neurosurg Psychiatry*, 65 (1): 56–59.

Koudouni, A. and Orologas, A. (2004). 'Contribution of aerobic exercise to the improvement of quality of life in persons suffering from multiple sclerosis'. *Mult Scler*, 10 (7032): S132.

Kraemer, W.J. *et al.*, (2002). 'American College of Sports Medicine position stand. Progression models in resistance training for healthy adults'. *Med Sci Sports Exerc*, 34 (2): 364–380.

Kraemer, W.J. and Ratamess, N.A. (2004). 'Fundamentals of resistance training: progression and exercise prescription'. *Med Sci Sports Exerc*, 36 (4): 674–688.

Kraft, G., Alquist, A. and Lateur, B. (1996). 'Effects of resistive exercise on strength in multiple sclerosis (MS)'. *Arch Phys Med Rehabil*, 77 984.

Krupp, L.B., Alvarez, L.A., LaRocca, N.G. and Scheinberg, L.C. (1988). 'Fatigue in multiple sclerosis'. *Arch Neurol*, 45 (4): 435–437.

Kurtzke, J.F. (2005). 'Epidemiology and etiology of multiple sclerosis'. *Phys Med Rehabil Clin N Am*, 16 (2): 327–349.

Lambert, C.P., Archer, R.L. and Evans, W.J. (2001). 'Muscle strength and fatigue during isokinetic exercise in individuals with multiple sclerosis'. *Med Sci Sports Exerc*, 33 (10): 1613–1619.

Lassmann, H., Bruck, W. and Lucchinetti, C.F. (2007). 'The immunopathology of multiple sclerosis: an overview'. *Brain Pathol*, 17 (2): 210–218.

Le-Page C., Bourdoulous, S., Beraud, E., Couraud, P.O., Rieu, M. and Ferry, A. (1996). 'Effect of physical exercise on adoptive experimental auto-immune encephalomyelitis in rats'. *Eur J Appl Physiol Occup Physiol*, 73 (1–2): 130–135.

Le-Page C., Ferry, A. and Rieu, M. (1994). 'Effect of muscular exercise on chronic relapsing experimental autoimmune encephalomyelitis'. *J Appl Physiol*, 77 (5): 2341–2347.

Liguori, M., Marrosu, M.G., Pugliatti, M., Giuliani, F., De, R.F., Cocco, E., Zimatore, G.B., Livrea, P. and Trojano, M. (2000). 'Age at onset in multiple sclerosis'. *Neurol Sci*, 21 (4 Suppl 2): S825–S829.

Lublin, F.D. and Reingold, S.C. (1996). 'Defining the clinical course of multiple sclerosis: results of an international survey. National Multiple Sclerosis Society (USA) Advisory Committee on Clinical Trials of New Agents in Multiple Sclerosis'. *Neurology*, 46 (4): 907–911.

Marsh, H., Alexander, J. and Costello, E. (1986). 'Short-term exercise programme effect on physicak work capacity'. *Arch Phys Med Rehabil*, 67 (9): 644.

McCullagh, R., Fitzgerald, A.P., Murphy, R.P. and Cooke, G. (2008). 'Long-term benefits of exercising on quality of life and fatigue in multiple sclerosis patients with mild disability: a pilot study'. *Clin Rehabil*, 22 (3): 206–214.

McDonald, W.I., Compston, A., Edan, G., Goodkin, D., Hartung, H.P., Lublin, F.D., McFarland, H.F., Paty, D.W., Polman, C.H., Reingold, S.C., Sandberg-Wollheim, M., Sibley, W., Thompson, A., van den Noort, S., Weinshenker, B.Y., Wolinsky, J.S. (2001). 'Recommended diagnostic criteria for multiple sclerosis: guidelines from the International Panel on the diagnosis of multiple sclerosis'. *Ann Neurol*, 50 (1): 121–127.

Miller, A. and Dishon, S. (2006). 'Health-related quality of life in multiple sclerosis: the impact of disability, gender and employment status'. Qual.Life Res., 15 (2): 259–271.

Miller, D.H. and Leary, S.M. (2007). 'Primary-progressive multiple sclerosis'. *Lancet Neurol*, 6 (10): 903–912.

Morris, M.E., Cantwell, C., Vowels, L. and Dodd, K. (2002). 'Changes in gait and fatigue from morning to afternoon in people with multiple sclerosis'. *J Neurol Neurosurg Psychiatry*, 72 (3): 361–365.

Mostert, S. and Kesselring, J. (2002). 'Effects of a short-term exercise training program on aerobic fitness, fatigue, health perception and activity level of subjects with multiple sclerosis'. *Mult Scler*, 8 (2): 161–168.

Motl, R.W. and Gosney, J.L. (2008). 'Effect of exercise training on quality of life in multiple sclerosis: a meta-analysis'. *Mult Scler*, 14 (1): 129–135.

Ng, A.V., Miller, R.G., Gelinas, D. and Kent-Braun, J.A. (2004). 'Functional relationships of central and peripheral muscle alterations in multiple sclerosis'. *Muscle Nerve*, 29 (6): 843–852.

Oken, B.S., Kishiyama, S., Zajdel, D., Bourdette, D., Carlsen, J., Haas, M., Hugos, C., Kraemer, D.F., Lawrence, J. and Mass, M. (2004). 'Randomized controlled trial of yoga and exercise in multiple sclerosis'. *Neurology*, 62 (11): 2058–2064.

Olsen, L.R., Mortensen, E.L. and Bech, P. (2004). 'Prevalence of major depression and stress indicators in the Danish general population'. *Acta Psychiatr Scand*, 109 (2): 96–103.

Ozenci, V., Kouwenhoven, M. and Link, H. (2002). 'Cytokines in multiple sclerosis: methodological aspects and pathogenic implications'. *Mult Scler*, 8 (5): 396–404.

O'Connell, R., Murphy, R.M., Hutchinson, M., Cooke, G. and Coote, S. (2003). 'A controlled study to assess the effects of aerobic training on patients with multiple sclerosis'. 14th International World Confederation for Physical Therapy, Barcelona RR-PL-2105.

Petajan, J.H., Gappmaier, E., White, A.T., Spencer, M.K., Mino, L. and Hicks, R.W. (1996). 'Impact of aerobic training on fitness and quality of life in multiple sclerosis'. *Annals of Neurology*, 39 (4): 432–441.

Petajan, J.H. and White, A.T. (1999). 'Recommendations for physical activity in patients with multiple sclerosis'. *Sports Med*, 27 (3): 179–191.

Pilz, G., Wipfler, P., Ladurner, G. and Kraus, J. (2008). 'Modern multiple sclerosis treatment – what is approved, what is on the horizon'. *Drug Discov Today*, 13 (23–24): 1013–1025.

Pittock, S.J. and Rodriguez, M. (2008). 'Benign multiple sclerosis: a distinct clinical entity with therapeutic implications'. *Curr Top Microbiol Immunol*, 318 1–17.

Ponichtera, J.A., Rodgers, M.M., Glaser, R.M. and Mathews T (1992). 'Concentric and eccentric isokinetic lower extremity strength in persons with multiple sclerosis'. *J Orthop Sports Phys Ther*, 16 114–122.

Ponichtera-Mulcare, J.A. (1993). 'Exercise and multiple sclerosis'. *Med Sci Sports Exerc*, 25 (4): 451–465.

Ponichtera-Mulcare, J.A., Mathews T, Barret PJ and Gupta SC (1997). 'Change in aerobic fitness of patients with multiple sclerosis during a 6 month training program'. *Sports Med Train Rehabil*, 7 265–272.

Poser, C.M. and Ronthal, M. (1991). 'Exercise and Alzheimers's disease, Parkinson's disease, and multiple sclerosis'. *The Physician and Sports Medicine*, 19: 85–92.

Rampello, A., Franceschini, M., Piepoli, M., Antenucci, R., Lenti, G., Olivieri, D. and Chetta, A. (2007). 'Effect of Aerobic Training on Walking Capacity and Maximal Exercise Tolerance in Patients With Multiple Sclerosis: A Randomized Crossover Controlled Study'. *Phys Ther*, 87 (5): 545–555.

Rasova, K., Havrdova, E., Brandejsky, P., Zalisova, M., Foubikova, B. and Martinkova, P. (2006). 'Comparison of the influence of different rehabilitation programmes on clinical, spirometric and spiroergometric parameters in patients with multiple sclerosis'. *Mult Scler*, 12 (2): 227–234.

Rice, C.L., Vollmer, T.L. and Bigland-Ritchie, B. (1992). 'Neuromuscular responses of patients with multiple sclerosis'. *Muscle Nerve*, 15 (10): 1123–1132.

Rietberg, M., Brooks, D., Uitdehaag, B. and Kwakkel, G. (2005). 'Exercise therapy for multiple sclerosis'. *Cochrane Database Syst Rev* (1): CD003980.

Rodgers, M.M., Mulcare, J.A., King, D.L., Mathews, T., Gupta, S.C. and Glaser, R.M. (1999). 'Gait characteristics of individuals with multiple sclerosis before and after a 6-month aerobic training program'. *J Rehabil Res Dev*, 36 (3): 183–188.

Romberg, A., Virtanen, A. and Ruutiainen, J. (2005). 'Long-term exercise improves functional impairment but not quality of life in multiple sclerosis'. *J Neurol*, 252 839–845.

Romberg, A., Virtanen, A., Ruutiainen, J., Aunola, S., Karppi, S.L., Vaara, M., Surakka, J., Pohjolainen, T. and Seppanen, A. (2004). 'Effects of a 6-month exercise program on patients with multiple sclerosis: a randomized study'. *Neurology*, 63 (11): 2034–2038.

Rossi, S., Furlan, R., De Chiara, V., Musella, A., Lo Giudice, T., Mataluni, G., Cavasinni, F., Cantarella, C., Bernardi, G., Muzio, L., Martorana, A., Martino, G. and Centonze, D. (2009). 'Exercise attenuates the clinical, synaptic and dendritic abnormalities of experimental autoimmune encephalomyelitis'. *Neurobiol Dis*, 36 (1): 51–59.

Rovaris, M., Confavreux, C., Furlan, R., Kappos, L., Comi, G. and Filippi, M. (2006). 'Secondary progressive multiple sclerosis: current knowledge and future challenges'. *Lancet Neurol*, 5 (4): 343–354.

Savci, S., Inal-Inc, Arikan, H., Guclu-Gunduz, A., Cetisli-Korkmaz, N., Armutlu, K. and Karabudak, R. (2005). 'Six-minute walk distance as a measure of functional exercise capacity in multiple sclerosis'. *Disabil Rehabil*, 27 (22): 1365–1371.

Schapiro RT, Petajan, J.H. and Kosich D (1988). 'Role of cardiovascular fitess in miltiple sclerosis: a pilot study'. *J Neurol Rehabil*, 2 43–49.

Schulz, K.H., Gold, S.M., Witte, J., Bartsch, K., Lang, U.E., Hellweg, R., Reer, R., Braumann, K.M. and Heesen, C. (2004). 'Impact of aerobic training on immune-endocrine parameters, neurotrophic factors, quality of life and coordinative function in multiple sclerosis'. *J Neurol Sci*, 225 (1–2): 11–18.

Schwid, S.R., Thornton, C.A., Pandya, S., Manzur, K.L., Sanjak, M., Petrie, M.D., McDermott, M.P. and Goodman, A.D. (1999). 'Quantitative assessment of motor fatigue and strength in MS'. *Neurology*, 53 (4): 743–750.

Sharma, K.R., Kent-Braun, J., Mynhier, M.A., Weiner, M.W. and Miller, R.G. (1995). 'Evidence of an abnormal intramuscular component of fatigue in multiple sclerosis'. *Muscle Nerve*, 18 (12): 1403–1411.

Smith, R.M., Adeney-Steel, M., Fulcher, G. and Longley, W.A. (2006). 'Symptom change with exercise is a temporary phenomenon for people with multiple sclerosis'. *Archives of Physical Medicine and Rehabilitation*, 87 (5): 723–727.

Snook, E.M. and Motl, R.W. (2008). 'Physical activity behaviors in individuals with multiple sclerosis: roles of overall and specific symptoms, and self-efficacy'. *J Pain Symptom Manage*, 36 (1): 46–53.

Sobocki, P., Pugliatti, M., Lauer, K. and Kobelt, G. (2007). 'Estimation of the cost of MS in Europe: extrapolations from a multinational cost study'. *Mult Scler*, 13 (8): 1054–1064.

Sosnoff, J., Motl, R.W., Snook, E.M. and Wynn, D. (2009). 'Effect of a 4-week period of unloaded leg cycling exercise on spasticity in multiple sclerosis'. *Neuro Rehabilitation*, 24 (4): 327–331.

Surakka, J., Romberg, A., Ruutiainen, J., Aunola, S., Virtanen, A., Karppi, S.L. and Maentaka, K. (2004). 'Effects of aerobic and strength exercise on motor fatigue in men and women with multiple sclerosis: a randomized controlled trial'. *Clin Rehabil*, 18 (7): 737–746.

Sutherland, G. and Andersen, M.B. (2001). 'Exercise and multiple sclerosis: physiological, psychological, and quality of life issues'. *J Sports Med Phys Fitness*, 41 (4): 421–432.

Sutherland, G., Andersen, M.B. and Stoove, M.A. (2007). 'Can aerobic exercise training affect health-related quality of life for people with multiple sclerosis'. *J Sport Exerc Psych*, 23 (2): 122–135.

Tantucci, C., Massucci, M., Piperno, R., Grassi, V. and Sorbini, C.A. (1996). 'Energy cost of exercise in multiple sclerosis patients with low degree of disability'. *Mult Scler*, 2 (3): 161–167.

Taylor, N.F., Dodd, K.J., Prasad, D. and Denisenko, S. (2006). 'Progressive resistance exercise for people with multiple sclerosis'. *Disabil Rehabil*, 28 (18): 1119–1126.

Thoumie, P. and Mevellec, E. (2002). 'Relation between walking speed and muscle strength is affected by somatosensory loss in multiple sclerosis'. *J Neurol Neurosurg Psychiatry*, 73 (3): 313–315.

van den Berg, M., Dawes, H., Wade, D.T., Newman, M., Burridge, J., Izadi, H. and Sackley, C.M. (2006). 'Treadmill training for individuals with multiple sclerosis: a pilot randomised trial'. *J Neurol Neurosurg Psychiatry*, 77 (4): 531–533.

White, A.T., Wilson, T.E., Davis, S.L. and Petajan, J.H. (2000). 'Effect of precooling on physical performance in multiple sclerosis'. *Mult Scler*, 6 (3): 176–180.

White, L.J. and Dressendorfer, R.H. (2004). 'Exercise and multiple sclerosis'. *Sports Med*, 34 (15): 1077–1100.

White, L.J., McCoy, S.C., Castellano, V., Gutierrez, G., Stevens, J.E., Walter, G.A. and Vandenborne, K. (2004). 'Resistance training improves strength and functional capacity in persons with multiple sclerosis'. *Mult Scler*, 10 (6): 668–674.

White, L.J., Castellano, V. and McCoy, S.C. 'Cytokine responses to resistance training in people with multiple sclerosis'. *J Sports Sci*, 24 (8): 911–914.

13

PARKINSON DISEASE

Gammon M. Earhart

Introduction

Parkinson disease (PD) is a progressive, neurodegenerative disease that affects between 1 and 2 percent of individuals over 65 years of age and 3–5 percent of those aged 85 or older (Fahn, 2003). PD is the second most common neurodegenerative disorder after Alzheimer's disease. Currently, approximately six million people are affected by PD worldwide (Viartis, 2008). PD was originally attributed to neuronal loss within the substantia nigra pars compacta, and a concomitant loss of dopamine. PD is now thought to be a multi-system disorder that involves not only the dopaminergic system, but other neurotransmitter systems, whose role may become more prominent as the disease progresses (Perry *et al.*, 1991). There are four cardinal features of PD: rest tremor, rigidity, bradykinesia and postural instability, all of which are motor symptoms. However, PD also may include any combination of a myriad of non-motor symptoms including autonomic disruptions, orthostatic hypotension, sweating dysfunction, pain, sensory symptoms, cognitive changes, sleep disorders, fatigue, loss of motivation, anxiety and depression (Fahn, 2003). Both motor and non-motor aspects of PD may impact upon the ability of those with PD to participate in exercise and/or the effects that exercise might have on those with PD.

Exercise and primary prevention

Emerging evidence suggests that greater levels of physical activity may be associated with a reduced risk of developing PD (Thacker *et al.*, 2008). The relative risk of developing PD among individuals who regularly exercised moderately, compared to those who did no exercise, was reduced by 40 percent. Moderate exercise was defined as ≥ 16 MET-h/wk for men and ≥ 11.5 MET-h/wk for women and included activities like cycling, swimming, jogging/running, tennis and aerobics. Light physical activity, which included walking and dancing, was not associated with a reduced risk of PD. Evidence from animal models of PD also suggests that exercise can have neuroprotective effects. In 2001, Tillerson *et al.* demonstrated a decrease in the extent of dopamine terminal degeneration in a toxin-induced rat model of parkinsonism as a result of forced use of the affected limb. The following year, they reported that forced non-use of the affected limb exacerbated neuronal degeneration (Tillerson *et al.*, 2002). The suggestions that physical activity may be protective and that physical inactivity might potentiate neuronal loss were groundbreaking. Since this time, additional studies of exercise effects on animals have yielded mixed results. Some demonstrate neuroprotective effects from exercise (Mabandla *et al.*, 2004; Faherty *et al.*, 2005; Howells *et al.*, 2005; Yoon *et al.*, 2007), while others demonstrate enhancement of physical function with no evidence of neuroprotection (Al-Jarrah *et al.*, 2007; O'Dell *et al.*, 2007). There are, to date, no definitive studies that examine whether or not exercise in humans with PD has a neuroprotective effect, though several trials are underway that will attempt to determine whether exercise modifies disease progression. This chapter reviews what is presently known about the effects of exercise on physical function, disease severity and quality of life in PD and provides evidence-based recommendations regarding the design and delivery of exercise programmes for individuals with PD.

Current evidence regarding exercise effects in PD

While it is currently unclear whether or not exercise can have disease-modifying effects, there is much evidence in the literature documenting the benefits of exercise with respect to general physical function and disease-specific measures. Most studies of exercise to date have focused on relatively small groups of individuals with mild to moderate disease (Hoehn & Yahr stages 1–3) and have examined short-term interventions. In addition, nearly all exercise studies have tested individuals in their fully medicated state and, as such, the effects of exercise on PD may be confounded by the potential masking of symptoms by medications. Very few studies have employed large samples or examined the long-term effects of exercise, and there is a clear need for additional long-term research with large samples that are tested off medication. The section that follows describes the evidence for the effects of exercise on general physical function, with a focus on gait, balance and falls, activities of daily living (ADLs) and depression among people with PD. The subsequent section describes the evidence for the effects of exercise on disease-specific symptoms such as disease severity, the cardinal symptoms of PD and health-related quality of life. Figure 13.1 shows average effect sizes for several of the measures discussed in the following paragraphs.

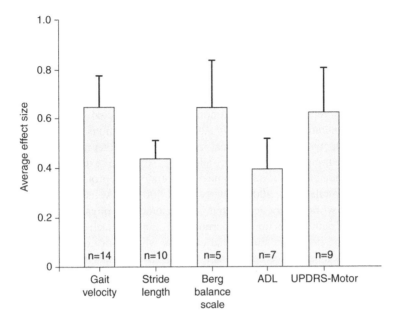

FIGURE 13.1 Average effect sizes (± SEs) obtained via review of the literature on the effects of exercise on various symptoms of PD. Values of n reported in the lower portion of each bar denote the number of studies used to obtain each average.

Effects of exercise on functional outcomes in PD

Gait

Among all the effects of exercise on function in PD, the benefits to gait are arguably the most well-substantiated by the literature (Figure 13.1). Parkinsonian gait is characterized by short, shuffling steps and reduced gait velocity, both of which can be improved with exercise. Summary effect sizes for stride length and gait velocity as assessed by de Goede *et al.* (2001) were 0.46 and 0.49, respectively. Effect sizes for gait velocity may actually be even larger, with an average value of greater than 0.6 (Figure 13.1). Improvements in stride length and velocity have been noted following aerobic training, treadmill exercise training, physical therapy, multiple-task training, dance and Tai Chi. Some studies have suggested that treadmill exercise training may be superior to conventional approaches for improving gait in PD (Miyai *et al.*, 2000, 2002). Gains noted with treadmill exercise training could be attributed to several different mechanisms including cardiopulmonary adaptations, walking pace retraining (with the treadmill serving as an external pacemaker), enhancements in corticomotor excitability (Fisher *et al.*, 2008) and motor learning. For a more thorough discussion please see Herman *et al.* (2009).

Freezing, defined as 'an episodic inability (lasting seconds) to generate effective stepping' (Giladi and Nieuwboer, 2008), is another aspect of gait performance in PD that may be addressed via exercise. However, evidence regarding the effects of exercise on freezing is limited. A physical therapy programme focused on improving balance, postural control, walking and learning new strategies to overcome freezing resulted in significant improvements in freezing as assessed by the Freezing of Gait questionnaire (Brichetto *et al.*, 2006). Small but significant reductions in freezing were also noted following a three-week home-based exercise programme that incorporated gait training using external cues (Nieuwboer *et al.*, 2007). However, the effects were greatly reduced at the 6-week follow-up. Small, non-significant improvements in freezing were also noted following participation in traditional exercise classes or tango dance classes (Hackney *et al.*, 2007). Freezing during turning may be reduced immediately following a period of walking on a rotating treadmill (Hong and Earhart, 2008).

Balance and falls

A review of the literature revealed moderate evidence to support the beneficial effects of exercise on balance in PD (Figure 13.1). Many studies have noted significant improvements in balance tasks following exercise (for review see Goodwin *et al.*, 2008; Dibble *et al.*, 2009a). Improvements have been noted in the Berg Balance Scale, Functional Reach Test, Timed Up and Go, Tinetti Balance Assessment Tool, computerized posturography and other measures. These improvements have followed a variety of interventions including treadmill exercise training, resistance exercise training, dance, Tai Chi, whole body vibration and exercises specifically targeted to train balance.

Despite moderate evidence for the benefits of exercise on balance, there is limited information regarding the effects of exercise on falls in PD. Two studies have examined number of falls before and after exercise, with neither reporting a significant change (Protas *et al.*, 2005; Ashburn *et al.*, 2007). However, one study did report a significant reduction in near-falls after exercise, as assessed by a falls diary (Ashburn *et al.*, 2007).

Activities of daily living

Individual studies show mixed results with respect to the effectiveness of exercise in improving ADLs. However, a meta-analysis suggests that exercise can convey improvements in ADLs, with a summary effect size across seven studies being 0.40 (de Goede *et al.*, 2001; Figure 13.1). Significant improvements assessed by the ADL section of the Unified Parkinson Disease Rating Scale (UPDRS) have been recently noted following intensive inpatient rehabilitation (Ellis *et al.*, 2008). To improve ADLs, it has been recommended that functionally meaningful tasks be trained and that the training take place in the home environment of the patient (Kwakkel *et al.*, 2007). The effects of exercise are likely task- and perhaps even context-specific and as such the tasks trained may not generalize to related activities or to contexts that are not directly trained.

Depression

Depression is more common in individuals with PD than in those without and the effects of exercise on depression in PD have been investigated in a few studies. No randomized, controlled studies to date have reported significant improvements in depression as a result of exercise (Goodwin *et al.*, 2008; Tanaka *et al.*, 2009). These studies, however, looked at exercise periods of two months or less. In contrast, one open long-term rehabilitation trial of 20 weeks duration reported significant improvements in depression following physical rehabilitation (Pellecchia *et al.*, 2004).

Effects of exercise on disease-specific outcomes in PD

Disease severity

Disease severity is most often assessed using the UPDRS (Goetz *et al.*, 2007). The UPDRS includes four separate scales for nonomotor (scale I) and motor (scale II) experiences of daily living, motor examination (scale III) and motor complications (scale IV). These individual scales can be summed to obtain a total score, or used individually to obtain sub-scores. Sub-scores on the UPDRS-III motor examination are often reported as an outcome measure in studies examining the effects of exercise in those with PD (Figure 13.1). While many studies have reported improvements in UPDRS total or motor scores with exercise, many others have not (for review see Kwakkel *et al.*, 2007). The summary effect size across several studies of physical therapy programmes was 0.22 and was not statistically significant (de Goede *et al.*, 2001). However, more recent studies evaluating treadmill training suggest that aerobic exercise may improve UPDRS scores (Toole *et al.*, 2005; Herman *et al.*, 2007; Skidmore *et al.*, 2008; Fisher *et al.*, 2008; Schenkman *et al.*, 2008).

Many of the significant changes reported in UPDRS in the literature are smaller than the minimal clinically important change of five points in the motor score for individuals in Hoehn & Yahr stages 1–3 (Schrag *et al.*, 2006). Some studies, however, do report changes larger than the minimal clinically important change (Herman *et al.*, 2007). A limitation of most exercise studies is that patients have been tested on medications, which, as noted previously, may mask or ameliorate many of the symptoms of PD, and, may thus reduce the magnitude of change noted on the UPDRS with exercise. In addition, the majority of exercise studies have spanned relatively short intervals of time, i.e. six months or less, and very few have examined UPDRS scores over longer periods which may be more indicative of disease progression. There is currently no definitive evidence to suggest that exercise modifies disease progression, but there are many randomized controlled studies of exercise underway that will hopefully soon provide additional information in this regard (Keus *et al.*, 2009).

Cardinal symptoms of PD

With respect to the four cardinal symptoms of PD, there is little or no evidence to support the effects of habitual exercise on resting tremor or rigidity, but more evidence to support exercise training effects on bradykinesia and postural instability. No studies have reported any changes in tremor as a result of exercise training. One study noted improved rigidity in a group of 16 people with PD following a program of physical therapy, which included stretching exercises intended to address rigidity, as well as many other components to address balance, gait and functional mobility (Pacchetti *et al.*, 2000). However, another study of range of motion exercises noted no change in rigidity (Hurwitz, 1989). Few studies have addressed the effects of exercise on bradykinesia specifically, but several studies report increased speed of movement as assessed via functional tasks such as moving from sit to stand, ascending and descending stairs or gait. A cued, task-specific exercise training programme, as well as a conventional exercise programme, increased peak velocities of movement and decreased movement time during sit to stand (Mak and Hui-Chan, 2008). Faster performance on sit to stand timed tests and on stair climbing has also consistently been reported following resistance exercise training (for review see Falvo *et al.*, 2008). There is moderate evidence to indicate that exercise can improve gait speed, as noted in the previous section on gait. Improvements in gait speed have been noted following a variety of interventions including treadmill exercise training, cued gait training, resistance exercise training and multi-faceted physical therapy programmes (for reviews see Goodwin *et al.*, 2008; Kwakkel *et al.*, 2007; de Goede *et al.*, 2001).

A recent systematic review provided moderate evidence that habitual exercise can result in improvements in postural instability. This is distinct from improvements in performance on balance tasks. The International Classification of Functioning, Disability and Health (ICF), a framework for the description of health and health-related states published by the World Health Organization (WHO, 2002), categorizes balance tasks as Activity, whereas postural instability is in the Body Structure and Function category (Dibble *et al.*, 2009a). The most commonly used assessment tool for postural instability in randomized controlled trials is the Sensory Organization Test (SOT). Improvements in SOT performance have been noted following treadmill exercise training (Toole *et al.*, 2005) and balance training combined with high-intensity resistance exercise (Hirsch *et al.*, 2003).

Quality of life

A synthesis of evidence across studies suggests that quality of life (QoL) may improve with exercise, with an estimated standardized effect size of 0.27 (Goodwin *et al.*, 2008). Once again, however, evidence is mixed and various outcome measures are used to assess QoL. These measures include PD-specific tools like the PDQ-39 and generic tools like the Sickness Impact Profile (SIP) and EuroQOL (EQ-5D). Significant improvements in QoL as assessed by PD-specific tools have been reported following treadmill exercise training (Herman *et al.*, 2007), dance (Hackney and Earhart, 2009c), physical therapy (Brichetto *et al.*, 2006; Pellecchia *et al.*, 2004), Nordic pole walking (van Eijkeren *et al.*, 2008) and resistance exercise (Dibble *et al.*, 2009b). Improvements in QoL, as assessed by generic tools, have been reported following physical therapy (Ellis *et al.*, 2008) and group aerobic and strengthening exercise (Rodrigues de Paula *et al.*, 2006).

Structuring an exercise programme for people with PD

In designing an exercise programme for an individual with PD, there are several factors to consider. These should include the goals of the individual, his or her current fitness level, medications and comorbid conditions. Exercise is best implemented when participants are in the 'on' state, i.e. at a time when their medications are working well. Current formal recommendations for exercise in those with PD include incorporation of: 1) dynamic balance activities, 2) teaching and practice of specific movement strategies for functional tasks, 3) training for joint mobility and muscle power, and 4) the use of external cues (Keus *et al.*, 2007). In addition, one should consider incorporating aerobic exercise in a programme for individuals with PD. This section reviews the evidence regarding the effects of specific modes of exercise in PD and provides evidence-based recommendations for the design and delivery of such programmes. Consideration is given to traditional exercise approaches, such as aerobic exercise and resistance training, as well as alternative approaches such as dance and Tai Chi.

Aerobic exercise

Documented beneficial effects of aerobic exercise for individuals with PD include improved exercise capacity, UPDRS scores, ADLs, balance and QoL. While there are many forms of aerobic exercise, including cycling, walking/running, swimming, tennis/racquetball and aerobics/calisthenics, the majority of studies to date have employed treadmill exercise training as the form of aerobic exercise intervention (for review see Herman *et al.*, 2009). In contrast, there are no studies to date that have examined the effects of swimming on PD. Given the preponderance of treadmill exercise training studies, it is difficult to separate the effects of aerobic exercise from the effects of treadmill exercise. However, considering the multiple beneficial effects of treadmill exercise training that have been documented, the use of treadmill training seems quite appropriate for individuals with PD. Treadmill exercise training has been shown to be feasible, safe and efficacious with respect to disease severity QoL and gait with carry-over of effects demonstrated several weeks or months after the cessation of training (Miyai *et al.*, 2002; Pelosin *et al.*, 2007;

Herman *et al.*, 2007). Evidence suggests that individuals with PD can tolerate high intensity treadmill exercise training (Fisher *et al.*, 2008) but should be closely monitored for autonomic function (Skidmore *et al.*, 2008). Innappropriate candidates would include individuals with uncontrolled cardiac conditions or who those are unable to walk (with or without assistance). It is not necessary to unload the patient with a body weight support device, but a harness used simply to aid in the prevention of falls is advisable. A treadmill exercise training programme, or other aerobic exercise programme, should include a minimum of three sessions per week and each session should be at least 30 minutes in duration. The Centers for Disease Control and Prevention (CDC) advises that healthy older adults should aim for 150 minutes per week of moderate intensity or 75 minutes per week of vigorous intensity aerobic exercise (CDC, 2008). These recommendations are also likely to be appropriate for people with PD.

Resistance exercise training

Skeletal muscle weakness may be a secondary cause of bradykinesia (Berardelli *et al.*, 2001) and/or a primary symptom of PD (Kakinuma *et al.*, 1998). In addition, skeletal muscle weakness is a contributing factor to postural instability (Nallegowda *et al.*, 2004). As such, resistance exercise should be included in the management of PD as there is sufficient evidence in the literature to support the beneficial effects of the exercise modality (Goodwin *et al.*, 2008). To date, most approaches to resistance exercise for PD have been relatively conservative compared to recommendations for resistance exercise prescription in healthy older adults. While the evidence is limited, those with PD appear to be able to tolerate high intensity resistance exercise (Dibble *et al.*, 2006, 2009b) and demonstrate strength gains similar to those of age-matched individuals without PD (Scandalis *et al.*, 2001). As noted earlier in the chapter, resistance exercise has also been associated with improvements in quality of life, gait, balance and functional mobility. Specifically, improvements have been noted in six-minute walk distance, navigating stairs and moving from sit to stand. Resistance exercise training may also be associated with reduced oxidative stress in people with PD (Bloomer *et al.*, 2008), which could have implications for disease modification as oxidative stress has been implicated in the death of substantia nigra neurons in PD (Henchcliffe and Beal, 2008; Schapira, 2008). Future clinical investigations should further investigate the impact of high intensity resistance exercise and clinicians/health professionals should ensure that they prescribe exercise of sufficient intensity to promote optimal strength gains and functionally meaningful improvements.

Current recommendations for resistance exercise in individuals with PD are lacking, but recommendations for healthy older adults are available. These include an exercise training frequency of 2–3 times per week, a repetition maximum (RM) loading range of 8–12 RM, and 3-minute rest intervals for novice exercisers. More advanced exercisers should increase the frequency to 4–5 times per week with an eventual emphasis on a 1–6 RM loading range and rest intervals held constant (Falvo *et al.*, 2008). The appropriateness of these recommendations for individuals with PD has yet to be established, but available evidence to date suggests that these guidelines should be feasible for people with PD. However, careful attention should be paid to the development and management of fatigue in this population.

Balance training

Exercise training has been observed to improve performance on many different balance tests as noted earlier in the chapter (Dibble *et al.*, 2009a). A broad variety of approaches can be taken to improve balance performance. For example, treadmill exercise training can impart improved balance performance, as can resistance exercise, though these interventions may not be specifically designed to target balance but instead may be primarily targeting gait or muscle strength, respectively. Balance-specific approaches in the literature are rare, as most studies reporting improved balance examined multi-faceted approaches that included balance exercises along with other strategies in a comprehensive physical therapy intervention. The lack of task-specific exercise training in balance studies may be related to our limited understanding of the mechanisms underlying postural instability in PD. A synthesis of the literature suggests that some physical activity or exercise, regardless of whether it is specifically focused on improving balance, can promote enhanced balance performance in individuals with mild to moderate PD. However, advances in the area of task-specific balance training may lead to targeted interventions that are more successful than general physical activity at improving balance. Specific recommendations about the dose of balance therapy needed to evoke positive changes are lacking. Randomized, controlled studies have ranged from 3–12 weeks, with 2–10 sessions per week and a total of 6–24 hours of intervention (Dibble *et al.*, 2009a). Once again, it is likely that individuals with PD can tolerate intense balance training programmes similar to those implemented for healthy elderly individuals.

Alternative exercise approaches

Dance is an alternative approach to exercise that may be ideally suited to those with PD, as it can address each of the key areas that have been recently identified by Keus *et al.* (2007) as being important for exercise programme design in this patient group. Dance is an activity performed to music which can provide an external cue to facilitate movement, thus addressing the first recommended component which is the use of external cues. In addition, dance involves the teaching and practice of specific movement strategies, the second recommended component of a PD-specific exercise programme. Dance also incorporates dynamic balance challenges, the third recommended component, as participants must respond to continual changes in the environment. Finally, dance can result in improved cardiovascular function, a testament to the fact that, if done with sufficient intensity, dance is an excellent form of aerobic exercise (Belardinelli *et al.*, 2008; Peidro *et al.*, 2002). Several studies have now reported significant improvements in balance, six-minute walk distance and gait velocity in groups with PD who participated in Argentine tango or waltz/foxtrot classes (Hackney *et al.*, 2007; Hackney and Earhart, 2009a, 2009b). Two studies have also noted improvements in QoL with dance (Westheimer, 2007; Hackney and Earhart, 2009c). For a comprehensive review of the literature regarding dance and PD please see Earhart (2009). While improvements have been seen with as little as 15 hours of dance within a two-week period, evidence suggests that longer interventions (10–13 weeks) convey greater benefits. More work is needed to determine the optimal schedule for dance programmes but guidelines derived from the available literature suggest a frequency of 2–3 times per week for 1–1.5 hours per session. Dance sessions should ideally be sufficiently intense to elevate heart rate to the levels discussed previously for aerobic exercise. In addition, special consideration should be given to the instruction of the dance classes, as the individual(s) leading the class must be knowledgeable regarding PD and be able to work within the movement abilities of participants.

Tai Chi is another alternative exercise approach that has been examined in several studies with mixed results (for review see Lee *et al.*, 2008). Results have been varied with regard to UPDRS scores, gait and QoL, with some studies reporting improvements and others demonstrating no change in these measures. Only two studies to date have specifically reported balance outcomes, and both noted reduced falls or improved balance (Marjama-Lyons *et al.*, 2002; Hackney and Earhart, 2008). Many of the Tai Chi studies are limited by a small sample size and some also lack a control group. It is also unclear whether Tai Chi is superior to traditional exercise, as one study found no differences between a conventional exercise group and a Tai Chi group (Cheon *et al.*, 2006). There are no studies to date that have examined the effects of yoga on PD.

Additional considerations

In addition to the approaches outlined above, there are many exercise programmes available that have been designed specifically for people with PD (Argue, 2000; Hamburg, 2003; Cianci, 2006; Zid, 2007) but these have yet to be rigorously tested to determine their efficacy. Newly emerging programmes focus on constrain-focused agility exercise for people with PD (King and Horak, 2009). Programmes such as this offer a strong scientific framework and include principles that can be incorporated into ongoing, long-term exercise programmes designed to delay mobility disability. A programme of this type may include task-specific agility exercise to drive neuroplasticity and exercise to reduce mobility constraints. Specific constraints that can be targeted include rigidity, bradykinesia, freezing, inflexible selection of motor programmes, impaired sensory integration and reduced executive function and attention. The principles focus on self-initiated movement, big and quick movements, large and flexible centre of mass control, reciprocal and coordinated arm and leg movements, and rotational movement of the torso over pelvis and pelvis over legs. Movements from Tai Chi, kayaking, boxing, lunges, agility training and Pilates can be included. Programmes of this nature, with a constraint-specific approach, are just being developed and have yet to be implemented and tested.

In addition to exercise, consideration should also be given to the use of cues during exercise training and to the teaching of movement strategies. A complete review of cueing and movement strategy instruction is beyond the scope of this chapter, as these techniques are not forms of exercise but are techniques that may be employed along with exercise to enhance functional gains. However, it is noteworthy that exercise incorporating cues has been shown to improve gait (Sidaway *et al.*, 2006), timed balance tests and balance confidence (Nieuwboer *et al.*, 2007). The use of cues and teaching of movement strategies is supported by the literature and has been recommended by the Practice Recommendations Development Group. Please see Keus *et al.* (2007) for a more complete discussion of these issues. Several reviews are also available that cover the use of external cues in greater detail (Nieuwboer, 2008; Lim *et al.*, 2005; Rubinstein *et al.*, 2002).

Adherence/maintenance

As with any population, those with PD need to continue exercising to maintain the benefits obtained. Some studies have demonstrated carry-over of exercise effects for several weeks following completion of an exercise intervention (Herman *et al.*, 2007; Hackney and Earhart, 2010). However, little is known about the longer-term effects of exercise and the appropriate maintenance schedules needed to maintain benefits. Numerous reviews of the literature cite this lack of information about long-term effects of exercise and the need to better understand exercise dose-response relationships (Crizzle and Newhouse, 2006; Kwakkel *et al.*, 2007; Goodwin *et al.*, 2008). As longer-term studies are implemented, promoting participation and adherence to exercise will be critical. Exercise programmes that are done in a group setting may enhance motivation of participants and encourage them to continue participating over long periods of time (O'Brien *et al.*, 2008). In addition, programmes that are community based and geographically convenient for participants are more likely to promote adherence. Finally, consideration should be given to developing programmes that provide exercise opportunities for people with PD and their caregivers alike to maximize benefits to both groups and enhance motivation to continue.

Summary and conclusions

Current evidence suggests that exercise may be beneficial for improving gait, balance, strength, activities of daily living and quality of life in individuals with

PD. There is currently not sufficient evidence to support the benefits of exercise on falls, depression or modification of the disease process. There is also a lack of information about the effects of exercise on individuals in different disease stages, as most studies to date have focused on individuals in Hoehn & Yahr stages 1–3, with a preponderance of participants in stage 2. As exercise has moved to the forefront as an area ripe for research in PD, there are currently several long-term randomized controlled trials underway. As such, much more will likely be learned about the effects of exercise on PD health outcomes in the coming years. In the interim, there is sufficient evidence to support the inclusion of exercise as a key component in the management of PD. Exercise programmes designed for individuals with PD should ideally include components that address aerobic training, resistance training, balance training and gait training. Exercise training programmes should be implemented at intensities similar to those for individuals of similar age without PD, but with close monitoring for development of fatigue and to ensure the safety of participants, in order to optimize benefits. Long-term involvement in exercise, and involvement from the early stages of the disease, should be encouraged to optimize and maintain function as much as possible in the face of this progressive disease.

References

Al-Jarrah, M., Pothaskos, K., Novikova, L., Smirnova, I. V., Kurz, M. J., Stehno-Bittel, L. and Lau, Y. S. (2007). Endurance exercise promotes cardiorespiratory rehabilitation without neurorestoration in the chronic mouse model of parkinsonism with severe neurodegeneration. *Neuroscience*, 149(1), 28–37.

Argue, J. (2000). *Parkinson's Disease and the Art of Moving.* Oakland, CA: New Harbinger Publications.

Ashburn, A. Fazakarley, L., Ballinger, C., Pickering, R., McLellan, L. D. and Fitton, C. (2007). A randomised control trial of a home based exercise programme to reduce the risk of falling among people with Parkinson's disease. *Journal of Neurology, Neurosurgery, and Psychiatry*, 78(7), 678–684.

Belardinelli, R., Lacalaprice, F., Ventralla, C., Volpe, L. and Faccenda, E. (2008). Waltz dancing in patients with chronic heart failure: a new form of exercise training. *Circulation: Heart Failure*, 1, 107–114. Available at: http://circheartfailure.ahajournals. org/cgi/content/short/1/2/107. [Accessed 26 May 2009].

Berardelli, A., Rothwell, J. C., Thompson, P. D. and Hallett, M. (2001). Pathophysiology of bradykinesia in Parkinson's disease. *Brain*, 124(11), 2131–2146.

Bloomer, R. J., Schilling, B. K., Karlage, R. E., Ledoux, M. S., Pfeiffer, R. F. and Callegari, J. (2008). Effect of resistance training on blood oxidative stress in Parkinson's disease. *Medicine and Science in Sports Exercise*, 40(8), 1385–1389.

Brichetto, G., Pelosin, E., Marchese, R. and Abbruzzese, G. (2006). Evaluation of physical therapy in parkinsonian patients with freezing of gait: a pilot study. *Clinical Rehabilitation*, 20(1), 31–35.

Centers for Disease Control and Prevention (CDC) (2008). *How much physical activity do adults need?* Available at: http://www.cdc.gov/physicalactivity/everyone/guidelines/ adults.html. [Accessed 28 July 2009].

Cheon, S. M., Sung, H. R., Ha, M. S. and Kim, J. W. (2006). Tai Chi for physical and mental health of patients with Parkinson's disease. In: *Proceedings of the first international conference of tai chi for health*. Seoul, Republic of Korea, 68 (abstract).

Cianci, H. (2006). *Parkinson's Disease: Fitness Counts*. 3rd edn. Miami, FL: National Parkinson Foundation.

Crizzle, A. M. and Newhouse, I. J. (2006). Is physical exercise beneficial for persons with Parkinson's disease? *Clinical Journal of Sport Medicine*, 16(5), 422–425.

de Goede, C. J. T., Keus, S., Kwakkel, G. and Wagenaar, R. C. (2001). The effects of physical therapy in Parkinson's disease: a research synthesis. *Archives of Physical Medicine and Rehabilitation*, 82, 509–515.

Dibble, L. E., Hale, T. F., Marcus, R. L., Droge, J., Gerber, J. P. and LaStayo, P. C. (2006). High-intensity resistance training amplifies muscle hypertrophy and functional gains in persons with Parkinson's disease. *Movement Disorders*, 21(9), 1444–1452.

Dibble, L. E. Addison, O. and Papa, E. (2009a). The effect of exercise on balance in persons with Parkinson's disease: a systematic review across the disability spectrum. *Journal of Neurologic Physical Therapy*, 33(1), 14–26.

Dibble, L. E., Hale, T. F., Marcus, R. L., Gerber, J. P. and LaStayo, P. C. (2009b). High intensity eccentric resistance training decreases bradykinesia and improves quality of life in person with Parkinson's disease: A preliminary study. *Parkinsonism Relat Disord*, 15(10), 752–757.

Earhart, G. M. (2009). Dance as therapy for individuals with Parkinson disease. *European Journal of Physical Rehabil Med*, 45(2), 231–238.

Ellis, T., Katz, D. I., White, D. K., DePiero, T. J., Hohler, A. D., Saint-Hillaire, M. (2008). Effectiveness of an inpatient multidisciplinary rehabilitation program for people with Parkinson's disease. *Physical Therapy*, 88(7), 577–583.

Faherty, C. J., Raviie Shepherd K., Herasimtschuk, A. and Smeyne, R. J. (2005). Environmental enrichment in adulthood eliminates neuronal death in experimental Parkinsonism. *Brain Research: Molecular Brain Research*, 134(1), 170–179.

Fahn, S. (2003). Description of Parkinson's disease as a clinical syndrome. *Annals of the New York Academy of Science*, 991, 1–14.

Falvo, M. J., Schilling, B. K. and Earhart, G. M. (2008). Parkinson's disease and resistive exercise: rationale, review, and recommendations. *Movement Disorders*, 23(1), 1–11.

Fisher, B. E., Wu, A. D., Salem, G. J. Song, J., Lin, C.-H., Yip, J., Cen, S., Gordon, J., Jakowec, M. and Petzinger, G. (2008). The effect of exercise training in improving motor performance and corticomotor excitability in people with early Parkinson's disease. *Archives of Physical Medicine and Rehabilitation*, 89(7), 1221–1229.

Giladi, N. and Nieuwboer, A. (2008). Understanding and treating freezing of gait in parkinsonism, proposed working definition, and setting the stage. *Movement Disorders*, 23(S2), S423–S425.

Goetz, C. G., Fahn, S., Martinez-Martin, P., Poewe, W., Sampaio, C., Stebbins, G. T., Stern, M. B., Tilley, B. C., Dodel, R., Dubois, B., Holloway, R., Jankovic, J., Kulisevsky, J., Lang, A. E., Lees, A., Leurgans, S., LeWitt, P. A., Nyenhuis, D., Olanow, C. W., Rascol, O., Schrag, A., Teresi, J. A., Van Hilten, J. J. and LaPelle, N. (2007). Movement Disorder Society-sponsored revision of the Unified Parkinson's Disease Rating Scale (MDS-UPDRS): Process, format, and clinimetric testing plan. *Movement Disorders*, 22(1), 41–47.

Goodwin, V. A., Richards, S. H., Taylor, R. S., Taylor, A. H. and Campbell, J. L. (2008). The effectiveness of exercise intervention for people with Parkinson's disease: a systematic review and meta-analysis. *Movement Disorders*, 23(5), 631–640.

Hackney, M. E., Kantorovich, S., Levin, R. and Earhart, G. M. (2007). Effects of tango on functional mobility in Parkinson's disease: a preliminary study. *Journal of Neurologic Physical Therapy*, 31(4), 173–179.

Hackney, M. E. and Earhart, G. M. (2008). Tai Chi improves balance and mobility in people with Parkinson disease. *Gait and Posture*, 28, 456–460.

Hackney, M. E. and Earhart, G. M. (2009a). Effects of dance on movement control in Parkinson's disease: a comparison of Argentine tango and American ballroom. *Journal of Rehabiliation Medicine*, 41(6), 475–481.

Hackney, M. E. and Earhart, G. M. (2009b). Short duration, intensive tango dancing for Parkinson disease: an uncontrolled pilot study. *Complementary Therapies in Medicine*, 17(4), 203–207.

Hackney, M. E. and Earhart, G. M. (2009c). Alternative forms of exercise and health-related quality of life in Parkinson disease. *Parkinsonism and Related Disorders*, 15(9), 644–648.

Hackney, M. E. and Earhart, G. M. (2010). Effects of dance on gait and balance in Parkinson disease: a comparison of partnered and non-partnered dance movement. *Neurorehabil Neural Repair*, 24(4), 384–392.

Hamburg, J. (2003). *Motivating Moves for People with Parkinson's Disease*. The Parkinson's Disease Foundation, New York City.

Henchcliffe, C. and Beal, M. F. (2008). Mitochondrial biology and oxidative stress in Parkinson disease pathogenesis. *Nature Clinical Practice Neurology*, 4(11), 600–609.

Herman, T., Giladi, N., Gruendlinger, L. and Hausdorff, J. M. (2007). Six weeks of intensive treadmill training improves gait and quality of life in patients with Parkinson's disease: a pilot study. *Archives of Physical Medicine and Rehabilitation*, 88(9), 1154–1158.

Herman, T., Giladi, N. and Hausdorff, J. M. (2009). Treadmill training for the treatment of gait disturbances in people with Parkinson's disease: a mini-review. *Journal of Neural Transmission*, 116, 307–318.

Hirsch, M. A., Toole, T., Maitland, C. G. and Rider, R. A. (2003). The effects of balance training and high-intensity resistance training on persons with idiopathic Parkinson's disease. *Archives of Physical Medicine and Rehabilitation*, 84(8), 1109–1117.

Hong, M. and Earhart, G. M. (2008). Rotating treadmill training reduces freezing in Parkinson disease: preliminary observations. *Parkinsonism and Related Disorders*, 14(4), 359–363.

Howells, F. M., Russell, V. A., Mabandla, M. V. and Kellaway, L. A. (2005). Stress reduces the neuroprotective effect of exercise in a rat model for Parkinson's disease. *Behavioural Brain Research*, 165(2), 210–220.

Hurwitz, A. (1989). The benefit of a home exercise program for ambulatory Parkinson's disease patients. *Journal of Neuroscience Nursing*, 21(3), 180–184.

Kakinuma, S., Nogaki, H., Pramanik, B. and Morimatsu, M. (1998). Muscle weakness in Parkinson's disease: isokinetic study of the lower limbs. *European Neurology*, 39(4), 218–222.

Keus, S. H., Bloem, B. R., Hendriks, E. J., Bredero-Cohen, A. B. and Munneke, M. (2007). Practice Recommendations Development Group. Evidence-based analysis of physical therapy in Parkinson's disease with recommendations for practice and research. *Movement Disorders*, 22(4), 451–460.

King, L. A. and Horak, F. B. (2009). Delaying mobility disability in people with Parkinson's disease using a sensorimotor agility exercise program. *Physical Therapy*, 89(4), 384–393.

Kwakkel, G., de Goede, C. J. T. and van Wegen, E. E. H. (2007). Impact of physical therapy for Parkinson's disease: a critical review of the literature. *Parkinsonism and Related Disorders*, 13, S478–S487.

Lee, M. S., Lam, P. and Ernst, E. (2008). Effectiveness of tai chi for Parkinson's disease: A critical review. *Parkinsonism and Related Disorders*, 14, 589–594.

Lim, I., van Wegen, E., de Goede, C., Deutekom, M., Nieuwboer, A., Willems, A., Jones, D., Rochester, L. and Kwakkel, G. (2005). Effects of external rhythmical cueing on gait in patients with Parkinson's disease: a systematic review. *Clinical Rehabilitation*, 19(7), 695–713.

Mabandla, M., Kellaway, L., St Clair Gibson, A. and Russell, V. A. (2004) Voluntary running provides neuroprotection in rats after 6-hydroxydopamine injection into the medial forebrain bundle. *Metabolic Brain Disease*, 19(1–2), 43–50.

Mak, M. K. and Hui-Chan, C. W. (2008). Cued task-specific training is better than exercise in improving sit-to-stand in patients with Parkinson's disease: a randomized controlled trial. *Movement Disorders*, 23(4), 501–509.

Marjama-Lyons, J., Smith, L., Myal, B., Nelson, J., Holliday, G. and Seracino, D. (2002). Tai Chi and reduced rate of falling in Parkinson's disease: a single blinded pilot study. *Movement Disorders*, 17, S70–S71.

Miyai, I., Fujimoto, Y., Ueda, Y., Yamamoto, H., Nozaki, S., Saito, T. and Kang, J. (2000) Treadmill training with body weight support: its effect on Parkinson's disease. *Archives of Physical Medicine and Rehabilitation*, 81(7), 849–852.

Miyai, I., Fujimoto, Y., Yamamoto, H., Ueda, Y., Saito, T., Nozaki, S. and Kang, J. (2002). Long-term effect of body weight-supported treadmill training in Parkinson's disease: a randomized controlled trial. *Archives of Physical Medicine and Rehabilitation*, 83(10), 1370–1373.

Nallegowda, M., Singh, U., Handa, G., Khanna, M., Wadhwa, S., Yadav, S. L., Kumar, G. and Behari, M. (2004). Role of sensory input and muscle strength in maintenance of balance, gait, and posture in Parkinson's disease: a pilot study. *American Journal of Physical Medicine and Rehabilitation*, 83(12), 898–908.

Nieuwboer, A. (2008). Cueing for freezing of gait in patients with Parkinson's disease: a rehabilitation perspective. *Movement Disorders*, 23(S2), S475–481.

Nieuwboer, A., Kwakkel, G., Rochester, L., Jones, D., van Wegen, E., Willems, A. M., Chavret, F., Hetherington, V., Baker, K. and Lim, I. (2007). Cueing training in the home improves gait-related mobility in Parkinson's disease: the RESCUE trial. *Journal of Neurology, Neurosurgery and Psychiatry*, 78(2), 134–140.

O'Brien, M., Dodd, K. J. and Bilney, B. (2008). A qualitative analysis of a progressive resistance exercise programme for people with Parkinson's disease. *Disability and Rehabilitation*, 30(18), 1350–1357.

O'Dell, S. J., Gross, N. B., Fricks, A. N., Casiano, B. D., Nguyen, T. B. and Marchall, J. F. (2007). Running wheel exercises enhances recovery from nigrostriatal dopamine injury without inducing neuroprotection. *Neuroscience*, 144, 1141–1151.

Pacchetti, C., Mancini, F., Aglieri, R., Fundaro, C., Martignoni, E. and Nappi, G. (2000). Active music therapy in Parkinson's disease: an integrative method for motor and emotional rehabilitation. *Psychosomatic Medicine*, 62(3), 386–393.

Pediro, R. M., Osses, J., Caneva, J., Brion, G., Angelino, A., Kerbage, S., Garcia, Ben M. and Pesce, R. (2002). Tango: modificaciones cardiorrespiratorias durante el baile. *Revista Argentina de Cardiologia*, 70, 358–363.

Pellecchia, M. T., Grasso, A., Biancardi, L. G., Squillante, M., Bonavita, V. and Barone, P. (2004). Physical therapy in Parkinson's disease: an open long-term rehabilitation trial. *Journal of Neurology*, 251(5), 595–598.

Pelosin, E., Faelli, E., Lofrano, F., Avanzino, L., Marinelli, L., Bove, M., Ruggeri, P. and Abbruzzese, G. (2007). Treadmill training improves functional ability and cardiopulmonary capacity in stable Parkinson's disease. *Movement Disorders*, 22(S16), S175.

Perry, E. K., McKeith, I., Thompson, P., Marshall, E., Kerwin, J., Jabeen, S., Edwardson, J. A., Ince, P., Blessed, G. and Irving, D. (1991). Topography, extent, and clinical relevance of neurochemical deficits in dementia of Lewy body type, Parkinson's disease, and Alzheimer's disease. *Annals of the New York Academy of Science*, 640, 197–202.

Protas, E. J., Mitchell, K., Williams, A., Qureshy, H., Caroline, K. and Lai, E. C. (2005). Gait and step training to reduce falls in Parkinson's disease. *Neurological Rehabilitation*, 20(3), 183–190.

Rodrigues de Paula, F., Teixeira-Salmela, L. F., Coehlo de Morais Faria, C. D., Rocha de Brito, P. and Cardoso, F. (2006). Impact of an exercise program on physical, emotional, and social aspects of quality of life of individuals with Parkinson's disease. *Movement Disorders*, 21(8), 1073–1077.

Rubinstein, T. C., Giladi, N. and Hausdorff, J. M. (2002). The power of cueing to circumvent dopamine deficits: a review of physical therapy treatment of gait disturbances in Parkinson's disease. *Movement Disorders*, 17(6), 1148–1160.

Scandalis, T. A., Bosak, A., Berliner, J. C., Helman, L. L. and Wells, M. R. (2001). Resistance training and gait function in patients with Parkinson's disease. *American Journal of Physical Medicine and Rehabilitation*, 80(1), 38–43.

Schapira, A. H. V. (2008). Mitochondria in the aetiology and pathogenesis of Parkinson's disease. *Lancet Neurology*, 7, 97–109.

Schenkman, M., Hall, D., Kumar, R. and Kohrt, W. M. (2008). Endurance exercise training to improve economy of movement of people with Parkinson's disease: three case reports. *Physical Therapy*, 88(1), 63–76.

Schrag, A., Scampino, C., Counsell, N. and Poewe, W. (2006). Minimal clinically important change on the unified Parkinson's disease rating scale. *Movement Disorders*, 21(8), 1200–1207.

Sidaway, B., Anderson, J., Danielson, G., Martin, L. and Smith, G. (2006). Effect of long-term gait training using visual cues in patients with Parkinson disease. *Physical Therapy*, 86(2), 186–194.

Skidmore, F. M., Patterson, S. L., Shulman, L. M., Sorkin, J. D. and Macko, R. F. (2008). Pilot safety and feasibility study of treadmill aerobic exercise in Parkinson's disease with gait impairment. *Journal of Rehabilitation Research and Development*, 45(1), 117–124.

Tanaka, K., Quadros, A. C. Jr, Santos, R. F., Stella, F., Gobbi, L. T. and Gobbi, S. (2009). Benefits of physical exercise on executive functions in older people with Parkinson's disease. *Brain and Cognition*, 69(2), 435–441.

Thacker, E. L., Chen, H., Patel, A. V., McCullough, M. L., Calle, E. E., Thun, M. J., Schwarzchild, M. A. and Ascherio, A. (2008). Recreational physical activity and risk of Parkinson's disease. *Movement Disorders*, 23(1), 69–74.

Tillerson, J. L., Cohen, A. D., Philhower, J., Miller, G. W., Zigmond, M. J. and Schallert, T. (2001). Forced limb-use effects on the behavioral and neurochemical effects of 6-hydroxydopamine. *Journal of Neuroscience*, 21(12), 4427–4435.

Tillerson, J. L., Cohen, A. D., Caudle, W. M., Zigmon, M. J., Schalelrt, T. and Miller, G. W. (2002). Forced nonuse in unilateral parkinsonian rats exacerbates injury. *Journal of Neuroscience*, 22(15), 6790–6799.

Toole, T., Maitland, C. G., Earl, W., Hubmann, M. F. and Lynn, P. (2005). The effects of loading and unloading treadmill walking on balance, gait, fall risk, and daily function in Parkinsonism. *NeuroRehabilitation*, 20(4), 307–322.

van Eijkeren, F. J., Reijmers, R. S., Kleinveld, M. J., Minten, A., Bruggen, J. P. and Bloem, B. R. (2008). Nordic walking improves mobility in Parkinson's disease. *Movement Disorders*, 23(15), 2239–2243.

Viartis. (2006–2009). *Prevalence of Parkinson's disease*. Available at: http://viartis.net/parkinsons.disease/prevalence.htm. [Accessed 2 March 2009].

Westheimer, O. (2008). Why dance for Parkinson's disease. *Topics in Geriatric Rehabilitation*, 24(2), 127–140.

World Health Organization (WHO) (2002). *Towards a common language for functioning, disability, and health. ICF*. Available at: http://www.who.int/classifications/icf/training/icfbeginnersguide.pdf. [Accessed 21 February 2010].

Yoon, M. C., Shin, M. S., Kim, T. S., Kim, B. K., Ko, I. G., Sung, Y. H., Kim, S. E., Lee, H. H., Kim, Y. P. and Kim, C. J. (2007). Treadmill exercise suppresses nigrostriatal dopamiergic neuronal loss in 6-hydroxydopamine-induced Parkinson's rats. *Neuroscience Letters*, 423(1), 12–17.

Zid, D. (2007). *Delay the Disease: Exercise and Parkinson's Disease*. Columbus, OH: Columbus Health Work Productions.

14

TYPE 2 DIABETES

Stephan F. E. Praet, Robert Rozenberg and Luc J. C. Van Loon

Introduction

Estimates of global diabetes prevalence and projections for the future indicate that diabetes prevalence will rise from 285 million today to more than 438 million by 2030 representing as much as 7.8 per cent of the global adult population (IDF 2009). This is already resulting in an increasing number of patients with pancreatic β-cell dysfunction who need exogenous insulin therapy at a relatively early stage in life (Detournay *et al.*, 2005). The latter implies that, also diabetes related complications, like retinopathy, neuropathy, myocardial infarction and stroke, will be experienced more frequently in the future. The increasing incidence of overt clinical complications in a vastly expanding diabetes population will impose an enormous burden on our healthcare system. Even though a genetic predisposition for pancreatic β-cell dysfunction may be present (Sladek *et al.*, 2007; Saxena *et al.*, 2007; Prokopenko *et al.*, 2009; Cauchi *et al.*, 2008), obesity and a sedentary lifestyle are both independently associated with diabetes and diabetes-related co-morbidities and considered to be the foundation of type 2 diabetes (Sullivan *et al.*, 2005; van Hoek *et al.*, 2008; Lyssenko and Groop, 2009).

Type 2 diabetes: metabolic stress leading to metabolic dysfunction

Metabolic stress: a chronic positive energy balance

The aetiology of insulin resistance and pancreatic β-cell dysfunction has been studied extensively and it has become clear that the key component in the development of type 2 diabetes is inactivity in combination with overeating. In energetic terms this means a chronic positive energy balance or from a physiological point of view chronic metabolic stress (Stumvoll *et al.*, 2005; Kahn *et al.*, 2006;

Eriksson, 2007). A persistent caloric overload will cause adipocyte 'overfilling' with triacylglycerol in mainly visceral adipose tissue, producing large and dysfunctional adipocytes. This adipocyte dysfunction is characterized by insulin resistance, impairing lipolysis and the ability to clear circulating triacylglycerol. This reduced buffering capacity for fatty acids results in a greater release of free fatty acids and glycerol from adipose tissue into the circulation. The impaired fat oxidative capacity is accompanied by a reduced ability to switch to glucose oxidation in type 2 diabetes, resulting in a state of reduced metabolic flexibility. Persistent high plasma free fatty acid and triacylglycerol levels lead to ectopic fat deposition in skeletal muscle (Boden and Chen, 1995; Boden, 1997) and liver tissue (Kabir *et al.*, 2005) inducing insulin resistance in these tissues and completing the 'downward spiral'.

Adipocyte dysfunction

Besides insulin resistance, adipocyte dysfunction is also associated with the release of adipokines (e.g. tumour necrosis factor α (TNF-α), interleukin-6 (IL-6), monocyte chemoattractant protein-1 (MCP-1), leptin, retinol binding protein-4 (RBP-4), etc.). These adipokines induce an inflammatory response of the adipose tissue. Inflammation of adipose tissue is regarded an important (etiological) factor in the pathogenesis of insulin resistance and its metabolic complications such as dyslipidemia, hypertension, and heart disease (Rasouli and Kern, 2008). Secretion of cytokines, particularly MCP-1 by adipocytes, endothelial cells, monocytes and muscle cells, initiates macrophage recruitment and amplifies insulin resistance of the adipocyte (Xu *et al.*, 2003; Varma *et al.*, 2009).

It is also known that type 2 diabetes is associated with microvascular rarefaction (loss of small blood vessels), down-regulation of counterregulatory angiogenic responses and low oxygen pressure in adipose tissue (Pasarica *et al.*, 2009). These observations in animals suggest that adipose tissue hypoxia forms an important factor in adipocyte dysfunction. Although it remains difficult to discern cause from consequence, both adipocyte dysfunction and inflammation, hypoxia, apoptosis and necrosis, as well as disturbances in adipose tissue blood flow appear to play a major role in obesity-related impairments in adipokine expression/secretion and subsequent insulin resistance (Franssen *et al.*, 2008; Goossens, 2008).

Myocyte dysfunction

Several studies indicate that aforementioned inadequacy of 'overloaded' dysfunctional adipocytes to clear circulating fatty acids is associated with ectopic fat deposition in the myocyte (Russell *et al.*, 2003b; van Loon and Goodpaster, 2006; van Loon *et al.*, 2004). In accordance, myocytes overloaded with intramyocellular lipids (IMCL) show clear signs of impaired insulin signalling (van Loon and Goodpaster, 2006). Type 2 diabetes patients also demonstrate a reduced expression of genes involved in the mitochondrial oxidative metabolism. Whether this reduction has a genetic or environmental origin has yet to be determined. A key regulatory factor for oxidative metabolism is PPARg coactivator-1a (PGC-1a). Several studies indicate that PGC-1a is responsible for transcriptional control of many of these genes and stimulates oxidative phosphorylation, mitochondrial biogenesis and the generation of type 1 muscle fibres (Lin *et al.*, 2002; Mootha *et al.*, 2003; Patti *et al.*, 2003; Schrauwen, 2007). In accordance, PGC-1a in skeletal muscle is reduced in type 2 diabetes (Lin *et al.*, 2002; Mootha *et al.*, 2003; Patti *et al.*, 2003; Schrauwen, 2007). Interestingly, both acute exercise (Russell *et al.*, 2005) and endurance exercise training (Russell *et al.*, 2003a) increase PGC-1a expression, suggesting an environmental basis for the altered expression of mitochondrial enzymes in type 2 diabetes patients.

Ectopic intra-hepatocelluar fat storage and hepatocyte dysfunction

Another preferential site for ectopic fat storage is the liver (Taylor, 2008). Fat deposition in hepatocytes, so-called intrahepatic lipids (IHL), is currently considered an essential factor in hepatic insulin resistance (Ryysy *et al.*, 2000; Perseghin *et al.*, 2007) and hepatic inflammation, initiating non-alcoholic fatty liver disease (Cai *et al.*, 2005). Fatty liver insulin resistance results in a decreased insulin-mediated suppression of hepatic glucose output and further raises plasma triacylglycerol concentrations. Once established, the increased insulin secretion necessary to maintain plasma glucose levels will further increase liver fat deposition (Taylor, 2008), adding to the vicious circle of type 2 diabetes as summarized in both Figures 14.1 and 14.2.

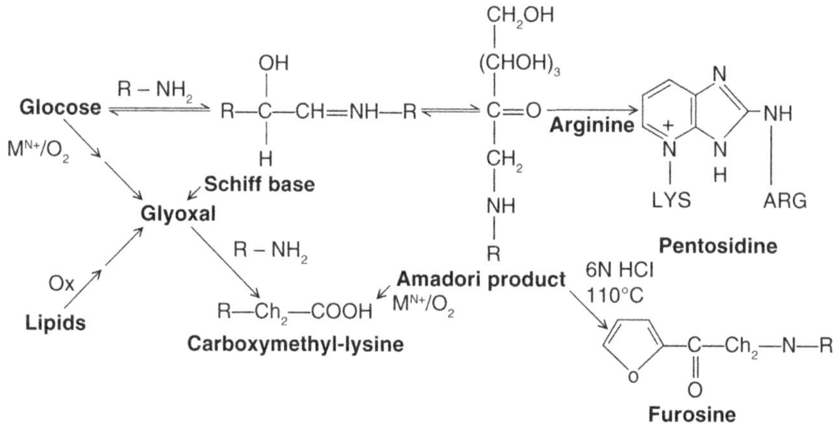

FIGURE 14.1 Hypothesized biochemical relationship between glucose, cross-linking in collagen (R-NH2) by glycation and lipid peroxidation. Adapted from Monnier *et al.*, 1999.

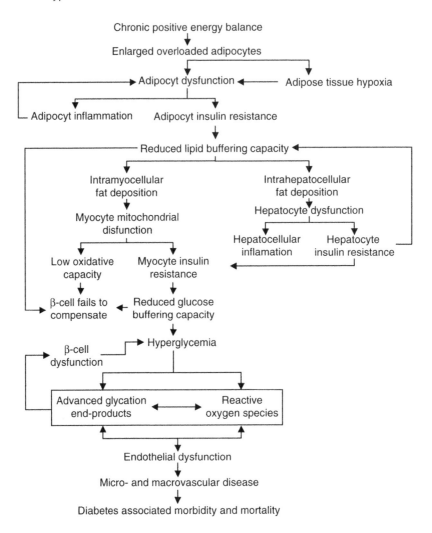

FIGURE 14.2 Schematic interpretation of the relations between the pathophysiologic processes associated with type 2 diabetes, as discussed in this chapter. Although still heavily debated, the described mechanisms in the pathogenesis of type 2 diabetes suggests a specific time sequence (Taylor, 2008). The eventually development of β-cell dysfunction is the result of 1) peripheral insulin resistance, which the β-cell is incapable of compensating, 2) the accumulation triacylglycerol in pancreatic islets and 3) advanced glycation end-products (AGE) and reactive oxygen species (ROS) generation.

Pancreatic β-cell dysfunction

In order to maintain metabolic homeostasis, peripheral insulin resistance forces pancreatic β-cells to boost insulin production to the point where insulin production becomes insufficient to fully compensate for the reduced peripheral insulin sensitivity in muscle-, liver- and/or fat tissue (Stumvoll *et al.*, 2005). Glucose-mediated insulin secretion is further suppressed by the exposure of β-cells to increased levels of fatty acids, derived from circulating and locally deposited triacylglycerol (Tushuizen *et al.*, 2007; Lee *et al.*, 1994). Once the β-cell fails, post-prandial hyperglycemia induces protein glycation and the formation of reactive oxygen species. The latter is believed to cause further damage to cellular components of insulin production and initiates β-cell apoptosis.

Hyperglycemia

The insulin resistant state

The World Health Organization (WHO) criteria state that type 2 diabetes can be diagnosed if fasting plasma glucose levels are equal or above 7.0 mmol/L or if 2 h following an 75 g oral glucose tolerance test (OGTT) plasma glucose concentration rises above 11.1 mmol/L (1999). These diagnostic cut-off points have been based on epidemiological studies that have examined the risk of developing retinopathy over a range of plasma glucose levels (WHO/IDF, 2006). However, even in 'high-risk' obese subjects without blood glucose abnormalities during an OGTT, real-life hyperglycemia was already detectable for almost 14 per cent of a 24-hour period (Costa *et al.*, 2007). These so-called post-prandial hyperglycemic spikes are an early feature of the insulin resistant state even in the absence of formal intermediate hyperglycemia, as defined by the WHO (WHO/IDF, 2006). We have demonstrated that hyperglycemia is present for as much as 8–13 hours per day under strictly standardized, but otherwise free-living conditions. Although long-term studies are lacking, these hyperglycemic episodes are considered to cause the development of vascular complications in prediabetic states (Ceriello, 2005; Baron, 2001). The complex pathophysiological background will be explained in the following paragraphs.

The final pathway in type 2 diabetes leading to micro- and macrovascular disease

Advanced glycation end-products

High circulating plasma glucose levels initiates binding of glucose to amino-acids in proteins, especially the positively charged amine group in lysine, hydroxyl-lysine and arginine is sensitive to glycation. The first, still reversible step in the glycation reaction generates so-called Amadori-products. In the following steps irreversible advanced glycogen end-products (AGE) will be formed (Goh and

Cooper, 2008; Monnier *et al.*, 2008). Glycation leads to protein degeneration. A well-known example is the glycation of hemoglobine resulting in HbA_{1c}. Given the omnipresence of proteins throughout the body, glycation has been observed in almost any organ system. AGE are not exclusively associated with type 2 diabetes, but have a more general role in many degenerative processes typical seen in ageing. Chronic exposure to Amadori-products and AGE is believed to cause vasculopathy (Goldin *et al.*, 2006), glomerulopathy (Hogan *et al.*, 1992, Nishikawa *et al.*, 2000) and may also induce nerve cell damage (Vincent *et al.*, 2007).

Oxidative stress

Reactive oxygen species (ROS) occur in normal functioning cells. ROS, mainly superoxide anion ($O_2^{\cdot-}$), hydroxyl ($OH^\cdot$) and peroxyl radicals (H_2O_2, $ROO^\cdot$) are produced in the electron transport chain as a by-product of the ATP-generation process. Despite their potentially destructive effects, ROS are essential in the defense mechanisms of macrophages and other immune cells and can have insulin-mimicking effects, suggesting an intra-cellular signal function. From this viewpoint ROS are a sensor for 'energy overloading' of a cell and, as such, facilitates the insulin action cascade (Eriksson, 2007; Goldstein *et al.*, 2005; van Hoek *et al.*, 2008; Loh *et al.*, 2009).

   Due to aforementioned pathophysiological interactions seen in type 2 dia-betes, both adipocytes, myocytes and hepatocytes become stacked with energy substrates. This 'overload' increases mitochondrial respiratory chain activity, uncoupled oxidation and consequently ROS generation. The process is probably intensified by inflammation, AGE and/or the hypoxic environment. An imbal-ance between ROS generation and the cellular anti-oxidant defence system, or oxidative stress in adipocytes, myocytes, hepatocytes, β-cells and endothelium is regarded an important trigger in the onset and progression of type 2 diabe-tes (Rosen *et al.*, 2001; Eriksson, 2007; Goldstein *et al.*, 2005; Ha *et al.*, 2008; Loh *et al.*, 2009; Mullarkey *et al.*, 1990). The generation of ROS is further stimu-lated by AGE through a receptor mediated process (RAGE: receptor for AGE) (Mullarkey *et al.*, 1990; Schmidt *et al.*, 1994; Schmidt *et al.*, 1996). The combined effects of ROS and AGE in type 2 diabetes are termed glucolipotoxicity.

Exercise as a treatment strategy in type 2 diabetes

Introduction

Since a chronic positive energy balance is the most important foundation for the development of type 2 diabetes, exercise seems to be an obvious treatment strat-egy. Indeed, exercise does not only enhance insulin sensitivity (Boule *et al.*, 2001; Ibanez *et al.*, 2005; Devlin *et al.*, 1987; Fenicchia *et al.*, 2004; Koopman *et al.*, 2005; Yassine *et al.*, 2009), but also promotes weight loss (Shaw *et al.*, 2006; Franz *et al.*, 2007; Nield *et al.*, 2008; Jakicic *et al.*, 2008; Jakicic *et al.*, 1999;

Jakicic *et al.*, 2003; Jeffery *et al.*, 2003; Ewbank *et al.*, 1995; Ibanez *et al.*, 2005), restores muscle mass and exercise capacity (Castaneda *et al.*, 2002), improves endothelial function (Cohen *et al.*, 2008), enhances anti-oxidant systems (Covas *et al.*, 2002; Brites *et al.*, 1999; Powers *et al.*, 1999), lowers blood pressure (Castaneda *et al.*, 2002; Stewart *et al.*, 2002), corrects dyslipidemia (Arora *et al.*, 2009; Krook *et al.*, 2003; Balducci *et al.*, 2004; Bruce and Hawley, 2004; Cauza *et al.*, 2006) and reduces psychosocial stress (Arora *et al.*, 2009).

Exercise to enhance insulin sensitivity

Both a single bout of endurance (Devlin *et al.*, 1987) as well as resistance type exercise (Fenicchia *et al.*, 2004; Koopman *et al.*, 2005) have been shown to increase whole-body insulin sensitivity and/or improve oral glucose tolerance. The effects of exercise on skeletal muscle insulin sensitivity are attributed to 1) the up-regulation and prolonged activation of skeletal muscle GLUT-4 expression (Garcia-Roves *et al.*, 2003; Sriwijitkamol *et al.*, 2007) 2) improved nitric oxide-mediated skeletal muscle blood flow (Maiorana *et al.*, 2003) 3) increased skeletal muscle blood flow following cessation of exercise (Bisquolo *et al.*, 2005) 4) depletion of liver and muscle glycogen stores (Pencek *et al.*, 2005; Price *et al.*, 1999; Dela *et al.*, 1995; Garcia-Roves *et al.*, 2003) 5) reduced hormonal stimulation of hepatic glucose output (Segal *et al.*, 1991) 6) and the normalization of blood lipids (Bruce and Hawley, 2004) and induction of weight loss. The glucoregulatory benefits of an exercise training programme are not only represented by the sum of the effects of each successive bout of exercise (Koopman *et al.*, 2006a; Koopman *et al.*, 2005; Dela *et al.*, 1995), but in addition, more prolonged endurance exercise training is accompanied by structural adaptive responses and lasting improvements in insulin sensitivity in both young (Dela *et al.*, 1992), elderly (Kahn *et al.*, 1990) and/or insulin resistant subjects (Dela *et al.*, 1995; Dela *et al.*, 1994, Perseghin *et al.*, 1996, Rogers *et al.*, 1988). An example of these long-term adaptations is the up-regulation of mitochondrial enzyme activity with endurance training, improving whole-body oxygen uptake capacity (Mandroukas *et al.*, 1986; Henriksson, 1992), although this particular response may be attenuated in more advanced and older type 2 diabetes patients (Cauza *et al.*, 2005; Wagner *et al.*, 2006; Schneider *et al.*, 1984; Howorka *et al.*, 1997; De Feyter *et al.*, 2007). Long-term resistance type exercise interventions have also been reported to improve glucose tolerance (Sigal *et al.*, 2007) and/or whole body insulin sensitivity (Dunstan *et al.*, 2002; Fenicchia *et al.*, 2004; Holten *et al.*, 2004).

Exercise to induce weight loss

It has been well established that dietary interventions are essential in a successful weight management programme to treat type 2 diabetes. However, several systematic reviews report that exercise combined with dietary interventions result in greater weight reductions, more effective long-term weight maintenance in obese patients (Shaw *et al.*, 2006; Franz *et al.*, 2007) and improvements in glycemic control in type 2 diabetes (Nield *et al.*, 2008). Furthermore, cross-sectional and post hoc analyses of prospective studies indicate that physical activity prevents weight regain after weight loss in a dose dependent manner (Jakicic *et al.*, 2008; Jakicic *et al.*, 1999; Jakicic *et al.*, 2003; Jeffery *et al.*, 2003; Ewbank *et al.*, 1995).

Besides increasing energy expenditure, exercise training is demonstrated to induce hunger/satiety feelings and lowers daily food intake (King *et al.*, 2007). Animal studies indicate that exercise-induced signals from muscle and adipose tissue, such as fatty acids, lactate and IL-6, may alter hypothalamic pathways regulating energy homeostasis and energy intake (Patterson and Levin, 2008). As such, future studies should aim to unravel the complex interaction of dietary modulation with different exercise modalities and intensities on expression and release of certain myokines, adipokines and gut hormones that have been shown to regulate energy homeostasis and basal metabolic rate. The latter approach is likely to improve our understanding of the large interindividual variability following combined exercise and dietary interventions aimed at durable weight loss and cardiometabolic health benefits in obesity and type 2 diabetes.

Exercise to treat diabetic myopathy

Exercise training is demonstrated to improve oxidative capacity and overall cardiorespiratory fitness (Ozdirenc *et al.*, 2004; McGavock *et al.*, 2004; Boule *et al.*, 2003; Jakicic *et al.*, 2009). This suggests that, although the cause of diabetic myopathy is not yet to be resolved as explained before, exercise is able to reverse the myocyte dysfunction. Several explanations for the beneficial effect of exercise on diabetic myopathy can be theorized. If the diabetic myopathy is due to low habitual physical activity level, exercise may improve overall muscle function similar as in non-diabetic sedentary subjects. Exercise training is proven to stimulate the expression of key regulators of muscle protein synthesis (Farrell, 2001; Koopman *et al.*, 2006b), this finding is demonstrated in early (Dunstan *et al.*, 2002) and advanced-stage type 2 diabetes patients (Castaneda *et al.*, 2002; De Feyter *et al.*, 2007). The aforementioned improvements in insulin sensitivity and anti-oxidant systems associated with exercise may reverse the downward spiral of type 2 diabetes and its complications. Since muscle biopsies following exercise intervention studies in type 2 diabetes patients are scarce (Wang *et al.*, 2009), future exercise intervention studies should ideally include muscle tissue analyses.

Exercise to treat endothelial dysfunction and hypertension

Endothelial dysfunction is principally defined as an impaired vasodilatory response to acetylcholine or a reduced bio-availability of NO and is believed to be an early event in artherogenic disease (Moyna and Thompson, 2004; Ding and Triggle,

2005). Although the exact mechanisms are still unknown (Ribisl et al., 2007), endothelial dysfunction has recently been suggested as a common factor that links insulin resistance to the impaired oxygen transport and uptake in peripheral skeletal muscle tissue of type 2 diabetes patients (Mohler et al., 2006; Scheuermann-Freestone et al., 2003). However, physical activity has been reported to improve endothelial function both in middle-aged and elderly individuals, in patients with type 1 or type 2 diabetes, as well as those with signs of cardiovascular disease (Vona et al., 2004; Fuchsjager-Mayrl et al., 2002; Hambrecht et al., 2000; Moyna and Thompson, 2004). Several intervention studies have shown that acute exercise increases vascular wall-shear stress, improving the balance between vasodilation (NO) and (e.g. endothelin-1 and angiotensin II) vasoconstrictor pathways (Thijssen et al., 2008; Thijssen et al., 2007). These pathways are also likely to be responsible for the known exercise training-induced reduction in blood pressure (Thijssen et al., 2007). Several meta-analyses have shown that an exercise intervention in obese and insulin resistant patients is able to reduce systolic blood pressure by 5–7 mmHg (Pescatello et al., 2004; Thomas et al., 2006). Although both resistance and endurance type exercise training seem to lower mean arterial blood pressure to a similar extent in type 2 diabetes populations (Snowling and Hopkins, 2006), further research is needed to explore their isolated contribution and mechanism(s) of action in insulin resistant populations.

Exercise to treat dyslipidaemia

Research studies indicate that exercise interventions of sufficient volume and intensity may modulate post-prandial lipid handling (Stich and Berlan, 2004; Boon et al., 2007; Paglialunga and Cianflone, 2007) and increases in physical activity, with (Halle et al., 1999; Dunstan et al., 1997; Pi-Sunyer et al., 2007) or without dietary intake restriction (Krook et al., 2003; Balducci et al., 2004), have been demonstrated to improve fasting blood lipid levels in type 2 diabetes. Furthermore, a period of 5–6 months of aerobic exercise combined with resistance training induces regional changes in fat and lean muscle mass in obese type 2 diabetes patients, despite an unaltered body weight, using dual energy x-ray absorptiometry (DEXA) and MRI (De Feyter et al., 2007; Sigal et al., 2007). Future studies should aim to unravel the mechanisms of action and modulating effects of different modes of exercise training on post-absorptive and post-prandial lipid handling in type 2 diabetes patients (Pastromas et al., 2007). A recent study indicates that isocaloric bouts of higher intensity exercise may result in more abdominal fat loss in type 2 diabetes patients compared to lower intensity exercise (Hansen et al., 2007). Ideally, dietary intake and hormonal responses should be monitored to differentiate the impact of isocaloric exercise bouts of different volumes and intensities on both post-prandial glycemica and/or lipidemia.

Exercise prescription in type 2 diabetes

Initial considerations

The American College of Sports Medicine (ACSM, 2006) recommends exercise testing before exposing type 2 diabetes patients to more vigorous exercise programmes (i.e. > 6 metabolic equivalent tasks (METs)) (ACSM, 2006). The American Diabetes Association (ADA) and the U.S. Preventive Services Task Force advise exercise testing to detect silent myocardial ischaemia if 10-years' cardiovascular risk exceeds 10 per cent (ACSM, 2006; Fowler-Brown *et al.*, 2004; Sigal *et al.*, 2006). The UK Prospective Diabetes type 2 Study (UKPDS) Risk Engine (www.dtu.ox.ac.uk) provides an accurate estimation of a patient's risk for coronary heart disease (Stevens *et al.*, 2001). Although a stress-ECG is not the most sensitive diagnostic tool to detect SMI (Nesto *et al.*, 1988) and predict coronary events (Nesto, 1999), it can be argued that, when trying to minimize the risk of a coronary event, it is still the most cost-effective tool (Cosson *et al.*, 2004). An exercise stress test is also able to detect autonomic cardiac dysfunction (i.e. chronotropic incompetence (Elhendy *et al.*, 2003; Khan *et al.*, 2005) and impaired heart rate recovery (Myers *et al.*, 2007; Cheng *et al.*, 2003) as well as exercise-related hypertension. On top of this, exercise testing provides objective information on the patient's fitness level. This information can be used to determine safe exercise intensity levels and tune an exercise programme for the individual type 2 diabetes patient (Fang *et al.*, 2005; Praet and van Loon, 2007).

Prevention of overload injuries in exercise training

Type 2 diabetes patients are not only subjected to cardiorespiratory deconditioning (Fang *et al.*, 2005) but also to musculoskeletal deconditioning (Volpato *et al.*, 2002; Sayer *et al.*, 2005; Andersen *et al.*, 2004; Petrofsky *et al.*, 2005). It can be theorized that severely deconditioned patients (i.e. <75 per cent of predicted $\dot{V}O_{2max}$) first need resistance training to strengthen myotendinous structures before starting intensive endurance training. The latter concept is supported by resistance type exercise studies that report long-term programme adherence between 68 per cent (Dunstan *et al.*, 2006) and 72 per cent (Dunstan *et al.*, 2005), without concomitant musculoskeletal overuse injuries. Starting with low intensity exercises and gradually increasing the exercise training load (with supervision on the correct execution of the exercises) will help to prevent injuries.

Hypoglycaemia prevention

Only in patients treated with exogenous insulin and/or insulin secretagogues, physical activity can cause hypoglycemia, especially at peak exogenous insulin levels and prolonged physical activity. Current ADA and ACSM guidelines suggest that extra carbohydrate should be ingested (Table 14.1) if preexercise glucose levels are below 5.0 mmol/L (ADA) and/or reduce the administered dose of exogenous insulin or insulin secretagogue to avoid hypoglycemia for individuals on exogenous insulin and/or insulin secretagogue treatment (Sigal *et al.*, 2006; ACSM, 2006). Other types of treatment, including incretin-mimicking drugs, are unlikely to cause hypoglycemia. Patients should avoid injecting insulin into exercising limbs (risk of rapid absorption), and an abdominal injection is preferred. Finally, both patients and supervisors should be aware of signs and symptoms of hypoglycaemia: fatigue, fainting, feeling faint, sweat, tremor, dizziness, hunger and poor coordination.

Influence of other drugs

Obese patients and patients with type 2 diabetes frequently take diuretics, β-blockers, ACE inhibitors, aspirin and lipid-lowering agents. In most patients, these medications will not interfere with the physical activities they choose to perform, but patients and healthcare providers should be aware of potential problems to minimize their impact. Diuretics, especially in higher doses, can interfere with fluid and electrolyte balance and may cause muscle cramps (Mosenkis and Townsend, 2005). β-blockers can blunt the adrenergic symptoms of hypoglycemia, thereby increasing risk of hypoglycemia unawareness (Sigal *et al.*, 2006; Sigal *et al.*, 1999; Sigal *et al.*, 1994). In general, β-blockers reduce maximal exercise capacity by ±10 per cent through their negative inotropic and chronotropic effects (Sigal *et al.*, 1994; Beloka *et al.*, 2008). However, most people with type 2 diabetes do not exercise at very high workload intensities, so this reduction in maximum capacity is generally not problematic (Sigal *et al.*, 2006). In people with coronary artery disease, β-adrenergic blockade actually increases exercise capacity by reducing coronary ischemia and improving stroke volume and cardiac output (Vanhees *et al.*, 1984). As such, only in hypertensive patients with a limited exercise capacity due to β-blocker induced chronotropic incompetence, different types of anti-hypertensive medication, such as ACE-inhibitors or AII-antagonist, may need to be considered.

TABLE 14.1 Carbohydrate supplementation to prevent exercise-related hypoglycemia

Planned type of exercise	Capillary blood glucose	Extra carbohydrate
30 min low intensity	< 5 mmol/l	10–15 gram
	> 5 mmol/l	none
30–60 min moderate intensity	< 5 mmol/l	30–45 gram
	5–10 mmol/l	15 gram
	10–16 mmol/l	none
60 min moderate intensity	< 5 mmol/l	45 gram
	5–10 mmol/l	30–45 gram
	10–16 mmol/l	15 gram

Exercise modality

Aerobic exercise training

Aerobic exercise training has been shown to improve insulin sensitivity in both young (Dela *et al.*, 1992), elderly (Kahn *et al.*, 1990) and/or insulin resistant individuals (Dela *et al.*, 1995; Dela *et al.*, 1994, Perseghin *et al.*, 1996, Rogers *et al.*, 1988) and may be considered the exercise modality of choice when trying to correct the disturbed energy balance associated with type 2 diabetes. Aerobic exercise intensity tends to be a more important exercise training parameter than exercise duration in healthy athletes (Laursen *et al.*, 2002; Laursen *et al.*, 2005; Tabata *et al.*, 1996; Tanisho and Hirakawa, 2009). Furthermore, higher intensity aerobic exercise appears to be more effective in improving glycemic control than isocaloric lower intensity training (Earnest, 2008; Praet *et al.*, 2008a). It can be theorized that short high-intensive intervals provide sufficient stress to the muscular system, without overloading the cardiopulmonary system. However, for safety reasons, high intensity exercise may not be appropriate for severely deconditioned type 2 diabetes patients when first engaging in an exercise programme and may induce hyperglycemic events post-exercise in untrained type 2 diabetes patients, caused by an exercise-induced catecholamine response (Nagasawa *et al.*, 1991; Manders *et al.*, 2009). Hence, a slow progressive start to an exercise programme, tailored to the physical fitness of the patient, may help to prevent adverse events and hyperglycemic reactions. More work is warranted to investigate the proposed benefits of high intensity aerobic exercise over other exercise modalities as a means to improve glycemic control in type 2 diabetes patients. Furthermore, although high intensity aerobic exercise might allow fast improvements in whole-body oxidative capacity, it might not be advantageous in relation to other exercise modalities over an extended time frame (Hansen *et al.*, 2009).

Resistance exercise training

Interestingly, studies investigating the effect of resistance exercise training demonstrate significant improvements in insulin sensitivity and body composition that are comparable with aerobic exercise (Castaneda *et al.*, 2002; Arora *et al.*, 2009; Ibanez *et al.*, 2005; Hansen *et al.*, 2007; Chomentowski *et al.*, 2009; Donnelly *et al.*, 2009, Dunstan *et al.*, 2002; Fenicchia *et al.*, 2004, Holten *et al.*, 2004; Sigal *et al.*, 2007). Resistance exercise can increase muscle mass (Fenicchia *et al.*, 2004) and prevent the loss of muscle mass following energy intake restriction (Chaston *et al.*, 2007; Chomentowski *et al.*, 2009; Donnelly *et al.*, 2009), especially in elderly obese subjects (Chomentowski *et al.*, 2009) and elderly patients with type 2 diabetes (Park *et al.*, 2007). Increases in muscle mass improve whole-body glucose disposal potential. Furthermore, the addition of resistance exercises to a programme might improve adherence as a programme with strict aerobic exercise routines may not be well tolerated (Praet *et al.*, 2008b), probably due to muscle weakness, cardiovascular co-morbidities and reduced exercise tolerance associated with type 2 diabetes (Sayer *et al.*, 2005; Ribisl *et al.*, 2007). In practice, combining resistance exercise training with aerobic exercise training is recommended and studies confirm the synergistic combination of both types of training (Sigal *et al.*, 2007; Marcus *et al.*, 2008). Figure 14.3 represents a model that may reflect a role for resistance type exercise training in weight management (Donnelly *et al.*, 2009).

Tailoring an exercise programme

Current guidelines

Current guidelines from the ADA, the European Association for the Study of Diabetes (EASD), the American College of Physicians (ACP) and the ACSM firmly emphasize the therapeutic strength of exercise. The ADA states that 'to improve glycemic control, assist with weight maintenance, and reduce risk of CVD, at least 150 min/week of moderate-intensity aerobic physical activity is recommended and/ or at least 90 min/week of vigorous aerobic exercise, … distributed over at least 3 days/week and with no more than 2 consecutive days without physical activity'. Since 2006, the ADA guidelines explicitly mention and recognize that 'people with type 2 diabetes should be encouraged to perform resistance exercise 3 times a week, targeting all major muscle groups, progressing to 3 sets of 8–10 repetitions at a weight that cannot be lifted more than 8–10 times' (Sigal *et al.*, 2006; American Diabetes Association, 2009). The ACSM recommends 20–60 minutes endurance exercise 3–4 times/week at an intensity of 50–80 per cent $\dot{V}O_{2max}$/heart rate reserve, striving to accumulate a minimum of 1000 kcal/week of physical activity. If weight loss is required, the ACSM advises 250–300 min/wk or 2000 kcal/wk of physical activity (Donnelly *et al.*, 2009). For resistance training the ACSM advocates 1 set of exercise for the major muscle groups minimal 2 times a week using 10–15 repetitions progressing to 15–20 repetitions (ACSM, 2006). The lack of well-controlled prospective randomized controlled trials explains the differences in exercise recommendations, the absence of detailed information and the absence of differentiation for various subgroups of type 2 diabetes patients.

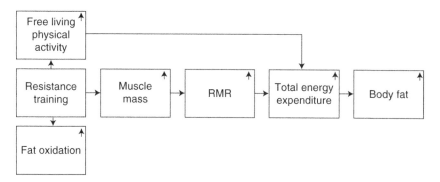

FIGURE 14.3 Conceptual model of resistance training and the potential effect on energy expenditure. A conceptual model that includes both the energy expenditure from increased muscle mass and the potential energy expenditure from increased activities of daily living. (RMR = resting metabolic rate.) Figure based on Donnelly *et al.*, 2009.

TABLE 14.2 Generic exercise recommendations for type 2 diabetes patients, based on current guidelines from the American Diabetes Association (ADA), the European Association for the Study of Diabetes (EASD), the American College of Physicians (ACP) and the American College of Sports Medicine (ACSM). Further specified based on available evidence, discussed in this chapter. CVR, cardiovascular risk; BMI, body mass index; T2DM, type 2 diabetes; W_{max}, maximum power output during cycle ergometry testing; 1-RM, 1 repetition maximum strength; reps, repetitions; AET, aerobic exercise training; RET, resistance exercise training for 7–10 different muscle groups; INT, interval training. Adapted from Praet and van Loon (2007)

Recommendations

ECG-stress testing	Baseline fitness	$\dot{V}O_{2max}$ (L.min-1) (direct or estimated)		Exercise programme START (0 – 6 months)			Exercise programme MAINTENANCE (> 6 months)		
				Freq.	Intensity	Volume	Freq.	Intensity	Volume
T2DM<2 yrs	<2 if > 2 CVR-factors otherwise optional	<100% pred. $\dot{V}O_{2peak}$	AET	1×/wk	50 → 65% W_{max}	30 min	3×/wk	65 → 75% W_{max}	45 → 60 min
			RET	2×/wk	60 → 70% 1-RM	2 sets of 8–12 reps	2×/wk	70 → 85% 1-RM	3 sets of 8–12 reps
			INT		80 → 100% W_{max}	4 → 10×(30' in/60' out)		60 → 80% W_{max}	6 → 10×(45' in/90' out)
			DIET	if BMI>30: energy restricted			if BMI>30: energy restricted		
		>100% pred. $\dot{V}O_{2peak}$	AET	3×/wk	60 → 70% W_{max}	45 min	3×/wk	70 → 80% W_{max}	60 → 75 min
			RET	1×/wk	60 → 70% 1-RM	3 sets of 8–12 reps	1×/wk	70 → 85% 1-RM	3 sets of 8–12 reps
			INT		80 → 100% W_{max}	6 → 10×(30' in/60' out)		70 → 85% W_{max}	10 → 15×(45' in/90' out)
			DIET	if BMI>30: energy restricted			if BMI>30: energy restricted		

	ECG-stress testing	Baseline fitness		Exercise programme START		Exercise programme MAINTENANCE	
T2DM 2–5 yrs	if >2 CVR-factors otherwise optional	<100% pred. $\dot{V}O_{2peak}$	AET	2×/wk 50→60% W_{max}	30 min	2×/wk 50→60% W_{max}	45→60 min
			RET	2×/wk 60→70% 1-RM	2 sets of 8–12 reps	2×/wk 70→85% 1-RM	3 sets of 8–12 reps
			INT	80→100% W_{max}	4→8×(30' in/60' out)	60→80% W_{max}	4→8×(45' in/90' out)
			DIET	if BMI>30: energy restricted		if BMI>30: energy restricted	
		>100% pred. $\dot{V}O_{2peak}$	AET	3×/wk 60→70% W_{max}	45 min	2–3×/wk 60→70% W_{max}	60→75 min
			RET	1×/wk 60→70% 1-RM	2 sets of 8–12 reps	1–2×/wk 70→85% 1-RM	2→3 sets of 8–12 reps
			INT	80→100% W_{max}	6→10×(30' in/60' out)	70→90% W_{max}	6→10×(45' in/90' out)
			DIET	if BMI>30: energy restricted		if BMI>30: energy restricted	
T2DM >5 yrs	preferably, unless contraindicated	<100% pred. $\dot{V}O_{2peak}$	AET	0–1×/wk 50→60% W_{max}	30 min	1×/wk 50→60% W_{max}	30→45 min
			RET	2–3×/wk 50→60% 1-RM	2–3 sets of 8–12 reps	3×/wk 60→75% 1-RM	3 sets of 8–12 reps
			INT	70→90% W_{max}	4→8×(30' in/60' out)	80→100% W_{max}	8→12×(30' in/60' out)
			DIET	if BMI>30: energy restricted		if BMI>30: energy restricted	
		>100% pred. $\dot{V}O_{2peak}$	AET	1–2×/wk 50→60% W_{max}	30 min	2×/wk 60→70% W_{max}	45 min
			RET	1–2×/wk 60→70% 1-RM	2 sets of 8–12 reps	2×/wk 70→80% 1-RM	2®3 sets of 8–12 reps
			INT	90→110% W_{max}	4→8×(30' in/60' out)	100→120% W_{max}	8→12×(30' in/60' out)
			DIET	if BMI>30: energy restricted		if BMI>30: energy restricted	

Continued

TABLE 14.2 *continued*

	ECG-stress testing	Baseline fitness		Exercise programme START		Exercise programme MAINTENANCE	
Elderly T2DM (age > 70 yrs)	preferably, unless contraindicated	<100% pred. $\dot{V}O_{2peak}$	AET	1×/wk 50 → 60% W_{max}	30 min	1×/wk 50 → 60% W_{max}	45 → 60 min
			RET	2×/wk 60 → 70% 1-RM	2→3 sets of 8–12 reps	3×/wk 70 → 80% 1-RM	2®3 sets of 8–12 reps
			INT	70 → 90% W_{max}	4 → 8×(30' in/60' out)	80 → 100% W_{max}	8 → 12×(30' in/60' out)
			DIET	if BMI<30: dietary support		if BMI<30: dietary support	
		>100% pred. $\dot{V}O_{2peak}$	AET	1×/wk 50 → 60% W_{max}	45 min	2×/wk 50 → 60% W_{max}	45 min
			RET	2×/wk 60 → 70% 1-RM	2 sets of 8–12 reps	2×/wk 70 → 80% 1-RM	2®3 sets of 8–12 reps
			INT	90 → 110% W_{max}	4 → 8×(30' in/60' out)	100 → 120% W_{max}	8 → 12×(30' in/60' out)
			DIET	if BMI>30: energy restricted		if BMI>30: energy restricted	

The following paragraphs provide evidence-based recommendations for an effective exercise intervention programme for type 2 diabetes patients (also refer to Table 14.2). However, there are still many different combinations possible, the choice for a specific programme depends on specific long-term goals, the level of motivation, fitness level, prevalence of macro- and microvascular co-morbidities, body composition, qualitative muscle strength. Furthermore, orthopaedic limitations should be taken into consideration.

Duration

Several studies have shown that the energy equivalent of a single bout of aerobic exercise represents the major determinant of the exercise-induced changes in weight reduction (Hansen *et al.*, 2007; Donnelly *et al.*, 2009) and blood glucose homeostasis (Larsen *et al.*, 1999; Larsen *et al.*, 1997; Di Loreto *et al.*, 2005). The current consensus is that to obtain durable metabolic improvements through exercise, the absolute minimum dose of weekly energy expenditure should be 4.2 MJ (~1000 kcal) (Di Loreto *et al.*, 2005; American College of Sports Medicine, 2006). This is in accordance with exercise programmes of 60–90 minutes per week that have shown a beneficial effect on markers of type 2 diabetes (i.e. fasting glucose of OGTT) or its associated risk factors (blood pressure, weight, dyslipidemia, endothelial vasodilatation response) (Taylor, 2007; Moyna and Thompson, 2004; Cauza *et al.*, 2006; Zoppini *et al.*, 2006). Nevertheless, for optimal results, the weekly energy expenditure should probably be twice as high (O'Donovan *et al.*, 2005; Di Loreto *et al.*, 2005; Donnelly *et al.*, 2009) and lower exercise intensities should be compensated for by an increase in exercise duration.

Frequency

When normalized for exercise duration, different exercise frequencies (i.e. 2–7 times a week) seem to induce similar changes. However, it can be theorized that both intensive interval training and resistance exercise training need an adaptation period of 48 hours. Hence, a frequency of 2–3 times a week is commonly used in interval and resistance training programmes (Ibanez *et al.*, 2005; Dunstan *et al.*, 2006; Dunstan *et al.*, 2005; Cohen *et al.*, 2008; Tanisho and Hirakawa, 2009; Fenicchia *et al.*, 2004).

Intensity

For aerobic exercise training, research indicates that a minimum of 50–60 per cent peak oxygen consumption ($\dot{V}O_{2peak}$), heart rate reserve (HRR) or peak power output (PPO) is needed to improve type 2 diabetes markers and associated risk factors (Zoppini *et al.*, 2006; De Feyter *et al.*, 2007; Cauza *et al.*, 2006; Swain and Franklin, 2002; American College of Sports Medicine, 2006), whereas 70–80 per cent $\dot{V}O_{2peak}$/HRR/PPO represents the upper limit of tolerated exercise intensity (Taylor,

2007; Ligtenberg *et al.*, 1997; Zoppini *et al.*, 2006; American College of Sports Medicine, 2006). An alternative approach is to use ratings of perceived exertion (e.g. Borg RPE Scale). High intensive interval training (HIT) is very effective in enhancing cardiovascular fitness (Schjerve *et al.*, 2008; Warburton *et al.*, 2005) even in patients with severe chronic heart failure (Meyer *et al.*, 1997). HIT has been proven effective using approximately 100 per cent PPO or 80–100 per cent $\dot{V}O_{2peak}$, applied in a set of 5–10 repetitions of 20 seconds–4 minutes (Tanisho and Hirakawa, 2009; Tabata *et al.*, 1996; Tjonna *et al.*, 2008; Nemoto *et al.*, 2007). Using short, but intensive intervals of 30 seconds has proven safe and effective in patients with heart disease (Wisloff *et al.*, 2007; Rognmo *et al.*, 2004; Warburton *et al.*, 2005; Meyer *et al.*, 1997). The short duration is probably not sufficient to stress the heart, but is effective in stressing the skeletal muscle and eliciting an adaptative training response. For resistance exercise training, research shows beneficial effects on insulin sensitivity and diabetes associated risk factors with 5–7 exercises targeting the large muscle groups with 2–3 sets of 8–10 repetitions using a progressive resistance of 50–85 per cent van 1-RM (Dunstan *et al.*, 2006; Misra *et al.*, 2008, Ibanez *et al.*, 2005; Dunstan *et al.*, 2005; Cohen *et al.*, 2008; Castaneda *et al.*, 2002, Arora *et al.*, 2009).

Enhancing exercise programme adherence

The long-term programme adherence has been reported to vary substantially (10–80 per cent) (Balducci *et al.*, 2004; Praet *et al.*, 2008; Dunstan *et al.*, 2006). Low adherence rates threaten the clinical efficacy of even the most physiologically effective exercise intervention. Therefore, exercise interventions might benefit from psychological strategies such as motivational interviewing, booster sessions, restricting the travel time towards a training facility and providing the patient with feedback on physical activity levels. The level of supervision and motivational support increases programme adherence and it should be noted that aforementioned beneficial effect of exercise is based on studies investigating supervised exercise programmes (Dunstan *et al.*, 2005) Our research group found that the main reason of premature termination of the exercise intervention was the prevalence of tendinomuscular overuse injuries (De Feyter *et al.*, 2007). Close supervision and programme modification (i.e exercise type and intensity) based on preventive screening can be expected to reduce drop-out as mentioned earlier. By definition, most randomized clinical trials completely disregard a patient's free choice or preference for a specific type of exercise. Future intervention studies may show higher programme adherence when participants can choose from different exercise programmes.

Advanced stage type 2 diabetes patients

An expanding type 2 diabetes sub-group is the long-standing, insulin treated, type 2 diabetes patients. These patients generally suffer from severe exercise intolerance due to the combination of low oxidative capacity, micro- and macrovascular disease, neuropathy-related muscle weakness and/or sarcopenia. For this group the generic exercise programme is often too demanding. Implementing an intermediate exercise programme to bring the patient to a level at which they are able to participate in generic diabetes intervention programmes can overcome this problem. Such intermediate programmes should implement short high-intensity interval training and resistance training with only 1–2 set and 1–5 repetition exercises to increase muscle strength. These short exercises do not produce feelings of dyspnoea or discomfort and have been proven safe and effective in cardiac patients. The efficacy and safety of such intermediate programmes in long-standing type 2 diabetes patients with a high cardiovascular risk profile was recently confirmed in a small scale study by our research group (De Feyter *et al.*, 2007). Nevertheless, more large-scale trials are warranted since exercise intervention studies generally exclude this specific type 2 diabetes subpopulation.

Summary and conclusions

Structured exercise (with or without dietary and pharmacological intervention) is recognized in current guidelines as a cornerstone treatment for insulin resistance, achieving good glycemic control, and improving cardiovascular risk profile in type 2 diabetes patients. However, detailed information on optimal exercise training parameters is lacking (i.e. type of exercise, duration, frequency, intensity, level of supervision and support). Furthermore there is insufficient research data to differentiate between various patient subgroups (i.e. fitness level, disease stage, motivation, co-morbidity). Nevertheless, this chapter has presented exercise recommendations for type 2 diabetes patients on the basis of current evidence. Future research aimed at investigating optimal exercise modalities for different patient subgroups will provide further insight into the efficacy and cost effectiveness of exercise interventions in type 2 diabetes.

References

ACSM (2006). *ACSM's Guidelines For Exercise Testing and Prescription*, Seventh Edition. 207–211.

American Diabetes Association (2009). Executive summary: standards of medical care in diabetes. *Diabetes Care*, 32 Suppl 1: S6–12.

Andersen, H., Nielsen, S., Mogensen, C. E. and Jakobsen, J. (2004). Muscle strength in type 2 diabetes. *Diabetes*, 53: 1543–8.

Arora, E., Shenoy, S. and Sandhu, J. S. (2009). Effects of resistance training on metabolic profi le of adults with type 2 diabetes. *Indian J Med Res*, 129: 515–19.

Balducci, S., Leonetti, F., Di Mario, U. and Fallucca, F. (2004). Is a long-term aerobic plus resistance training program feasible for and effective on metabolic profiles in type 2 diabetic patients? *Diabetes Care*, 27: 841–2.

Baron, A. D. (2001). Impaired glucose tolerance as a disease. *Am J Cardiol*, 88: 16H–9H.

Beloka, S., Gujic, M., Deboeck, G., Niset, G., Ciarka, A., Argacha, J. F., Adamopoulos, D., van de Borne, P. and Naeije, R. 2008. beta-Adrenergic Blockade and Metabo-Chemoreflex Contributions to Exercise Capacity. *Med Sci Sports Exerc.*, 40: 1932–1938.

Bisquolo, V. A., Cardoso, C. G., Jr., Ortega, K. C., Gusmao, J. L., Tinucci, T., Negrao, C. E., Wajchenberg, B. L., Mion, D., Jr. and Forjaz, C. L. (2005). Previous exercise attenuates muscle sympathetic activity and increases blood flow during acute euglycemic hyperinsulinemia. *J Appl Physiol*, 98: 866–71.

Boden, G. (1997). Role of fatty acids in the pathogenesis of insulin resistance and NIDDM. *Diabetes*, 46: 3–10.

Boden, G. and Chen, X. (1995). Effects of fat on glucose uptake and utilization in patients with non-insulin-dependent diabetes. *J Clin Invest*, 96: 1261–8.

Boon, H., Blaak, E. E., Saris, W. H., Keizer, H. A., Wagenmakers, A. J. and van Loon, L. J. (2007). Substrate source utilisation in long-term diagnosed type 2 diabetes patients at rest, and during exercise and subsequent recovery. *Diabetologia*, 50: 103–12.

Boule, N. G., Haddad, E., Kenny, G. P., Wells, G. A. and Sigal, R. J. (2001). Effects of exercise on glycemic control and body mass in type 2 diabetes mellitus: a meta-analysis of controlled clinical trials. *JAMA*, 286: 1218–27.

Boule, N. G., Kenny, G. P., Haddad, E., Wells, G. A. and Sigal, R. J. (2003). Meta-analysis of the effect of structured exercise training on cardiorespiratory fitness in type 2 diabetes mellitus. *Diabetologia*, 46: 1071–81.

Brites, F. D., Evelson, P. A., Christiansen, M. G., Nicol, M. F., Basilico, M. J., Wikinski, R. W. and Llesuy, S. F. (1999). Soccer players under regular training show oxidative stress but an improved plasma antioxidant status. *Clin Sci (Lond)*, 96: 381–5.

Bruce, C. R. and Hawley, J. A. (2004). Improvements in insulin resistance with aerobic exercise training: a lipocentric approach. *Med Sci Sports Exerc*, 36: 1196–201.

Cai, D., Yuan, M., Frantz, D. F., Melendez, P. A., Hansen, L., Lee, J. and Shoelson, S. E. (2005). Local and systemic insulin resistance resulting from hepatic activation of IKK-beta and NF-kappaB. *Nat Med*, 11: 183–90.

Castaneda, C., Layne, J. E., Munoz-Orians, L., Gordon, P. L., Walsmith, J., Foldvari, M., Roubenoff, R., Tucker, K. L. and Nelson, M. E. (2002). A randomized controlled trial of resistance exercise training to improve glycemic control in older adults with type 2 diabetes. *Diabetes Care*, 25: 2335–41.

Cauchi, S., Meyre, D., Durand, E., Proenca, C., Marre, M., Hadjadj, S., Choquet, H., De Graeve, F., Gaget, S., Allegaert, F., Delplanque, J., Permutt, M. A., Wasson, J., Blech, I., Charpentier, G., Balkau, B., Vergnaud, A. C., Czernichow, S., Patsch, W., Chikri, M., Glaser, B., Sladek, R. and Froguel, P. (2008). Post genome-wide association studies of novel genes associated with type 2 diabetes show gene-gene interaction and high predictive value. *PLoS ONE*, 3: e2031.

Cauza, E., Hanusch-Enserer, U., Strasser, B., Kostner, K., Dunky, A. and Haber, P. (2005). Strength and endurance training lead to different post exercise glucose profiles in diabetic participants using a continuous subcutaneous glucose monitoring system. *Eur J Clin Invest*, 35: 745–51.

Cauza, E., Hanusch-Enserer, U., Strasser, B., Kostner, K., Dunky, A. and Haber, P. (2006). The metabolic effects of long term exercise in type 2 diabetes patients. *Wien Med Wochenschr*, 156: 515–19.

Ceriello, A. (2005). Postprandial hyperglycemia and diabetes complications: is it time to treat? *Diabetes*, 54: 1–7.

Chaston, T. B., Dixon, J. B. and O'Brien, P. E. (2007). Changes in fat-free mass during significant weight loss: a systematic review. *Int J Obes* (Lond), 31: 743–50.

Cheng, Y. J., Lauer, M. S., Earnest, C. P., Church, T. S., Kampert, J. B., Gibbons, L. W. and Blair, S. N. (2003). Heart rate recovery following maximal exercise testing as a predictor of cardiovascular disease and all-cause mortality in men with diabetes. *Diabetes Care*, 26: 2052–7.

Chomentowski, P., Dube, J. J., Amati, F., Stefanovic-Racic, M., Zhu, S., Toledo, F. G. and Goodpaster, B. H. (2009). Moderate exercise attenuates the loss of skeletal muscle mass that occurs with intentional caloric restriction-induced weight loss in older, overweight to obese adults. *J Gerontol A Biol Sci Med Sci*, 64: 575–80.

Cohen, N. D., Dunstan, D. W., Robinson, C., Vulikh, E., Zimmet, P. Z. and Shaw, J. E. (2008). Improved endothelial function following a 14-month resistance exercise training program in adults with type 2 diabetes. *Diabetes Res Clin Pract*, 79: 405–11.

Cosson, E., Paycha, F., Paries, J., Cattan, S., Ramadan, A., Meddah, D., Attali, J. R. and Valensi, P. (2004). Detecting silent coronary stenoses and stratifying cardiac risk in patients with diabetes: ECG stress test or exercise myocardial scintigraphy? *Diabet Med*, 21: 342–8.

Costa, B., Vizcaino, J., Pinol, J. L., Cabre, J. J. and Fuentes, C. M. (2007). Relevance of casual undetected hyperglycemia among high-risk individuals for developing diabetes. *Diabetes Res Clin Pract*, 78: 289–292.

Covas, M. I., Elosua, R., Fito, M., Alcantara, M., Coca, L. and Marrugat, J. (2002). Relationship between physical activity and oxidative stress biomarkers in women. *Med Sci Sports Exerc*, 34: 814–19.

De Feyter, H. M., Praet, S. F., van den Broek, N. M., Kuipers, H., Stehouwer, C. D., Nicolay, K., Prompers, J. J. and van Loon, L. J. (2007). Exercise training improves glycemic control in long-standing, insulin-treated type 2 diabetes patients. *Diabetes Care*, 30: 2511–13.

Dela, F., Larsen, J. J., Mikines, K. J., Ploug, T., Petersen, L. N. and Galbo, H. (1995). Insulin-stimulated muscle glucose clearance in patients with NIDDM. Effects of one-legged physical training. *Diabetes*, 44: 1010–20.

Dela, F., Mikines, K. J., Von Linstow, M., Secher, N. H. and Galbo, H. (1992). Effect of training on insulin-mediated glucose uptake in human muscle. *Am J Physiol*, 263: E1134–43.

Dela, F., Ploug, T., Handberg, A., Petersen, L. N., Larsen, J. J., Mikines, K. J. and Galbo, H. (1994). Physical training increases muscle GLUT4 protein and mRNA in patients with NIDDM. *Diabetes*, 43: 862–5.

Detournay, B., Raccah, D., Cadilhac, M. and Eschwege, E. (2005). Epidemiology and costs of diabetes treated with insulin in France. *Diabetes Metab*, 31: 3–18.

Devlin, J. T., Hirshman, M., Horton, E. D. and Horton, E. S. (1987). Enhanced peripheral and splanchnic insulin sensitivity in NIDDM men after single bout of exercise. *Diabetes*, 36: 434–9.

Di Loreto, C., Fanelli, C., Lucidi, P., Murdolo, G., De Cicco, A., Parlanti, N., Ranchelli, A., Fatone, C., Taglioni, C., Santeusanio, F. and De Feo, P. (2005). Make your diabetic patients walk: long-term impact of different amounts of physical activity on type 2 diabetes. *Diabetes Care*, 28: 1295–302.

Ding, H. and Triggle, C. R. (2005). Endothelial cell dysfunction and the vascular complications associated with type 2 diabetes: assessing the health of the endothelium. *Vasc Health Risk Manag*, 1: 55–71.

Donnelly, J. E., Blair, S. N., Jakicic, J. M., Manore, M. M., Rankin, J. W. and Smith, B. K. (2009). American College of Sports Medicine Position Stand. Appropriate physical activity intervention strategies for weight loss and prevention of weight regain for adults. *Med Sci Sports Exerc*, 41: 459–71.

Dunstan, D. W., Mori, T. A., Puddey, I. B., Beilin, L. J., Burke, V., Morton, A. R. and Stanton, K. G. (1997). The independent and combined effects of aerobic exercise and dietary fish intake on serum lipids and glycemic control in NIDDM. A randomized controlled study. *Diabetes Care*, 20: 913–21.

Dunstan, D. W., Daly, R. M., Owen, N., Jolley, D., De Courten, M., Shaw, J. and Zimmet, P. (2002). High-intensity resistance training improves glycemic control in older patients with type 2 diabetes. *Diabetes Care*, 25: 1729–36.

Dunstan, D. W., Daly, R. M., Owen, N., Jolley, D., Vulikh, E., Shaw, J. and Zimmet, P. (2005). Home-based resistance training is not sufficient to maintain improved glycemic control following supervised training in older individuals with type 2 diabetes. *Diabetes Care*, 28: 3–9.

Dunstan, D. W., Vulikh, E., Owen, N., Jolley, D., Shaw, J. and Zimmet, P. (2006). Community center-based resistance training for the maintenance of glycemic control in adults with type 2 diabetes. *Diabetes Care*, 29: 2586–91.

Earnest, C. P. (2008). Exercise interval training: an improved stimulus for improving the physiology of pre-diabetes. Med Hypotheses, 71: 752–61.

Elhendy, A., Mahoney, D. W., Khandheria, B. K., Burger, K. and Pellikka, P. A. (2003). Prognostic significance of impairment of heart rate response to exercise: impact of left ventricular function and myocardial ischemia. *J Am Coll Cardiol*, 42: 823–30.

Eriksson, J. W. (2007). Metabolic stress in insulin's target cells leads to ROS accumulation – a hypothetical common pathway causing insulin resistance. *FEBS Lett*, 581: 3734–42.

Ewbank, P. P., Darga, L. L. and Lucas, C. P. (1995). Physical activity as a predictor of weight maintenance in previously obese subjects. *Obes Res*, 3: 257–63.

Fang, Z. Y., Sharman, J., Prins, J. B. and Marwick, T. H. (2005). Determinants of exercise capacity in patients with type 2 diabetes. *Diabetes Care*, 28: 1643–8.

Farrell, P. A. (2001). Protein metabolism and age: influence of insulin and resistance exercise. *Int J Sport Nutr Exerc Metab*, 11 Suppl: S150–63.

Fenicchia, L. M., Kanaley, J. A., Azevedo, J. L., Jr., Miller, C. S., Weinstock, R. S., Carhart, R. L. and Ploutz-Snyder, L. L. (2004). Influence of resistance exercise training on glucose control in women with type 2 diabetes. *Metabolism*, 53: 284–9.

Fowler-Brown, A., Pignone, M., Pletcher, M., Tice, J. A., Sutton, S. F. and Lohr, K. N. (2004). Exercise tolerance testing to screen for coronary heart disease: a systematic review for the technical support for the U.S. Preventive Services Task Force. *Ann Intern Med*, 140: W9–24.

Franssen, F. M., O'Donnell, D. E., Goossens, G. H., Blaak, E. E. and Schols, A. M. (2008). Obesity and the lung: 5. Obesity and COPD. *Thorax*, 63: 1110–7.

Franz, M. J., Vanwormer, J. J., Crain, A. L., Boucher, J. L., Histon, T., Caplan, W., Bowman, J. D. and Pronk, N. P. (2007). Weight-loss outcomes: a systematic review and meta-analysis of weight-loss clinical trials with a minimum 1-year follow-up. *J Am Diet Assoc*, 107: 1755–67.

Fuchsjager-Mayrl, G., Pleiner, J., Wiesinger, G. F., Sieder, A. E., Quittan, M., Nuhr, M. J., Francesconi, C., Seit, H. P., Francesconi, M., Schmetterer, L. and Wolzt, M. (2002). Exercise training improves vascular endothelial function in patients with type 1 diabetes. *Diabetes Care*, 25: 1795–801.

Garcia-Roves, P. M., Han, D. H., Song, Z., Jones, T. E., Hucker, K. A. and Holloszy, J. O. (2003). Prevention of glycogen supercompensation prolongs the increase in muscle GLUT4 after exercise. *Am J Physiol Endocrinol Metab*, 285: E729–36.

Goh, S. Y. and Cooper, M. E. (2008). Clinical review: The role of advanced glycation end products in progression and complications of diabetes. *J Clin Endocrinol Metab*, 93: 1143–52.

Goldin, A., Beckman, J. A., Schmidt, A. M. and Creager, M. A. (2006). Advanced glycation end products: sparking the development of diabetic vascular injury. *Circulation*, 114: 597–605.

Goldstein, B. J., Mahadev, K. and Wu, X. (2005). Redox paradox: insulin action is facilitated by insulin-stimulated reactive oxygen species with multiple potential signaling targets. *Diabetes*, 54: 311–21.

Goossens, G. H. (2008). The role of adipose tissue dysfunction in the pathogenesis of obesity-related insulin resistance. *Physiol Behav*, 94: 206–18.

Ha, H., Hwang, I. A., Park, J. H. and Lee, H. B. (2008). Role of reactive oxygen species in the pathogenesis of diabetic nephropathy. *Diabetes Res Clin Pract*, 82 Suppl 1: S42–5.

Halle, M., Berg, A., Garwers, U., Baumstark, M. W., Knisel, W., Grathwohl, D., Konig, D. and Keul, J. (1999). Influence of 4 weeks' intervention by exercise and diet on low-density lipoprotein subfractions in obese men with type 2 diabetes. *Metabolism*, 48: 641–4.

Hambrecht, R., Gielen, S., Linke, A., Fiehn, E., Yu, J., Walther, C., Schoene, N. and Schuler, G. (2000). Effects of exercise training on left ventricular function and peripheral resistance in patients with chronic heart failure: A randomized trial. *JAMA*, 283: 3095–101.

Hansen, D., Dendale, P., Berger, J., van Loon, L. J. and Meeusen, R. (2007). The effects of exercise training on fat-mass loss in obese patients during energy intake restriction. *Sports Med*, 37: 31–46.

Hansen, D., Dendale, P., Jonkers, R. A., Beelen, M., Manders, R. J., Corluy, L., Mullens, A., Berger, J., Meeusen, R. and van Loon, L. J. (2009). Continuous low- to moderate-intensity exercise training is as effective as moderate- to high-intensity exercise training at lowering blood HbA(1c) in obese type 2 diabetes patients. *Diabetologia*, 52: 1789–97.

Henriksson, J. (1992). Effects of physical training on the metabolism of skeletal muscle. *Diabetes Care*, 15: 1701–11.

Hogan, M., Cerami, A. and Bucala, R. (1992). Advanced glycosylation endproducts block the antiproliferative effect of nitric oxide. Role in the vascular and renal complications of diabetes mellitus. *J Clin Invest*, 90: 1110–15.

Holten, M. K., Zacho, M., Gaster, M., Juel, C., Wojtaszewski, J. F. and Dela, F. (2004). Strength training increases insulin-mediated glucose uptake, GLUT4 content, and insulin signaling in skeletal muscle in patients with type 2 diabetes. *Diabetes*, 53: 294–305.

Howorka, K., Pumprla, J., Haber, P., Koller-Strametz, J., Mondrzyk, J. and Schabmann, A. (1997). Effects of physical training on heart rate variability in diabetic patients with various degrees of cardiovascular autonomic neuropathy. *Cardiovasc Res*, 34: 206–14.

Ibanez, J., Izquierdo, M., Arguelles, I., Forga, L., Larrion, J. L., Garcia-Unciti, M., Idoate, F. and Gorostiaga, E. M. (2005). Twice-weekly progressive resistance training decreases abdominal fat and improves insulin sensitivity in older men with type 2 diabetes. *Diabetes Care*, 28: 662–7.

IDF (2009). IDF Diabetes Atlas, 4th edn. Brussels, Belgium: International Diabetes Federation.

Jakicic, J. M., Jaramillo, S. A., Balasubramanyam, A., Bancroft, B., Curtis, J. M., Mathews, A., Pereira, M., Regensteiner, J. G. and Ribisl, P. M. (2009). Effect of a lifestyle intervention on change in cardiorespiratory fitness in adults with type 2 diabetes: results from the Look AHEAD Study. *Int J Obes (Lond)*, 33: 305–16.

Jakicic, J. M., Marcus, B. H., Gallagher, K. I., Napolitano, M. and Lang, W. (2003). Effect of exercise duration and intensity on weight loss in overweight, sedentary women: a randomized trial. *JAMA*, 290: 1323–30.

Jakicic, J. M., Marcus, B. H., Lang, W. and Janney, C. (2008). Effect of exercise on 24-month weight loss maintenance in overweight women. *Arch Intern Med*, 168: 1550–9; discussion 1559–60.

Jakicic, J. M., Winters, C., Lang, W. and Wing, R. R. (1999). Effects of intermittent exercise and use of home exercise equipment on adherence, weight loss, and fitness in overweight women: a randomized trial. *JAMA*, 282: 1554–60.

Jeffery, R. W., Wing, R. R., Sherwood, N. E. and Tate, D. F. (2003). Physical activity and weight loss: does prescribing higher physical activity goals improve outcome? *Am J Clin Nutr*, 78: 684–9.

Kabir, M., Catalano, K. J., Ananthnarayan, S., Kim, S. P., van Citters, G. W., Dea, M. K. and Bergman, R. N. (2005). Molecular evidence supporting the portal theory: a causative link between visceral adiposity and hepatic insulin resistance. *Am J Physiol Endocrinol Metab*, 288: E454–61.

Kahn, S. E., Hull, R. L. and Utzschneider, K. M. (2006). Mechanisms linking obesity to insulin resistance and type 2 diabetes. *Nature*, 444: 840–6.

Kahn, S. E., Larson, V. G., Beard, J. C., Cain, K. C., Fellingham, G. W., Schwartz, R. S., Veith, R. C., Stratton, J. R., Cerqueira, M. D. and Abrass, I. B. (1990). Effect of exercise on insulin action, glucose tolerance, and insulin secretion in aging. *Am J Physiol*, 258: E937–43.

Khan, M. N., Pothier, C. E. and Lauer, M. S. (2005). Chronotropic incompetence as a predictor of death among patients with normal electrograms taking beta blockers (metoprolol or atenolol). *Am J Cardiol*, 96: 1328–33.

King, N. A., Caudwell, P., Hopkins, M., Byrne, N. M., Colley, R., Hills, A. P., Stubbs, J. R. and Blundell, J. E. (2007). Metabolic and behavioral compensatory responses to exercise interventions: barriers to weight loss. *Obesity (Silver Spring)*, 15: 1373–83.

Koopman, R., Manders, R. J., Jonkers, R. A., Hul, G. B., Kuipers, H. and van Loon, L. J. (2006a). Intramyocellular lipid and glycogen content are reduced following resistance exercise in untrained healthy males. *Eur J Appl Physiol*, 96: 525–34.

Koopman, R., Manders, R. J., Zorenc, A. H., Hul, G. B., Kuipers, H., Keizer, H. A. and van Loon, L. J. (2005). A single session of resistance exercise enhances insulin sensitivity for at least 24 h in healthy men. *Eur J Appl Physiol*, 94: 180–7.

Koopman, R., Zorenc, A. H., Gransier, R. J., Cameron-Smith, D. and van Loon, L. J. (2006b). Increase in S6K1 phosphorylation in human skeletal muscle following resistance exercise occurs mainly in type II muscle fibers. *Am J Physiol Endocrinol Metab*, 290: E1245–52.

Krook, A., Holm, I., Pettersson, S. and Wallberg-Henriksson, H. (2003). Reduction of risk factors following lifestyle modification programme in subjects with type 2 (non-insulin dependent) diabetes mellitus. *Clin Physiol Funct Imaging*, 23: 21–30.

Larsen, J. J., Dela, F., Kjaer, M. and Galbo, H. (1997). The effect of moderate exercise on postprandial glucose homeostasis in NIDDM patients. *Diabetologia*, 40: 447–53.

Larsen, J. J., Dela, F., Madsbad, S. and Galbo, H. (1999). The effect of intense exercise on postprandial glucose homeostasis in type II diabetic patients. *Diabetologia*, 42: 1282–92.

Laursen, P. B., Blanchard, M. A. and Jenkins, D. G. (2002). Acute high-intensity interval training improves Tvent and peak power output in highly trained males. *Can J Appl Physiol*, 27: 336–48.

Laursen, P. B., Shing, C. M., Peake, J. M., Coombes, J. S. and Jenkins, D. G. (2005). Influence of high-intensity interval training on adaptations in well-trained cyclists. *J Strength Cond Res*, 19: 527–33.

Lee, Y., Hirose, H., Ohneda, M., Johnson, J. H., Mcgarry, J. D. and Unger, R. H. (1994). Beta-cell lipotoxity in the pathogenesis of non-insulin-dependent diabetes mellitus of obese rats: impairment in adipocyte-beta-cell relationships. *Proc Natl Acad Sci U S A*, 91: 10878–82.

Ligtenberg, P. C., Hoekstra, J. B., Bol, E., Zonderland, M. L. and Erkelens, D. W. (1997). Effects of physical training on metabolic control in elderly type 2 diabetes mellitus patients. *Clin Sci* (Lond), 93: 127–35.

Lin, J., Wu, H., Tarr, P. T., Zhang, C. Y., Wu, Z., Boss, O., Michael, L. F., Puigserver, P., Isotani, E., Olson, E. N., Lowell, B. B., Bassel-Duby, R. and Spiegelman, B. M. (2002). Transcriptional co-activator PGC-1 alpha drives the formation of slow-twitch muscle fibres. *Nature*, 418: 797–801.

Loh, K., Deng, H., Fukushima, A., Cai, X., Boivin, B., Galic, S., Bruce, C., Shields, B. J., Skiba, B., Ooms, L. M., Stepto, N., Wu, B., Mitchell, C. A., Tonks, N. K., Watt, M. J., Febbraio, M. A., Crack, P. J., Andrikopoulos, S. and Tiganis, T. (2009). Reactive oxygen species enhance insulin sensitivity. *Cell Metab*, 10: 260–72.

Lyssenko, V. and Groop, L. (2009). Genome-wide association study for type 2 diabetes: clinical applications. *Curr Opin Lipidol*, 20: 87–91.

Maiorana, A., O'driscoll, G., Taylor, R. and Green, D. (2003). Exercise and the nitric oxide vasodilator system. *Sports Med*, 33: 1013–35.

Manders, R. J., van Dijk, J. W. and van Loon, L. J. (2009). Low-intensity exercise reduces the prevalence of hyperglycemia in type 2 diabetes. *Med Sci Sports Exerc*, 42: 219–225.

Mandroukas, K., Krotkiewski, M., Holm, G., Stromblad, G., Grimby, G., Lithell, H., Wroblewski, Z. and Bjorntrop, P. (1986). Muscle adaptations and glucose control after physical training in insulin-dependent diabetes mellitus. *Clin Physiol*, 6: 39–52.

Marcus, R. L., Smith, S., Morrell, G., Addison, O., Dibble, L. E., Wahoff-Stice, D. and Lastayo, P. C. (2008). Comparison of combined aerobic and high-force eccentric resistance exercise with aerobic exercise only for people with type 2 diabetes mellitus. *Phys Ther*, 88: 1345–54.

McGavock, J., Mandic, S., Lewanczuk, R., Koller, M., Muhll, I. V., Quinney, A., Taylor, D., Welsh, R. and Haykowsky, M. (2004). Cardiovascular adaptations to exercise training in postmenopausal women with type 2 diabetes mellitus. *Cardiovasc Diabetol*, 3: 3.

Meyer, K., Samek, L., Schwaibold, M., Westbrook, S., Hajric, R., Beneke, R., Lehmann, M. and Roskamm, H. (1997). Interval training in patients with severe chronic heart failure: analysis and recommendations for exercise procedures. *Med Sci Sports Exerc*, 29: 306–12.

Misra, A., Alappan, N. K., Vikram, N. K., Goel, K., Gupta, N., Mittal, K., Bhatt, S. and Luthra, K. (2008). Effect of supervised progressive resistance-exercise training protocol on insulin sensitivity, glycemia, lipids, and body composition in Asian Indians with type 2 diabetes. *Diabetes Care*, 31: 1282–7.

Mohler, E. R. 3rd, Lech, G., Supple, G. E., Wang, H. and Chance, B. (2006). Impaired exercise-induced blood volume in type 2 diabetes with or without peripheral arterial disease measured by continuous-wave near-infrared spectroscopy. *Diabetes Care*, 29: 1856–9.

Monnier, V. M., Bautista, O., Kenny, D., Sell, D. R., Fogarty, J., Dahms, W., Cleary, P. A., Lachin, J. and Genuth, S. (1999). Skin collagen glycation, glycoxidation, and crosslinking are lower in subjects with long-term intensive versus conventional therapy of type 1 diabetes: relevance of glycated collagen products versus HbA1c as markers of diabetic complications. DCCT Skin Collagen Ancillary Study Group. Diabetes Control and Complications Trial. *Diabetes*, 48: 870–80.

Monnier, V. M., Sell, D. R., Dai, Z., Nemet, I., Collard, F. and Zhang, J. (2008). The role of the amadori product in the complications of diabetes. *Ann N Y Acad Sci*, 1126: 81–8.

Mootha, V. K., Lindgren, C. M., Eriksson, K. F., Subramanian, A., Sihag, S., Lehar, J., Puigserver, P., Carlsson, E., Ridderstrale, M., Laurila, E., Houstis, N., Daly, M. J., Patterson, N., Mesirov, J. P., Golub, T. R., Tamayo, P., Spiegelman, B., Lander, E. S., Hirschhorn, J. N., Altshuler, D. and Groop, L. C. (2003). PGC-1alpha-responsive genes involved in oxidative phosphorylation are coordinately downregulated in human diabetes. *Nat Genet*, 34: 267–73.

Mosenkis, A. and Townsend, R. R. (2005). Muscle cramps and diuretic therapy. *J Clin Hypertens* (Greenwich), 7: 134–5.

Moyna, N. M. and Thompson, P. D. (2004). The effect of physical activity on endothelial function in man. *Acta Physiol Scand*, 180: 113–23.

Mullarkey, C. J., Edelstein, D. and Brownlee, M. (1990). Free radical generation by early glycation products: a mechanism for accelerated atherogenesis in diabetes. *Biochem Biophys Res Commun*, 173: 932–9.

Myers, J., Tan, S. Y., Abella, J., Aleti, V. and Froelicher, V. F. (2007). Comparison of the chronotropic response to exercise and heart rate recovery in predicting cardiovascular mortality. *Eur J Cardiovasc Prev Rehabil*, 14: 215–21.

Nagasawa, J., Sato, Y. and Ishiko, T. (1991). Time course of in vivo insulin sensitivity after a single bout of exercise in rats. *Int J Sports Med*, 12: 399–402.

Nemoto, K., Gen-No, H., Masuki, S., Okazaki, K. and Nose, H. (2007). Effects of high-intensity interval walking training on physical fitness and blood pressure in middle-aged and older people. *Mayo Clin Proc*, 82: 803–11.

Nesto, R. W. (1999). Screening for asymptomatic coronary artery disease in diabetes. *Diabetes Care*, 22: 1393–5.

Nesto, R. W., Phillips, R. T., Kett, K. G., Hill, T., Perper, E., Young, E. and Leland, O. S., Jr. (1988). Angina and exertional myocardial ischemia in diabetic and nondiabetic patients: assessment by exercise thallium scintigraphy. *Ann Intern Med*, 108: 170–5.

Nield, L., Summerbell, C. D., Hooper, L., Whittaker, V. and Moore, H. (2008). Dietary advice for the prevention of type 2 diabetes mellitus in adults. *Cochrane Database Syst Rev*: CD005102.

Nishikawa, T., Edelstein, D. and Brownlee, M. (2000). The missing link: a single unifying mechanism for diabetic complications. *Kidney Int Suppl*, 77: S26–30.

O'Donovan, G., Kearney, E. M., Nevill, A. M., Woolf-May, K. and Bird, S. R. (2005). The effects of 24 weeks of moderate- or high-intensity exercise on insulin resistance. *Eur J Appl Physiol*, 95: 522–8.

Ozdirenc, M., Kocak, G. and Guntekin, R. (2004). The acute effects of in-patient physiotherapy program on functional capacity in type II diabetes mellitus. *Diabetes Res Clin Pract*, 64: 167–72.

Paglialunga, S. and Cianflone, K. (2007). Regulation of postprandial lipemia: an update on current trends. *Appl Physiol Nutr Metab*, 32: 61–75.

Park, S. W., Goodpaster, B. H., Strotmeyer, E. S., Kuller, L. H., Broudeau, R., Kammerer, C., De Rekeneire, N., Harris, T. B., Schwartz, A. V., Tylavsky, F. A., Cho, Y. W. and Newman, A. B. (2007). Accelerated loss of skeletal muscle strength in older adults with type 2 diabetes: the health, aging, and body composition study. *Diabetes Care*, 30: 1507–12.

Pasarica, M., Sereda, O. R., Redman, L. M., Albarado, D. C., Hymel, D. T., Roan, L. E., Rood, J. C., Burk, D. H. and Smith, S. R. (2009). Reduced adipose tissue oxygenation in human obesity: evidence for rarefaction, macrophage chemotaxis, and inflammation without an angiogenic response. *Diabetes*, 58: 718–25.

Pastromas, S., Terzi, A. B., Tousoulis, D. and Koulouris, S. (2007). Postprandial lipemia: An under-recognized atherogenic factor in patients with diabetes mellitus. *Int J Cardiol*, 126: 3–12.

Patterson, C. M. and Levin, B. E. (2008). Role of exercise in the central regulation of energy homeostasis and in the prevention of obesity. *Neuroendocrinology*, 87: 65–70.

Patti, M. E., Butte, A. J., Crunkhorn, S., Cusi, K., Berria, R., Kashyap, S., Miyazaki, Y., Kohane, I., Costello, M., Saccone, R., Landaker, E. J., Goldfine, A. B., Mun, E., Defronzo, R., Finlayson, J., Kahn, C. R. and Mandarino, L. J. (2003). Coordinated reduction of genes of oxidative metabolism in humans with insulin resistance and diabetes: Potential role of PGC1 and NRF1. *Proc Natl Acad Sci U S A*, 100: 8466–71.

Pencek, R. R., Fueger, P. T., Camacho, R. C. and Wasserman, D. H. (2005). Mobilization of glucose from the liver during exercise and replenishment afterward. *Can J Appl Physiol*, 30: 292–303.

Perseghin, G., Lattuada, G., De Cobelli, F., Ragogna, F., Ntali, G., Esposito, A., Belloni, E., Canu, T., Terruzzi, I., Scifo, P., Del Maschio, A. and Luzi, L. (2007). Habitual physical activity is associated with intrahepatic fat content in humans. *Diabetes Care*, 30: 683–8.

Perseghin, G., Price, T. B., Petersen, K. F., Roden, M., Cline, G. W., Gerow, K., Rothman, D. L. and Shulman, G. I. (1996). Increased glucose transport-phosphorylation and muscle glycogen synthesis after exercise training in insulin-resistant subjects. *N Engl J Med*, 335: 1357–62.

Pescatello, L. S., Franklin, B. A., Fagard, R., Farquhar, W. B., Kelley, G. A. and Ray, C. A. (2004). American College of Sports Medicine position stand. Exercise and hypertension. *Med Sci Sports Exerc*, 36: 533–53.

Petrofsky, J. S., Stewart, B., Patterson, C., Cole, M., Al Malty, A. and Lee, S. (2005). Cardiovascular responses and endurance during isometric exercise in patients with type 2 diabetes compared to control subjects. *Med Sci Monit*, 11: CR470–7.

Pi-Sunyer, X., Blackburn, G., Brancati, F. L., Bray, G. A., Bright, R., Clark, J. M., Curtis, J. M., Espeland, M. A., Foreyt, J. P., Graves, K., Haffner, S. M., Harrison, B., Hill, J. O., Horton, E. S., Jakicic, J., Jeffery, R. W., Johnson, K. C., Kahn, S., Kelley, D. E., Kitabchi, A. E., Knowler, W. C., Lewis, C. E., Maschak-Carey, B. J., Montgomery, B., Nathan, D. M., Patricio, J., Peters, A., Redmon, J. B., Reeves, R. S., Ryan, D. H., Safford, M., van Dorsten, B., Wadden, T. A., Wagenknecht, L., Wesche-Thobaben, J., Wing, R. R. and Yanovski, S. Z. (2007). Reduction in weight and cardiovascular disease risk factors in individuals with type 2 diabetes: one-year results of the look AHEAD trial. *Diabetes Care*, 30: 1374–83.

Powers, S. K., Ji, L. L. and Leeuwenburgh, C. (1999). Exercise training-induced alterations in skeletal muscle antioxidant capacity: a brief review. *Med Sci Sports Exerc*, 31: 987–97.

Praet, S. F., Jonkers, R. A., Schep, G., Stehouwer, C. D., Kuipers, H., Keizer, H. A. and van Loon, L. J. (2008a). Long-standing, insulin-treated type 2 diabetes patients with complications respond well to short-term resistance and interval exercise training. *Eur J Endocrinol*, 158: 163–72.

Praet, S. F. and van Loon, L. J. (2007). Optimizing the therapeutic benefits of exercise in type 2 diabetes. *J Appl Physiol*, 103: 1113–20.

Praet, S. F., van Rooij, E. S., Wijtvliet, A., Boonman-De Winter, L. J., Enneking, T., Kuipers, H., Stehouwer, C. D. and van Loon, L. J. (2008b). Brisk walking compared with an individualised medical fitness programme for patients with type 2 diabetes: a randomised controlled trial. *Diabetologia*, 51: 736–46.

Price, T. B., Rothman, D. L. and Shulman, R. G. (1999). NMR of glycogen in exercise. *Proc Nutr Soc*, 58: 851–9.

Prokopenko, I., Langenberg, C., Florez, J. C., Saxena, R., Soranzo, N., Thorleifsson, G., Loos, R. J., Manning, A. K., Jackson, A. U., Aulchenko, Y., Potter, S. C., Erdos, M. R., Sanna, S., Hottenga, J. J., Wheeler, E., Kaakinen, M., Lyssenko, V., Chen, W. M., Ahmadi, K., Beckmann, J. S., Bergman, R. N., Bochud, M., Bonnycastle, L. L., Buchanan, T. A., Cao, A., Cervino, A., Coin, L., Collins, F. S., Crisponi, L., de Geus, E. J., Dehghan, A., Deloukas, P., Doney, A. S., Elliott, P., Freimer, N., Gateva, V., Herder, C., Hofman, A., Hughes, T. E., Hunt, S., Illig, T., Inouye, M., Isomaa, B., Johnson, T., Kong, A., Krestyaninova, M., Kuusisto, J., Laakso, M., Lim, N., Lindblad, U., Lindgren, C. M., McCann, O. T., Mohlke, K. L., Morris, A. D., Naitza, S., Orr, M., Palmer, C. N., Pouta, A., Randall, J., Rathmann, W., Saramies, J., Scheet, P., Scott, L. J., Scuteri, A., Sharp, S., Sijbrands, E., Smit, J. H., Song, K., Steinthorsdottir, V., Stringham, H. M., Tuomi, T., Tuomilehto, J., Uitterlinden, A. G., Voight, B. F., Waterworth, D., Wichmann, H. E., Willemsen, G., Witteman, J. C., Yuan, X., Zhao, J. H., Zeggini, E., Schlessinger, D., Sandhu, M., Boomsma, D. I., Uda, M., Spector, T. D., Penninx, B. W., Altshuler, D., Vollenweider, P., Jarvelin, M. R., Lakatta, E., Waeber, G., Fox, C. S., Peltonen, L., Groop, L. C., Mooser, V., Cupples, L. A., Thorsteinsdottir, U., Boehnke, M., Barroso, I., van Duijn, C., Dupuis, J., Watanabe, R. M., Stefansson, K., McCarthy, M. I., Wareham, N. J., Meigs, J. B. and Abecasis, G. R. (2009). Variants in MTNR1B influence fasting glucose levels. *Nat Genet*, 41: 77–81.

Rasouli, N. and Kern, P. A. (2008). Adipocytokines and the metabolic complications of obesity. *J Clin Endocrinol Metab*, 93: S64–73.

Ribisl, P. M., Lang, W., Jaramillo, S. A., Jakicic, J. M., Stewart, K. J., Bahnson, J., Bright, R., Curtis, J. F., Crow, R. S. and Soberman, J. E. (2007). exercise capacity and cardiovascular/metabolic characteristics of overweight and obese individuals with type 2 diabetes. The Look AHEAD Study. *Diabetes Care*, 30: 2679–2684.

Rogers, M. A., Yamamoto, C., Hagberg, J. M., Martin, W. H., 3rd, Ehsani, A. A. and Holloszy, J. O. (1988). Effect of 6 d of exercise training on responses to maximal and sub-maximal exercise in middle-aged men. *Med Sci Sports Exerc*, 20: 260–4.

Rognmo, O., Hetland, E., Helgerud, J., Hoff, J. and Slordahl, S. A. (2004). High intensity aerobic interval exercise is superior to moderate intensity exercise for increasing aerobic capacity in patients with coronary artery disease. *Eur J Cardiovasc Prev Rehabil*, 11: 216–22.

Rosen, P., Nawroth, P. P., King, G., Moller, W., Tritschler, H. J. and Packer, L. (2001). The role of oxidative stress in the onset and progression of diabetes and its complications: a summary of a Congress Series sponsored by UNESCO-MCBN, the American Diabetes Association and the German Diabetes Society. *Diabetes Metab Res Rev*, 17: 189–212.

Russell, A. P., Feilchenfeldt, J., Schreiber, S., Praz, M., Crettenand, A., Gobelet, C., Meier, C. A., Bell, D. R., Kralli, A., Giacobino, J. P. and Deriaz, O. (2003a). Endurance training in humans leads to fiber type-specific increases in levels of peroxisome proliferator-activated receptor-gamma coactivator-1 and peroxisome proliferator-activated receptor-alpha in skeletal muscle. *Diabetes*, 52: 2874–81.

Russell, A. P., Gastaldi, G., Bobbioni-Harsch, E., Arboit, P., Gobelet, C., Deriaz, O., Golay, A., Witztum, J. L. and Giacobino, J. P. (2003b). Lipid peroxidation in skeletal muscle of obese as compared to endurance-trained humans: a case of good vs. bad lipids? *FEBS Lett*, 551: 104–6.

Russell, A. P., Hesselink, M. K., Lo, S. K. and Schrauwen, P. (2005). Regulation of metabolic transcriptional co-activators and transcription factors with acute exercise. *FASEB J*, 19: 986–8.

Ryysy, L., Hakkinen, A. M., Goto, T., Vehkavaara, S., Westerbacka, J., Halavaara, J. and Yki-Jarvinen, H. (2000). Hepatic fat content and insulin action on free fatty acids and glucose metabolism rather than insulin absorption are associated with insulin requirements during insulin therapy in type 2 diabetic patients. *Diabetes*, 49: 749–58.

Saxena, R., Voight, B. F., Lyssenko, V., Burtt, N. P., De Bakker, P. I., Chen, H., Roix, J. J., Kathiresan, S., Hirschhorn, J. N., Daly, M. J., Hughes, T. E., Groop, L., Altshuler, D., Almgren, P., Florez, J. C., Meyer, J., Ardlie, K., Bengtsson Bostrom, K., Isomaa, B., Lettre, G., Lindblad, U., Lyon, H. N., Melander, O., Newton-Cheh, C., Nilsson, P., Orho-Melander, M., Rastam, L., Speliotes, E. K., Taskinen, M. R., Tuomi, T., Guiducci, C., Berglund, A., Carlson, J., Gianniny, L., Hackett, R., Hall, L., Holmkvist, J., Laurila, E., Sjogren, M., Sterner, M., Surti, A., Svensson, M., Svensson, M., Tewhey, R., Blumenstiel, B., Parkin, M., Defelice, M., Barry, R., Brodeur, W., Camarata, J., Chia, N., Fava, M., Gibbons, J., Handsaker, B., Healy, C., Nguyen, K., Gates, C., Sougnez, C., Gage, D., Nizzari, M., Gabriel, S. B., Chirn, G. W., Ma, Q., Parikh, H., Richardson, D., Ricke, D. and Purcell, S. (2007). Genome-wide association analysis identifies loci for type 2 diabetes and triglyceride levels. *Science*, 316: 1331–6.

Sayer, A. A., Dennison, E. M., Syddall, H. E., Gilbody, H. J., Phillips, D. I. and Cooper, C. (2005). Type 2 diabetes, muscle strength, and impaired physical function: the tip of the iceberg? *Diabetes Care*, 28: 2541–2.

Scheuermann-Freestone, M., Madsen, P. L., Manners, D., Blamire, A. M., Buckingham, R. E., Styles, P., Radda, G. K., Neubauer, S. and Clarke, K. (2003). Abnormal cardiac and skeletal muscle energy metabolism in patients with type 2 diabetes. *Circulation*, 107: 3040–6.

Schjerve, I. E., Tyldum, G. A., Tjonna, A. E., Stolen, T., Loennechen, J. P., Hansen, H. E., Haram, P. M., Heinrich, G., Bye, A., Najjar, S. M., Smith, G. L., Slordahl, S. A., Kemi, O. J. and Wisloff, U. (2008). Both aerobic endurance and strength training programmes improve cardiovascular health in obese adults. *Clin Sci* (Lond), 115: 283–93.

Schmidt, A. M., Hori, O., Brett, J., Yan, S. D., Wautier, J. L. and Stern, D. (1994). Cellular receptors for advanced glycation end products. Implications for induction of oxidant stress and cellular dysfunction in the pathogenesis of vascular lesions. *Arterioscler Thromb*, 14: 1521–8.

Schmidt, A. M., Hori, O., Cao, R., Yan, S. D., Brett, J., Wautier, J. L., Ogawa, S., Kuwabara, K., Matsumoto, M. and Stern, D. (1996). RAGE: a novel cellular receptor for advanced glycation end products. *Diabetes*, 45 Suppl 3: S77–80.

Schneider, S. H., Amorosa, L. F., Khachadurian, A. K. and Ruderman, N. B. (1984). Studies on the mechanism of improved glucose control during regular exercise in type 2 (non-insulin-dependent) diabetes. *Diabetologia*, 26: 355–60.

Schrauwen, P. (2007). High-fat diet, muscular lipotoxicity and insulin resistance. *Proc Nutr Soc*, 66: 33–41.

Segal, K. R., Edano, A., Abalos, A., Albu, J., Blando, L., Tomas, M. B. and Pi-Sunyer, F. X. (1991). Effect of exercise training on insulin sensitivity and glucose metabolism in lean, obese, and diabetic men. *J Appl Physiol*, 71: 2402–11.

Shaw, K., Gennat, H., O'rourke, P. and Del Mar, C. (2006). Exercise for overweight or obesity. *Cochrane Database Syst Rev*: CD003817.

Sigal, R. J., Fisher, S. J., Halter, J. B., Vranic, M. and Marliss, E. B. (1999). Glucoregulation during and after intense exercise: effects of beta-adrenergic blockade in subjects with type 1 diabetes mellitus. *J Clin Endocrinol Metab*, 84: 3961–71.

Sigal, R. J., Kenny, G. P., Boule, N. G., Wells, G. A., Prud'homme, D., Fortier, M., Reid, R. D., Tulloch, H., Coyle, D., Phillips, P., Jennings, A. and Jaffey, J. (2007). Effects of aerobic training, resistance training, or both on glycemic control in type 2 diabetes: a randomized trial. *Ann Intern Med*, 147: 357–69.

Sigal, R. J., Kenny, G. P., Wasserman, D. H., Castaneda-Sceppa, C. and White, R. D. (2006). Physical activity/exercise and type 2 diabetes: a consensus statement from the American Diabetes Association. *Diabetes Care*, 29: 1433–8.

Sigal, R. J., Purdon, C., Bilinski, D., Vranic, M., Halter, J. B. and Marliss, E. B. (1994). Glucoregulation during and after intense exercise: effects of beta-blockade. *J Clin Endocrinol Metab*, 78: 359–66.

Sladek, R., Rocheleau, G., Rung, J., Dina, C., Shen, L., Serre, D., Boutin, P., Vincent, D., Belisle, A., Hadjadj, S., Balkau, B., Heude, B., Charpentier, G., Hudson, T. J., Montpetit, A., Pshezhetsky, A. V., Prentki, M., Posner, B. I., Balding, D. J., Meyre, D., Polychronakos, C. and Froguel, P. (2007). A genome-wide association study identifies novel risk loci for type 2 diabetes. *Nature*, 445: 881–5.

Snowling, N. J. and Hopkins, W. G. (2006). Effects of different modes of exercise training on glucose control and risk factors for complications in type 2 diabetic patients: a meta-analysis. *Diabetes Care*, 29: 2518–27.

Sriwijitkamol, A., Coletta, D. K., Wajcberg, E., Balbontin, G. B., Reyna, S. M., Barrientes, J., Eagan, P. A., Jenkinson, C. P., Cersosimo, E., Defronzo, R. A., Sakamoto, K. and Musi, N. (2007). Effect of acute exercise on AMPK signaling in skeletal muscle of subjects with type 2 diabetes: a time-course and dose-response study. *Diabetes*, 56: 836–48.

Stevens, R. J., Kothari, V., Adler, A. I. and Stratton, I. M. (2001). The UKPDS risk engine: a model for the risk of coronary heart disease in Type II diabetes (UKPDS 56). *Clin Sci (Lond)*, 101: 671–9.

Stewart, K. J., Moyna, N. M., Thompson, P. D., Jansson, P. A., Ding, H., Triggle, C. R., Avogaro, A., Fadini, G. P., Gallo, A., Pagnin, E., De Kreutzenberg, S., Umpierre, D., Stein, R., Phielix, E., Mensink, M., Giugliano, D., Ceriello, A. and Esposito, K. (2002). Exercise training and the cardiovascular consequences of type 2 diabetes and hypertension: plausible mechanisms for improving cardiovascular health. *JAMA*, 288: 1622–31.

Stich, V. and Berlan, M. (2004). Physiological regulation of NEFA availability: lipolysis pathway. *Proc Nutr Soc*, 63: 369–74.

Stumvoll, M., Goldstein, B. J. and van Haeften, T. W. (2005). Type 2 diabetes: principles of pathogenesis and therapy. *Lancet*, 365: 1333–46.

Sullivan, P. W., Morrato, E. H., Ghushchyan, V., Wyatt, H. R. and Hill, J. O. (2005). Obesity, inactivity, and the prevalence of diabetes and diabetes-related cardiovascular comorbidities in the U.S., 2000–2002. *Diabetes Care*, 28: 1599–603.

Swain, D. P. and Franklin, B. A. (2002). Is there a threshold intensity for aerobic training in cardiac patients? *Med Sci Sports Exerc*, 34: 1071–5.

Tabata, I., Nishimura, K., Kouzaki, M., Hirai, Y., Ogita, F., Miyachi, M. and Yamamoto, K. (1996). Effects of moderate-intensity endurance and high-intensity intermittent training on anaerobic capacity and VO_{2max}. *Med Sci Sports Exerc*, 28: 1327–30.

Tanisho, K. and Hirakawa, K. (2009). Training effects on endurance capacity in maximal intermittent exercise: comparison between continuous and interval training. *J Strength Cond Res*, 23: 2405–2410.

Taylor, J. D. (2007). The impact of a supervised strength and aerobic training program on muscular strength and aerobic capacity in individuals with type 2 diabetes. *J Strength Cond Res*, 21: 824–30.

Taylor, R. (2008). Pathogenesis of type 2 diabetes: tracing the reverse route from cure to cause. *Diabetologia*, 51: 1781–9.

Thijssen, D. H., Rongen, G. A., Smits, P. and Hopman, M. T. (2008). Physical (in)activity and endothelium-derived constricting factors: overlooked adaptations. *J Physiol*, 586: 319–24.

Thijssen, D. H., Rongen, G. A., van Dijk, A., Smits, P. and Hopman, M. T. (2007). Enhanced endothelin-1-mediated leg vascular tone in healthy older subjects. *J Appl Physiol*, 103: 852–7.

Thomas, D. E., Elliott, E. J. and Naughton, G. A. (2006). Exercise for type 2 diabetes mellitus. *Cochrane Database Syst Rev*, 3: CD002968.

Tjonna, A. E., Lee, S. J., Rognmo, O., Stolen, T. O., Bye, A., Haram, P. M., Loennechen, J. P., Al-Share, Q. Y., Skogvoll, E., Slordahl, S. A., Kemi, O. J., Najjar, S. M. and Wisloff, U. (2008). Aerobic interval training versus continuous moderate exercise as a treatment for the metabolic syndrome: a pilot study. *Circulation*, 118: 346–54.

Tushuizen, M. E., Bunck, M. C., Pouwels, P. J., Bontemps, S., van Waesberghe, J. H., Schindhelm, R. K., Mari, A., Heine, R. J. and Diamant, M. (2007). Pancreatic fat content and beta-cell function in men with and without type 2 diabetes. *Diabetes Care*, 30: 2916–21.

van Hoek, M., Dehghan, A., Witteman, J. C., van Duijn, C. M., Uitterlinden, A. G., Oostra, B. A., Hofman, A., Sijbrands, E. J. and Janssens, A. C. (2008). Predicting type 2 diabetes based on polymorphisms from genome-wide association studies: a population-based study. *Diabetes*, 57: 3122–8.

van Loon, L. J. and Goodpaster, B. H. (2006). Increased intramuscular lipid storage in the insulin-resistant and endurance-trained state. *Pflugers Arch*, 451: 606–16.

van Loon, L. J., Koopman, R., Manders, R., van der Weegen, W., van Kranenburg, G. P. and Keizer, H. A. (2004). Intramyocellular lipid content in type 2 diabetes patients compared with overweight sedentary men and highly trained endurance athletes. *Am J Physiol Endocrinol Metab*, 287: E558–65.

Vanhees, L., Fagard, R. and Amery, A. (1984). Influence of beta-adrenergic blockade on the hemodynamic effects of physical training in patients with ischemic heart disease. Am Heart J, 108: 270–5.

Varma, V., Yao-Borengasser, A., Rasouli, N., Nolen, G. T., Phanavanh, B., Starks, T., Gurley, C. M., Simpson, P. M., Mcgehee Jr, R. E., Kern, P. A. and Peterson, C. A. (2009). Muscle inflammatory response and insulin resistance: synergistic interaction between macrophages and fatty acids leads to impaired insulin action. *Am J Physiol Endocrinol Metab*, 296: 1300–1310.

Vincent, A. M., Perrone, L., Sullivan, K. A., Backus, C., Sastry, A. M., Lastoskie, C. and Feldman, E. L. (2007). Receptor for advanced glycation end products activation injures primary sensory neurons via oxidative stress. *Endocrinology*, 148: 548–58.

Volpato, S., Blaum, C., Resnick, H., Ferrucci, L., Fried, L. P. and Guralnik, J. M. (2002). Comorbidities and impairments explaining the association between diabetes and lower extremity disability: The Women's Health and Aging Study. *Diabetes Care*, 25: 678–83.

Vona, M., Rossi, A., Capodaglio, P., Rizzo, S., Servi, P., De Marchi, M. and Cobelli, F. (2004). Impact of physical training and detraining on endothelium-dependent vasodilation in patients with recent acute myocardial infarction. *Am Heart J*, 147: 1039–46.

Wagner, H., Degerblad, M., Thorell, A., Nygren, J., Stahle, A., Kuhl, J., Brismar, T. B., Ohrvik, J., Efendic, S. and Bavenholm, P. N. (2006). Combined treatment with exercise training and acarbose improves metabolic control and cardiovascular risk factor profile in subjects with mild type 2 diabetes. *Diabetes Care*, 29: 1471–7.

Wang, Y., Simar, D. and Fiatarone Singh, M. A. (2009). Adaptations to exercise training within skeletal muscle in adults with type 2 diabetes or impaired glucose tolerance: a systematic review. *Diabetes Metab Res Rev*, 25: 13–40.

Warburton, D. E., Mckenzie, D. C., Haykowsky, M. J., Taylor, A., Shoemaker, P., Ignaszewski, A. P. and Chan, S. Y. (2005). Effectiveness of high-intensity interval training for the rehabilitation of patients with coronary artery disease. *Am J Cardiol*, 95: 1080–4.

WHO/IDF (2006). *Definition and diagnosis of diabetes mellitus and intermediate hyperglycemia: report of a WHO/IDF consultation*. Geneva, Switzerland: World Health Organization.

Wisloff, U., Stoylen, A., Loennechen, J. P., Bruvold, M., Rognmo, O., Haram, P. M., Tjonna, A. E., Helgerud, J., Slordahl, S. A., Lee, S. J., Videm, V., Bye, A., Smith, G. L., Najjar, S. M., Ellingsen, O. and Skjaerpe, T. (2007). Superior cardiovascular effect of aerobic interval training versus moderate continuous training in heart failure patients: a randomized study. *Circulation*, 115: 3086–94.

World Health Organization Expert Committee (WHO) (1999). *Definition, Diagnosis and Classification of Diabetes Mellitus and Its Complications. Part 1: Diagnosis and Classification of Diabetes Mellitus*. Geneva, World Health Organization.

Xu, H., Barnes, G. T., Yang, Q., Tan, G., Yang, D., Chou, C. J., Sole, J., Nichols, A., Ross, J. S., Tartaglia, L. A. and Chen, H. (2003). Chronic inflammation in fat plays a crucial role in the development of obesity-related insulin resistance. *J Clin Invest*, 112: 1821–30.

Yassine, H. N., Marchetti, C. M., Krishnan, R. K., Vrobel, T. R., Gonzalez, F. and Kirwan, J. P. (2009). Effects of exercise and caloric restriction on insulin resistance and cardiometabolic risk factors in older obese adults – a randomized clinical trial. *J Gerontol A Biol Sci Med Sci*, 64: 90–5.

Zoppini, G., Targher, G., Zamboni, C., Venturi, C., Cacciatori, V., Moghetti, P. and Muggeo, M. (2006). Effects of moderate-intensity exercise training on plasma biomarkers of inflammation and endothelial dysfunction in older patients with type 2 diabetes. *Nutr Metab Cardiovasc Dis*, 16: 543–9.

15

OBESITY

Pedro J. Teixeira, R. James Stubbs, Neil A. King,
Stephen Whybrow and John E. Blundell

Introduction

Human obesity is not a new phenomenon but it was not until the past 25–30 years that it became a public health concern. In fact, the prevalence of children, adolescents and adults with excess weight has risen substantially in recent decades, not only in affluent societies but also in less developed countries around the globe (Hu, 2008a). Additionally, there is a higher recognition that obesity is associated with a number of health complications, notably type 2 diabetes, heart disease, hypertension and stroke, and some cancers (Must *et al.*, 1999; Gregg *et al.*, 2005). Obesity also affects people's perceived health-related quality of life, namely mobility, pain and physical functioning, among other areas (Yan *et al.*, 2004; Hassan *et al.*, 2003; Coakley *et al.*, 1998). Regrettably, in a society that has a financial (and perhaps also a moral) stake in encouraging thin bodies, and that increasingly discriminates against those who are heavier, the psychological burden of obesity, especially in women, has resulted in a 'normative discontent' with physical appearance, contributing to disrupted eating patterns and unnecessary psychological suffering (Puhl and Heuer, 2009). Obesity's burden on the economy, through increased health care costs and work absenteeism, is also a concern (Janssen *et al.*, 2009; Trogdon *et al.*, 2008; Wang *et al.*, 2008). However, recognizing that major environment changes are closely linked with the recent growth in obesity is a critical consideration (Sallis and Glanz, 2009; Barry *et al.*, 2009).

Obesity is generally defined by a level of body fat sufficient to negatively affect physiological systems and overall health. The Body Mass Index (BMI, in kg/m^2) is the standard criterion used for classification of overweight and obesity (WHO, 1998). Although it does not measure fat directly, BMI is a practical and reliable measure, and is strongly correlated with more specific indices of fatness such as fat percentage (Gallagher *et al.*, 1996; Gallagher *et al.*, 2000); in the general population, the overwhelming majority of people with obesity as defined by BMI also present with increased adiposity. Importantly, considerable evidence describes the pattern of BMI's relation with morbidity and mortality in different groups (Hu, 2008b), which explains why this rather simple index continues to be used in both clinical practice and research. Two obvious limitations of BMI are its lack of sensitivity to body tissues which are not fat (e.g. muscle mass) and its inability to help determine where the excess fat is located in body. To obviate the latter problem, additional measures are currently used, which quantify the relative location of fat in the body, in particular the amount that is deposited in the abdominal region (Sardinha and Teixeira, 2005). Table 15.1 shows how BMI and the waist circumference are currently recommended to classify individuals into cardiovascular and metabolic risk categories.

Energy balance and body weight

Energy balance is the main determinant of body weight (and body weight change) and is the sum of energy intake minus total energy expenditure. The control of energy balance is interconnected with other biological systems that influence motivation and behaviour, and is sensitive to certain changes in the external and internal environment (e.g. temperature, pregnancy or high rates of sustained energy turnover) and to changes in the environmental supply of energy and nutrients (Stubbs *et al.*, 2003; Stubbs *et al.*, 2005). The sensitivity of the energy balance control (i.e. the capacity of the system to recognize changes in the environment) can often be greater than its responsiveness (i.e. its tendency to alter behaviour in order to maintain the constancy of the internal environment).

TABLE 15.1 Classification of overweight and obesity by BMI, waist circumference, and associated disease risk

			Disease risk*	
			(Relative to normal weight and waist circumference)	
	BMI	*Obesity*	*Men≤40 in (≤102 cm)*	*Men>40 in (≤102 cm)*
	(kg/m²)	*Class*	*Women≤35 in (≤88cm)*	*Women>35 in (≤88cm)*
Underweight	<18.5		—	—
Normal	18.5–24.9		—	—
Overweight	25.0–29.9		Increased	High
Obesity	30.0–34.9	I	High	Very high
	35.0–39.9	II	Very high	Very high
Extreme obesity	≥40	III	Extremely high	Extremely high

*Disease risk for type 2 diabetes, hypertension, and CVD. From USDHHS, 2000.

Being overweight is likely to result from 'normal' feeding responses when exposed to a Western diet under modern sedentary conditions (Stubbs and Tolkamp, 2006). Certain external and internal influences can greatly perturb the system in such a way that food (energy and nutrient) intake or physical activity patterns become maladaptive. Other biobehavioural drives can override and distort the cues associated with feeding or activity, often resulting in positive energy balance (Blundell and Stubbs, 1998; Blundell, 1995; Stubbs and Tolkamp, 2006). In fact, there appears to be little evidence of regulatory signals that protect humans from slow, continuous weight gain under modern Western conditions.

On average, total daily energy expenditure is higher in the obese than in the lean (for a given level of lifestyle activity) because they have a higher fat-free mass, which is the main determinant of energy expenditure (Prentice and Jebb, 1995; Prentice *et al.*, 1989; Swinburn *et al.*, 2009), and energy expenditure per unit of fat-free mass is similar for the lean and obese. However, when body size is accounted for, by expressing energy expenditure per kg of body weight, energy expenditure tends to be similar or lower in the obese compared to the lean (Jebb and Prentice, 1995). It is not always so, but the capacity for physical activity, and especially for exercise, is far less in the obese than the lean, as reflected in submaximal and maximal oxygen uptake (fitness) tests (Broeder *et al.*, 1992). This has certain consequences for energy balance and weight control in that many overweight individuals already have energy expenditures towards the upper end of their ability to exercise, and there is limited scope to increase it further.

Physical activity, fitness and health in obesity

The health benefits of increased physical activity in overweight and obese individuals are now very well documented (Physical Activity Guidelines Advisory Committee, 2008; Shaw *et al.*, 2006; Donnelly *et al.*, 2009). Partially because of the effects that physical activity has on physical fitness and body composition, increased activity produces benefits in reducing obesity associated co-morbidities and all-cause mortality; it improves glucose tolerance and it protects against type 2 diabetes, coronary heart disease, hypertension, stroke, colon cancer and breast cancer (Physical Activity Guidelines Advisory Committee, 2008). While this appears to be the case, there are several specific aspects of physical activity as a moderator of health risk in obesity that are still unclear. Against this background it is worth considering the 'fat but fit' concept (Blair and Church, 2004).

Lack of activity ranks alongside smoking and obesity in the WHO estimates of long-term health risk for high income countries (Ezzati *et al.*, 2006). It has also been suggested that fatness (independent of fitness) is a greater risk for diabetes, while lack of fitness (independent of fatness) is a risk for cardiovascular disease (Blair and Church, 2004). From the evidence, it is also reasonable to conclude that, for cardiovascular health, it is better to be slightly overweight and fit than underweight and unfit (Wei *et al.*, 1999; Wei, 2008; Wei *et al.*, 2000, Lee and Blair, 2002; Fogelholm, 2010). However, one should be cautious in over-extrapolating the 'fat but fit' argument, since most Western adults are by evolutionary standards overweight *and* unfit. Generally speaking, the more overweight a person is the more unfit they are likely to become, and the less able they are to engage in risk-reducing physical activity (Physical Activity Guidelines Advisory Committee, 2008). The American College of Sports Medicine (ACSM) notes that there are health benefits associated with physical activity even if weight is not lost (Donnelly *et al.*, 2009). Although these effects are now uncontroversial, it is critical to emphasize that both weight and physical activity are important for long-term health (Fogelholm, 2010). Rather than clearly showing that one factor is more important than the other, evidence suggests that both have important and at least partially distinct effects in decreasing long-term risk status (e.g. (Hu *et al.*, 2003, Blair and Church, 2004, Haapanen-Niemi *et al.*, 2000, WHO, 1998)). It is also likely that obesity and inactivity interact with each other in determining health outcomes. However, the ACSM notes that, to date, there is inadequate evidence to determine whether physical activity prevents or attenuate detrimental changes in chronic disease risk during weight gain (Donnelly *et al.*, 2009).

A controversial issue is the way in which physical activity is measured (or not measured at all) in studies that examine its relation to obesity and health. As reasonably pointed out by Blair and Church, 'the majority of studies examining obesity and health have not adequately accounted for physical activity … investigators have often relied on simple self-report questionnaires in which inaccuracy can increase proportionally with the respondent's weight' (Blair and Church, 2004: 1232). They go on to argue that cardio-respiratory fitness is a more objective measure of physical activity, accounting for 70–80 per cent of the variance in detailed activity records. This may be an important caveat when considering the relation between obesity and health, especially if one believes that low fitness (and low activity levels) is the common denominator in the obesity–health relationship. In other words, by not measuring physical activity or cardiorespiratory fitness, investigators may have, for years, overestimated the negative effects of obesity *per se* on cardiovascular and metabolic health.

Physical activity and the composition and distribution of weight lost

Currently, it is clear that a positive dose-response relation exists between the total energy expenditure of exercise, whether endurance or resistance training, and the amount of total and regional fat loss (Donnelly *et al.*, 2009). Lean tissue sparing occurs when weight is lost through increased activity (Ballor, 1996; Layman *et al.*, 2005). Both fat and lean tissue are lost during weight loss, but the ratio of fat to lean tissue is, *inter alia*, dependent on rate of weight lost and initial body composition, and on the dose of physical activity (Elia *et al.*, 2003; Elia *et al.*, 1999).

It has variously been suggested that physical activity increases fat oxidation (e.g. Smith *et al.*, 2000). However, as with the issue of physical activity and reduction of visceral fat (see below), this should be viewed in the context of the energy balance equation (Elia *et al.*, 2003; Elia *et al.*, 1999). As discussed elsewhere in this chapter, it is clear that physical activity increases energy expenditure. It is also clear that compensation of energy intake for the energy expended during physical activity tends to be partial and slow, even if the physical activity is prolonged and intense; this will result in a negative energy balance. A negative energy balance is characterized by an increased mobilization of fat stores and necessarily associated with some increase in fat oxidation. Central obesity, characterized by a high waist circumference and/or a high waist-to-hip ratio, often caused by large visceral fat deposits, is associated with a cluster of metabolic risk factors for chronic diseases including cardiovascular disease and diabetes (Kissebah and Krakower, 1994; Wang *et al.*, 2005). Preferentially reducing visceral fat and altering fat distribution most likely offers greater health benefits than losing weight *per se*. However, it is currently unclear whether physical activity achieves this. At relatively moderate energy imbalances there is sometimes a loss of fat, a gain of lean tissue and little net change in body weight (Kay and Fiatarone Singh, 2006; Ohkawara *et al.*, 2007; Ross and Katzmarzyk, 2003; Wong *et al.*, 2004). It may be that a large part of this fat loss is from visceral stores (Ohkawara *et al.*, 2007). The present balance of the evidence suggests that exercise, especially at higher intensities, increases fat loss (Mayo *et al.*, 2003). Some of this will be visceral, especially in people where most of their excess fat is stored in that depot. Although it is unclear whether physical activity can plausibly be used in obesity management to impact specific fat depots, observational studies do suggest that for a given BMI, fitter people have less abdominal fat (Ross and Katzmarzyk, 2003; Wong *et al.*, 2004). It is clear from the above arguments that simple statements such as 'physical activity increases fat oxidation' or 'physical activity reduces visceral fat' need to be viewed in the context of a model that links energy intake and energy expenditure; together, these components determine the trajectory of energy balance and body weight.

Physical activity/exercise, weight loss and weight loss maintenance

This section reviews research which has evaluated exercise/physical activity to promote weight loss and/or weight maintenance after weight loss. A critical aspect to consider in this analysis is whether exercise/physical activity was used alone or in the context of a broader lifestyle intervention where dietary changes were also sought. Another important distinction is between studies where exercise/physical activity was supervised and effectively performed by participants or instead prescribed to be integrated into people's daily lives without supervision (common in behavioural weight management programmes). The former answer the question 'does exercise work?' under ideal or controlled conditions (*efficacy* studies) whereas the latter provide answers to questions such as 'will this strategy/intervention be useful in the real world?' or 'to whom/under which circumstances may it be effective?' (*effectiveness* studies). Different conclusions may come from these different types of studies, which is sometimes confusing for policy makers and lay audiences; we will try to make this distinction clear in the following sections. Most weight management studies have focused on overall weight change with interventions of variable duration, sometimes with a no-contact follow-up phase (also of variable duration). In other cases, interventions have specifically focused on the maintenance phase, analyzing strategies/programmes potentially useful to prevent weight regain *after weight loss*. We will address these two types of studies separately. The current available evidence is unfortunately not sufficient to adequately address age- and gender-related differences in the effects of exercise in obesity; as such, the following should primarily apply to overweight/obese adult men and women.

Weight loss

The task of analyzing the evidence on the role of exercise/physical activity in producing weight loss and maintenance is facilitated by several recent review papers and other summary reports (e.g. Fogelholm and Kukkonen-Harjula, 2000; Catenacci and Wyatt, 2007; Donnelly *et al.*, 2009; Shaw *et al.*, 2006; Wu *et al.*, 2009). One way to analyze the impact of exercise on weight loss is to compare outcomes of exercise-only interventions against a control group. Catenacci and Wyatt reviewed 16 RCTs (or groups within an RCT) with overweight and mildly obese participants, lasting 4 to 16 months in duration, where (unsupervised) exercise was targeted at the level of ~60–180 min/wk (Catenacci and Wyatt, 2007). In most studies, body weight was not the study's primary outcome (CVD risk factors were), which explains the generally low dose of exercise which was prescribed. Results from this review were consistent with previous reviews (Miller *et al.*, 1997; Garrow and Summerbell, 1995; Ballor and Keesey, 1991) showing that exercise groups lost 1–3 kg more than controls. In contrast, studies using supervised exercise have shown that, despite considerable individual variability, the mean magnitude of weight loss can be substantial and is generally compatible with the additional energy expended by exercise (Church *et al.*, 2009; Donnelly *et al.*, 2003; Ross *et al.*, 2000). In other words, exercise alone will produce weight loss in a magnitude comparable to dietary restriction of similar caloric deficit. However, adherence tends to be lower in many of these studies (~50 per cent attrition) suggesting that community-dwelling overweight/obese persons will often struggle to adopt and/or sustain such high levels of weekly exercise. The latest Position Statement from the ACSM on intervention strategies for weight loss also reviewed a number of studies on exercise for weight loss (Donnelly *et al.*, 2009). Their summary statement on this topic indicates that 'physical activity will promote clinically significant weight loss', specifically at higher doses, i.e., above 225 min/wk of moderately vigorous physical activity (associated with a loss of 5–7.5 kg) (NHLBI Evidence category B). Doses in the range of 150–200 min/wk are associated with ~2–3 kg losses (Donnelly *et al.*, 2009).

A combination of dietary changes and increases in exercise/physical activity is currently recommended for overweight and obese individuals trying to lose weight

(Donnelly *et al.*, 2009; Physical Activity Guidelines Advisory Committee, 2008) and two recent reviews provide support to the notion that including exercise/physical activity in a weight management programme offers additional benefit versus using dietary changes alone (Catenacci *et al.*, 2008; Wu *et al.*, 2009). Wu and colleagues reviewed 18 studies with overweight or obese (BMI<38 kg/m²) middle-aged adults with a minimum duration of 6 months and seven trials which lasted at least 2 years (up to 6 years), including intervention and follow-up (Wu *et al.*, 2009). With one exception, dropout rates were below 30 per cent. Figure 15.1 shows the standardized weight loss differences among the groups. Weighted mean group differences were 2.3 kg after 1–2 years of follow-up and 1.8 kg for the time frame longer than 2 years, favouring the diet plus exercise group (2 per cent body fat difference overall). Importantly, interventions longer than 1 year in duration were about 5 times more effective than shorter interventions (Wu *et al.*, 2009). Comparable results were found in a 2007 Cochrane review, namely a small but significantly greater weight loss (an additional 1.1 kg) favouring the exercise+diet group versus diet alone (Shaw *et al.*, 2006). In this review, a positive moderating effect of exercise intensity was found with a weighted +1.5 kg difference between the high and low intensity groups. Although the previous studies did not factor in the level of dietary restriction, other reports concluded that exercise is particularly effective under moderate dietary-induced energy imbalance conditions (Donnelly *et al.*, 2009); that is, if dietary restriction is severe, exercise will not provide additional weight loss. Summarizing their findings on this topic, the ACSM panel stated that 'physical activity combined with diet will increase weight loss' (Evidence category A) (Donnelly *et al.*, 2009).

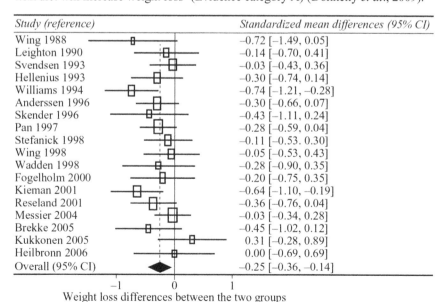

Study (reference)	Standardized mean differences (95% CI)
Wing 1988	−0.72 [−1.49, 0.05]
Leighton 1990	−0.14 [−0.70, 0.41]
Svendsen 1993	−0.03 [−0.43, 0.36]
Hellenius 1993	−0.30 [−0.74, 0.14]
Williams 1994	−0.74 [−1.21, −0.28]
Anderssen 1996	−0.30 [−0.66, 0.07]
Skender 1996	−0.43 [−1.11, 0.24]
Pan 1997	−0.28 [−0.59, 0.04]
Stefanick 1998	−0.11 [−0.53. 0.30]
Wing 1998	−0.05 [−0.53, 0.43]
Wadden 1998	−0.28 [−0.90, 0.35]
Fogelholm 2000	−0.20 [−0.75, 0.35]
Kieman 2001	−0.64 [−1.10, −0.19]
Reseland 2001	−0.36 [−0.76, 0.04]
Messier 2004	−0.03 [−0.34, 0.28]
Brekke 2005	−0.45 [−1.02, 0.12]
Kukkonen 2005	0.31 [−0.28, 0.89]
Heilbronn 2006	0.00 [−0.69, 0.69]
Overall (95% CI)	−0.25 [−0.36, −0.14]

−1   0   1
Weight loss differences between the two groups
P (for heterogeneity) = 0.4

FIGURE 15.1 Pooled standardized mean differences of weight loss between diet-plus-exercise and diet-only groups at the end of the study. See original reference for details on the studies listed. CI, Confidence Interval. From Wu *et al.*, 2009.

Weight loss maintenance (weight maintenance after weight loss)

Studies available to clarify whether the inclusion of exercise/physical activity is predictive of a superior ability to maintain weight loss can be divided into two groups: i) RCTs, either using exercise during the weight loss phase (versus diet alone) or using exercise during the maintenance phase (typically versus a control no contact group), and ii) non-randomized studies using observational, correlational, and/or retrospective designs. Although they generally show the same overall tendency – that exercise is beneficial – evidence is stronger for non-randomized designs than for RCTs, which could warrant caution in drawing conclusions regarding the role of exercise in long-term weight control. However, a closer inspection of the literature suggests that behavioural adherence is a critical moderating factor, negatively affecting RCTs versus non-RCTs. This is well exemplified in a study where 201 overweight women were assigned to different exercise arms based on energy expenditure and intensity level (Jakicic *et al.*, 2008). Predictably, while main effects of *prescribed* energy expenditure (2000 versus 1000 kcal/wk from exercise) were not observed, a retrospective analysis based on level of exercise/physical activity subjects reported *actually engaging in* at 24 months showed a clear dose-response relationship for exercise minutes and energy expenditure on weight loss; for instance, women reporting 300 min/wk or more of leisure-time physical activity lost and maintained more than three times the weight loss of women reporting 150 min/wk or less. More recently, the same trend was observed at the 3-year follow-up of a 1-year lifestyle intervention for overweight and moderately obese women, whether physical activity data was self-reported or objectively assessed by accelerometry (see Figure 15.2).

RCTs have typically shown modest, sometimes non-significant benefits in weight loss maintenance in the exercise groups, as highlighted in two comprehensive reviews on the topic (Fogelholm and Kukkonen-Harjula, 2000; Catenacci and Wyatt, 2007). The most recent of the two reviews (Catenacci and Wyatt, 2007) included four studies comparing exercise versus no exercise during the maintenance phase and eight studies evaluating the long-lasting effect of including an exercise (versus diet only) during the weight loss phase. The authors concluded that although only four of the twelve studies reported statistically significant benefits of exercise, 'exercise produced a weight difference that favoured the exercise group of, on average, –4.5 kg at longest follow-up.' (Catenacci and Wyatt, 2007: 523).

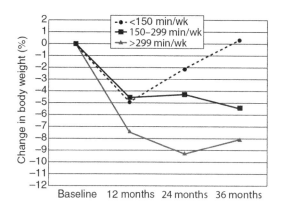

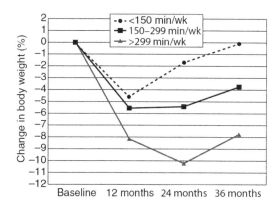

FIGURE 15.2 Weight loss and maintenance by physical activity categories in overweight women participating in behavioural obesity treatment (minutes/week of moderate and vigorous activity). In panel a), activity was assessed with the 7-day Physical Activity Recall (n=151), p<0.001 for ANOVA comparing body weight change at 36 months. In panel b), activity was assessed by accelerometry (GT3X Activity Monitor, Actigraph, Pensacola, FL) in a subset of women (n=60), p=0.017 for 36-months body weight change. Unpublished results from the PESO trial, including participants in both intervention and control groups (more details available in Silva *et al.*, 2008; Silva *et al.*, 2010a; Silva *et al.*, in press).

Non-randomized designs have more consistently showed improved weight maintenance if exercise/physical activity is present, especially at the highest adherence categories. This has been noted in several reviews and reports published in the last 15 years (Curioni and Lourenco, 2005; Miller *et al.*, 1997; Catenacci and Wyatt, 2007; Fogelholm and Kukkonen-Harjula, 2000; Donnelly *et al.*, 2009) and has been especially highlighted in studies from the US National Weight Control Registry, which relies exclusively on information from those already success-ful at maintaining weight previously lost; high levels of physical activity have been consistently reported by these weight maintenance 'experts', who average over 2500 kcal/wk of physical activity (see Catenacci and Wyatt, 2007). This is equivalent to 60–75 min/d of moderate intensity physical activity or 35–45 min/d of vigorous physical activity. However, the large individual variability should be noted, stressing that weight loss maintenance is clearly possible at lower exercise/ physical activity levels (Table 15.2). Taking all previous evidence into account, the 2009 Position Stand of the ACSM states that, after weight loss, weight main-tenance is likely to be associated with ~60 minutes walking per day at a moderate intensity (Donnelly *et al.*, 2009). As recently recommended (Stevens *et al.*, 2006), weight maintenance was defined by the ACSM panel as a weight fluctuation below 3 per cent. More recently, additional support for the role of physical activity in preventing weight gain, both before and after weight loss, has been provided by findings from the Nurses Health Study II (Mekary *et al.*, 2010) the Women's Health Study (Lee *et al.*, 2010) and the Doetinchem Cohort Study (May *et al.*, 2010).

TABLE 15.2 Frequency distribution of physical activity energy expenditure levels in the USA National Weight Control Registry between 1993 and 2004 (from Catenacci *et al.*, 2008)

Activity level (kcal/week)	1993–2004		
	M (%)	F (%)	All (%)
<500	12.7	16.0	15.2
500–999	10.0	10.2	10.1
1,000–1,499	10.3	11.0	10.8
1,500–1,999	8.6	10.4	10.0
2,000–2,499	9.3	10.0	9.9
2,500–2,999	8.4	9.4	9.1
3,000–3,499	9.8	7.2	7.9
3,500–3,999	5.6	6.2	6.0
4,000–4,499	6.0	4.6	4.9
4,500–4,999	4.1	3.6	3.7
>5,000	15.1	11.5	12.3

The critical issue of exercise adherence for successful long-term weight control is further exemplified in a study where participants were randomized to either 18 months of standard behaviour therapy including an exercise prescription of 1000 kcal/wk or to the same programme plus an incentive package (family support, exercise coaches and monetary rewards for meeting exercise goals), targeting 2500 kcal/wk (Jeffery *et al.*, 2003). The latter group reported a mean of 2317 kcal/wk in exercise energy expenditure compared to 1629 kcal/wk in the standard group, and mean weight loss and maintenance was 6.7 and 4.1 kg at 18 months, respectively. Despite the fact that it was an uncontrolled trial, it indicated that, when effectively executed, recommended exercise/physical activity will predict a significantly higher amount of weight loss which is maintained, in a dose-response manner (Ross and Janssen, 2001; Donnelly *et al.*, 2009). It is important to bear in mind that high individual variability in exercise/physical activity is present in virtually all published studies on this topic, which makes interpreting study outcomes using only mean values particularly limiting. Additionally, attrition rates in many reviewed studies were moderate to high, another important qualification when considering the practical implications of these findings.

Different types of exercise or physical activity

Most studies on exercise/physical activity and obesity evaluated structured aerobic exercise/physical activity (brisk walking, running, cycling, etc.). Compared to other forms of physical activity, this type of continuous, repetitive exercise induces larger energy expenditure rates and is typically easy to prescribe and monitor. Considering that these modalities are also largely accessible to the population and do not involve much learning on the part of study participants, the option is justifiable. However, other forms of exercise have been investigated, e.g. resistance or strength training and also less structured (informal) types of physical activity, especially walking within normal daily routines (e.g. daily chores, transportation, etc.). This is sometimes referred to as *lifestyle physical activity* (Donnelly *et al.*, 2009).

Regarding resistance exercise, a recent ACSM Position Stand (Donnelly *et al.*, 2009) suggests that while it increases fat-free mass and resting metabolism, reduces cardiovascular risk factors (even without weight loss) and may enhance fat loss when combined with aerobic exercise (versus resistance exercise alone), it is not an effective form to promote clinically significant weight reduction, if used in isolation or with a dietary intervention. The ACSM based this conclusion on category A level evidence (Donnelly *et al.*, 2009). These findings are most likely a consequence of resistance exercise's relatively low metabolic requirement (about 3–6 versus 6–12 kcal/h per kg of body weight for most aerobic activities) and lower fat oxidation rates, compared to continuous exercises involving large muscle masses. Insufficient evidence is presently available for evaluating the efficacy of resistance exercise for preventing weight regain or to draw conclusions on a potential dose–response relation with weight changes.

However, dietary energy-restricted programmes, which include resistance training within the prescribed exercise plan, may be especially suited to protect participants against concurrent muscle tissue loss (e.g. Kraemer *et al.*, 1999). The USDHHS 2008 Physical Activity Guidelines report committee concluded that the magnitude of weight loss observed with resistance exercise is typically less than 1 kg, stressing that, in some studies, increases in fat-free mass may have masked the true impact of this form of exercise on fat mass (Physical Activity Guidelines Advisory Committee, 2008).

Compared to aerobic or resistance exercise, lifestyle physical activity is more difficult to define and to measure in research studies. This is especially due to walking – the major component of lifestyle physical activity that is liable to substantial change induced by interventions – a form of activity which can be engaged in very purposefully (e.g. a Saturday morning brisk walk for exercise) or very informally (e.g. walking about during daily commuting). Objective measures of walking behaviour such as those derived from pedometers or accelerometers cannot distinguish between the different forms of walking. Additionally, people are typically not able to reliably recall all minutes of walking included in their day. Considering these limitations, most studies have used 'lifestyle interventions' (instead of actually measuring 'lifestyle physical activity') to promote increased walking and more active lives, and then measured the effects on BMI or weight.

Perhaps the best evidence available for the effects of walking on weight can be found in a 2007 review of pedometer-based interventions to increase walking physical activity (Bravata *et al.*, 2003). Twenty-six studies (eight RCTs) were included, with interventions lasting an average of 18 weeks with mostly overweight women (mean BMI of 30 kg/m^2). They showed a mean increase of 2183 steps/day over baseline and a significant mean decrease in BMI of 0.38 kg/m^2 (~1.2 per cent reduction); however, change in BMI and change in daily steps were not correlated (Bravata *et al.*, 2003). A limited number of studies which have directly compared interventions to increase walking with those aimed at increasing structured exercise (e.g. in aerobic classes) have generally found comparable results from both protocols on weight and other metabolic variables (e.g. Andersen *et al.*, 1999; Dunn *et al.*, 1999). Despite methodological limitations in evaluating the true effects of lifestyle physical activity on weight control and remaining questions as to the best lifestyle physical activity prescription, the aforementioned ACSM's Position Stand panel concluded that lifestyle physical activity is useful for weight management and also to 'counter the small energy imbalance responsible for obesity in most adults' (category B evidence) (Donnelly *et al.*, 2009).

Compensatory responses to exercise

The efficacy and effectiveness of exercise as a method of weight control was discussed in the previous section. In all of these studies, its success was ultimately based on body weight and the capacity to create and maintain a negative energy deficit. One reason why exercise fails to achieve a theoretically calculated weight loss is because of behavioural and metabolic responses that compensate for the exercise-induced increase in energy expenditure (see King *et al.*, 2007 for a more comprehensive review). When people take up exercise they could experience an increase in hunger and food intake; or they could become more sedentary during non-exercise periods; or metabolism could become downregulated or more efficient. This section discusses the evidence which could account for individual variability in exercise-induced weight changes and why some people fail to lose or maintain the theoretical weight loss. The information could be used to design more effective weight loss strategies – which are tailored to suit the individual. The phenomenon of compensatory adjustments to imposed changes in energy expenditure is not new; the work of Edholm in the 1950s suggested that energy expenditure and energy intake are not tightly regulated (Edholm *et al.*, 1955).

Compensatory responses can be categorized into physiological and behavioural. Physiological responses tend to be 'obligatory' and often occur as an automatic consequence of a reduction in tissue-related mass. For example, a decrease in fat and fat-free mass is typically accompanied by a reduction in resting metabolic rate (Elia, 1992) and the energy cost of exercise *per se* (Doucet *et al.*, 2003). They also tend to be predictable and constrained (as is the case with change in resting metabolic rate in relation to altered body composition). Behavioural responses are much more flexible and unpredictable (such as increased sleep, or a change in the non-exercise activity profiles) and tend to account for more of the variance in changes in energy balance that occurs in response to a change in activity profile.

There are very few studies that have characterized the physiological and behavioural compensatory responses to marked energy deficits. The data suggest that the largest component of compensation is through behaviour rather than physiology. Work by Johnstone *et al.* (2002) demonstrated that an increased rate of weight loss through dietary restriction will produce a 'compensatory' decrease in physical activity. It should be remembered that in addition to this active 'cross-talk' between reduced energy intake and physical activity energy expenditure, the obligatory changes mentioned above will also occur. These findings again point to the need to better quantify the aggregate effects of facultative (active) changes in behaviour *and* obligatory (or passive) changes in energy balance on overall predisposition to gain weight or success at losing it.

Measuring 'cross-talk' between energy intake and expenditure

It is important to note that in recent years much attention has focused on the role that diet composition plays in energy balance control in *ad libitum* feeding subjects. Far less attention has been paid to changes in energy expenditure in response to perturbed energy balance. Measuring interactions between energy intake and energy expenditure *as a consequence* of perturbed energy balance is a conceptual step further. We are only beginning to simultaneously measure changes in all components of energy balance in response to altered energy balance, in order to assess the rate and extent of mechanisms of weight control. One preliminary study has given us an initial, albeit imperfect assessment of the rate and extent of compensation of energy intake and energy expenditure in response to pertur- bations of energy balance due to altered diet and exercise (Stubbs *et al.*, 2004). Compensatory changes in energy intake and energy expenditure were in the oppo- site direction to the initial perturbation in energy balance (Figure 15.3).

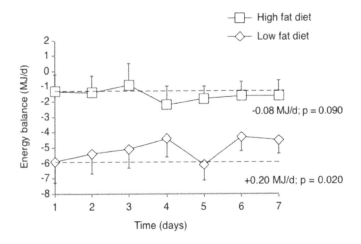

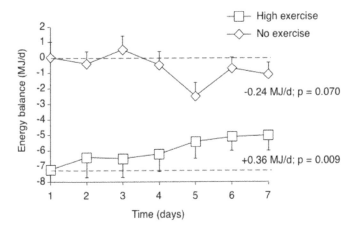

FIGURE 15.3 Convergence of energy balance over 7 days due to compensation of energy intake and expenditure in a study of 8 men subjected to diet and exercise- induced alterations of energy balance. From Stubbs *et al.*, (2004).

Compensation, however, tends not to occur at a linear rate as weight changes, since weight gain or loss tends to plateau. While these estimates may be provisional and imperfect, they do suggest that (i) 'cross-talk' between changes in energy intake and energy expenditure does exist, (ii) this cross-talk is stronger in relation to energy deficits than surfeits, and (iii) it takes weeks for significant compensatory changes in energy balance to occur in relation to a sustained perturbation of energy balance. In real life, several of these influences are likely to be superimposed on each other, making the determinants of both energy intake and energy expenditure multi-factorial. Interactions between the two will be similarly complex in both nature and their overall impact on energy balance, in the development and treatment of obesity.

Individual variability

Although little attention was given to Bouchard's work on variability in response to energy balance interventions more than 10 years ago (e.g. Bouchard, 1995), there has been a revitalized interest in the phenomenon of inter-individual variability in responses to exercise (King *et al.*, 2007). Some individuals will be predisposed to compensatory responses that render them resistant to the expected weight loss benefits. Even when exercise interventions are supervised, there is a wide range of weight loss responses, including weight gain (King *et al.*, 2008). However, when exercise is supervised people still experience beneficial physiological and psychological effects independent of any effect on body weight (King *et al.*, 2009b).

Behavioural compensatory response: energy intake and non-exercise energy expenditure

Most of the evidence shows that acute (single bout to one day) exercise-induced increases in energy expenditure generate little or no immediate effect on levels of hunger or daily energy intake (see Martins *et al.*, 2008 for a review). This means that in the very short term there is no compensation for exercise. When the exercise interventions and monitoring of food intake are extended, people typically show partial compensatory responses for relatively large increases in energy expenditure with an exercise intervention lasting 14 days (Whybrow *et al.*, 2008). The compensatory rise in food intake was on average about 30 per cent of the energy expended in exercise, but it was highly variable. These compensatory responses are accompanied by increases in the orexigenic drive measured by fasting hunger (King *et al.*, 2009a). However, because compensation is only partial it is important to note that such interventions lead to reductions in body weight – in lean or overweight subjects. Therefore, overall the evidence points to a weak coupling between activity energy expenditure and energy intake.

There is some evidence to demonstrate that the sensitivity of appetite regulation is better in physically active individuals (Long *et al.*, 2002), and can be improved via exercise training in sedentary individuals (Martins *et al.*, 2007). Exercise evoked an increase in orexigenic drive (overall increase in hunger which differed between individuals) but improved satiety signalling immediately after a meal. The combined strength of these two processes will determine the degree of compensation observed. In turn, the degree of compensation will determine how much weight is lost. Or, if there is over-compensation, how much weight is gained. Approximately 15 per cent of people gain weight with exercise (although it could vary from group to group) but the weight gain is almost entirely lean tissue. Generally there is an absolute decrease in body fat.

Some evidence has suggested that changes in non-exercise energy expenditure is an important contributor to the magnitude of weight gain in response to overfeeding and have a protective effect (Levine *et al.*, 1999). Alternatively, in conditions of imposed exercise, some individuals might compensate by decreasing non-exercise activity such that the net energy expenditure or total time spent active remains unaffected (Meijer *et al.*, 1999). One other behavioural factor that could be adjusted to compensate is sleep. However, this remains to be tested experimentally.

The challenge of behaviour change in overweight and obese persons

Meeting the exercise/physical activity recommended targets for weight control (as described in previous sections) may be considerably challenging for many people. It could be argued that many individuals, especially if they are moderately or severely obese, will find it difficult to include 30–60 minutes of moderate intensity activity in most days of their lives, at least initially. However, weight change is a function of the total sum of energy balance, not energy expenditure *per se*, and data from the US National Weight Control Registry (NWCR) (Catenacci *et al.*, 2008) clearly indicate that it is possible to lose *and maintain* substantial amounts of body weight with physical activity levels *below the recommended targets*. Again, this implies an energy balance approach to understanding weight control, namely combining increased energy expenditure with modifications in dietary intake (Kremers *et al.*, 2004; Schoeller, 2009). Indeed, a key message from the NWCR studies is that very few 'successful losers' use either dietary restraint or physical activity *in isolation* to keep their weight off. It is not the case that they found an adequate level of food energy intake *or* level of physical activity; instead, they found a feasible (and highly individual) way to *manage their daily energy balance*, resulting in successful weight loss maintenance.

The feasibility and efficacy of *any* physical activity prescription will depend on environmental and personal characteristics (e.g. features of appetite control or behavioural self-regulation), as well as on how successful an intervention is in accounting for and/or influencing true predictors (moderators, mediators) of change in exercise/physical activity and sedentary behaviours. In other words, individual response to exercise/physical activity programs is determined by a variety of factors which, to a large extent, are *independent* of the dose of exercise/physical activity that is prescribed. Thus, we believe that the time has come for research efforts to progressively shift from further determining the types and doses of exercise/physical activity which are most effective at the various stages of the 'weight management spectrum' (i.e. preventing primary weight gain, producing weight loss, avoiding weight regain) and be increasingly directed towards studying the reasons why so many overweight or at risk individuals are unable or unwilling to become more active, and especially investigating how can they be better supported in adopting physical activity for life with effective, ethically appropriate and cost-effective interventions. Research is also needed to further understand behavioural and physiological compensatory responses which may limit the efficacy of physical activity for weight control in non-responsive individuals.

Presently, what is known about predictors of exercise/physical activity and sedentary behaviours in the overweight/obese population is extremely limited, mostly derived from findings in the general, healthy population (e.g. Bauman *et al.*, 2002), and too much of the available research is cross-sectional and/or observational. General predictors of weight management outcomes have been summarized in previous review papers (Teixeira *et al.*, 2005; Elfhag and Rossner, 2005) and this research offers much needed insight into the mechanisms which are associated with improved weight loss and/or maintenance, namely those related to physical activity/exercise. Although a thorough discussion of these aspects is beyond the scope of this text, it is noteworthy that variables specifically related to motivation and self-regulation for exercise/physical activity appear to be predictors of success in weight control (e.g. Teixeira *et al.*, 2006). This is not surprising. In most environmental conditions, being motivated (e.g. for being physically active) will remain a necessary condition for effective and lasting individual behaviour change. We fully agree that the environment makes it increasingly difficult to live a physically active life – and widespread and substantial environmental changes will need to occur to revert this scenario. However, we also believe an adequately motivated person will in most cases find the best solution to meet his/her goals and pursue his life aspirations, including leading a healthful life (Deci and Ryan, 2000). It must be remembered that this 'person' is the same one thousands of healthy professionals consult with every day, around the world. Both the clinician and her patient cannot wait for societal and environmental change; they need assistance in their clinical decisions today and they deserve the best scientific research to provide it.

One predictor of exercise behaviours in obese persons, grounded on Social Cognitive Theory (Bandura, 2001), is exercise self-efficacy, usually associated with lower perceived barriers to be active (e.g. Teixeira *et al.*, 2006). Changes in both self-efficacy and perceived barriers (for exercise) have been found to predict long-term weight control (Teixeira *et al.*, 2010). Intrinsic motivation for exercise/physical activity, a hallmark of self-determined, highly volitional engagement with exercise/physical activity (including experiencing enjoyment and competence, valuing physical activity as important, and reduced feelings of pressure to be active), has been shown to predict long-term weight control in at least two independent studies (Teixeira *et al.*, 2006; Teixeira *et al.*, 2010) and to mediate moderate and vigorous physical activity in women, both in the short- (Silva *et al.*, 2010b) and in the long-term (Silva *et al.*, in press). Additionally, autonomous motivation also predicted improved eating behaviours in the context of weight control in women, a novel finding suggesting that exercise and eating may also 'cross-talk' at a motivational and self-regulatory level (Andrade *et al.*, 2010; Mata *et al.*, 2009; Kremers *et al.*, 2004). Autonomy, perceived competence, and intrinsic motivation are central concepts of self-determination theory, a framework for studying human motivation and action, which has proved promising in the field of behavioural medicine, including physical activity/exercise and weight control (Williams *et al.*, 1996; Williams *et al.*, 2005; Williams *et al.*, 2006 Wilson *et al.*, 2008). It has recently been adapted to weight control with positive results (Silva *et al.*, 2008, Silva *et al.*, in press). This is just one example of the use of behavioural theory to investigate exercise/physical activity adoption in this population, mostly at the individual level. Others need to be pursued at this and other levels (e.g. community, population) before solid progress in promoting physical activity in the overweight/obese can be achieved.

Summary

Exercise and physical activity are critical to effectively preventing and treating overweight and obesity. Overall weight loss achieved will depend on the amount of exercise actually completed; generally, the greater the volume of exercise performed (min/week; kcal/week), the greater the effect on body weight. Failure to comply with an exercise prescription is an important reason for the apparent modest effect of exercise in many long-term trials. However, even when compliance is >90 per cent, the potential benefit of the energy expended in exercise can be offset by compensatory responses, mainly driven by increases in hunger and food intake. This is highly variable from person to person and depends on genetic determination of physiological regulatory processes of energy balance. Some over-compensators will need additional help to manage their enhanced eating behaviour, highlighting the need for an energy balance approach to weight control. Difficulties with behavioural change in general, and especially with integrating new sustainable behavioural patterns into one's routines, are probably among the most important reasons why exercise fails to control body weight. Obstacles also exist in the built and socio-cultural environment. However, for an obese person, exercise is tremendously beneficial and widely recommended, even for the most severe cases (Blackburn *et al.*, 2010). In addition to weight management, exercise improves blood pressure and glucose control, predicts healthy body composition, promotes cardiovascular fitness and contributes to a range of beneficial outcomes in mental health and psychological well-being (Physical Activity Guidelines Advisory Committee, 2008).

References

Andersen, R. E., Wadden, T. A., Bartlett, S. J., Zemel, B., Verde, T. J. and Franckowiak, S. C. (1999). Effects of lifestyle activity vs structured aerobic exercise in obese women: a randomized trial. *JAMA*, 281, 335–340.

Andrade, A. M., Coutinho, S. R., Silva, M. N., Carraça, E. V., Mata, J., Melanson, K. J., Sardinha, L. B., Teixeira, P. J. (2010). The effect of physical activity on weight loss is mediated by eating self-regulation. *Patient Educ Couns*, 79: 320–326.

Barry, C. L., Brescoll V. L., Brownell, K. D. and Schlesinger, M. (2009). Obesity metaphors: how beliefs about the causes of obesity affect support for public policy. *Milbank Q*, 87, 7–47.

Ballor, D. L. (1996). Exercise training and body composition changes. In: Roche, A. F., Heymsfield, S. B. and Lohman, T. G. (eds) *Human Body Composition*. Champaign, IL: Human Kinetics Publishers.

Ballor, D. L. and Keesey, R. E. (1991). A meta-analysis of the factors affecting exercise-induced changes in body mass, fat mass and fat-free mass in males and females. *Int J Obes*, 15, 717–26.

Bandura, A. (2001). Social cognitive theory: an agentic perspective. *Annu Rev Psychol*, 52, 1–26.

Bauman, A. E., Sallis, J. F., Dzewaltowski, D. A. and Owen, N. (2002). Toward a better understanding of the influences on physical activity: the role of determinants, correlates, causal variables, mediators, moderators, and confounders. *Am J Prev Med*, 23, 5–14.

Blackburn, G. L., Wollner, S. and Heymsfield, S. B. (2010). Lifestyle interventions for the treatment of class III obesity: a primary target for nutrition medicine in the obesity epidemic. *Am J Clin Nutr*, 91, 289S-292S.

Blair, S. N. and Church, T. S. (2004). The fitness, obesity, and health equation: is physical activity the common denominator? *JAMA*, 292, 1232–4.

Blundell, J. E. (1995). The psychobiological approach to appetite and weight control. In: Brownell, K. D. and Fariburn, C. G. (eds) *Eating Disorders And Obesity: A Comprehensive Handbook*. New York, USA: The Guildford Press.

Blundell, J. E. and Stubbs, R. J. (1998). Diet composition and the control of food intake in humans. In: Bray, G. E., Bouchard, C. and James, W. P. T. (eds) *Handbook of Obesity*. New York: Marcel Dekker.

Bouchard, C. (1995). Individual differences in the response to regular exercise. *Int J Obes Relat Metab Disord*, 19 Suppl 4, S5–8.

Bravata, D. M., Sanders, L., Huang, J., Krumholz, H. M., Olkin, I. and Gardner, C. D. (2003). Efficacy and safety of low-carbohydrate diets: a systematic review. *JAMA*, 289, 1837–50.

Broeder, C. E., Burrhus, K. A., Svanevik, L. S. and Wilmore, J. H. (1992). The effects of aerobic fitness on resting metabolic rate. *Am J Clin Nutr*, 55, 795–801.

Catenacci, V. A., Ogden, L. G., Stuht, J., Phelan, S., Wing, R. R., Hill, J. O. and Wyatt, H. R. (2008). Physical activity patterns in the National Weight Control Registry. *Obesity (Silver Spring)*, 16, 153–61.

Catenacci, V. A. and Wyatt, H. R. (2007). The role of physical activity in producing and maintaining weight loss. *Nat Clin Pract Endocrinol Metab*, 3, 518–29.

Church, T. S., Martin, C. K., Thompson, A. M., Earnest, C. P., Mikus, C. R. and Blair, S. N. (2009). Changes in weight, waist circumference and compensatory responses with different doses of exercise among sedentary, overweight postmenopausal women. *PLoS One*, 4, e4515.

Coakley, E. H., Kawachi, I., Manson, J. E., Speizer, F. E., Willet, W. C. and Colditz, G. A. (1998). Lower levels of physical functioning are associated with higher body weight among middle-aged and older women. *Int J Obes Relat Metab Disord*, 22, 958–65.

Curioni, C. C. and Lourenco, P. M. (2005). Long-term weight loss after diet and exercise: a systematic review. *Int J Obes (Lond)*, 29, 1168–74.

Deci, E. L. and Ryan, R. M. (2000). The 'what' and 'why' of goal pursuits: Human needs and the self-determination of behavior. *Psychological Inquiry*, 11, 227–268.

Donnelly, J. E., Blair, S. N., Jakicic, J. M., Manore, M. M., Rankin, J. W. and Smith, B. K. (2009). American College of Sports Medicine Position Stand. Appropriate physical activity intervention strategies for weight loss and prevention of weight regain for adults. *Med Sci Sports Exerc*, 41, 459–71.

Donnelly, J. E., Hill, J. O., Jacobsen, D. J., Potteiger, J., Sullivan, D. K., Johnson, S. L., Heelan, K., Hise, M., Fennessey, P. V., Sonko, B., Sharp, T., Jakicic, J. M., Blair, S. N., Tran, Z. V., Mayo, M., Gibson, C. and Washburn, R. A. (2003). Effects of a 16-month randomized controlled exercise trial on body weight and composition in young, overweight men and women: the Midwest Exercise Trial. *Arch Intern Med*, 163, 1343–50.

Doucet, E., Imbeault, P., St-Pierre, S., Almeras, N., Mauriege, P., Despres, J. P., Bouchard, C. and Tremblay, A. (2003). Greater than predicted decrease in energy expenditure during exercise after body weight loss in obese men. *Clin Sci (Lond)*, 105, 89–95.

Dunn, A., Marcus, B., Kampert, J., Garcia, M., Kohl, H. and Blair, S. (1999). Comparison of lifestyle and structured interventions to increase physical activity and cardiorespiratory fitness. *Journal of American Medical Association*, 281, 327–334.

Edholm, O. G., Fletcher, J. G., Widdowson, E. M. and McCance, R. A. (1955). The energy expenditure and food intake of individual men. *Br J Nutr*, 9, 286–300.

Elfhag, K. and Rossner, S. (2005). Who succeeds in maintaining weight loss? A conceptual review of factors associated with weight loss maintenance and weight regain. *Obes Rev*, 6, 67–85.

Elia, M. (1992). Energy expenditure in the whole body. *Energy Metabolism*, 19–29.

Elia, M., Stratton, R. and Stubbs, R. J. (2003). Techniques for the study of energy balance in man. *Proceedings of the Nutrition Society*, 62, 529–537.

Elia, M., Stubbs, R. J. and Henry, C. J. (1999). Differences in fat, carbohydrate, and protein metabolism between lean and obese subjects undergoing total starvation. *Obes Res*, 7, 597–604.

Ezzati, M., Vander Hoorn, S., Lopez, A. D., Danaei, G., Rodgers, A., Mathers, C. D. and Murray, C. J. L. (2006). Comparative quantification of mortality and burden of disease attributable to selected risk factors. In: Lopez, A., Mathers, C., Ezzati, M., Jamison, D. T. and Murray, C. J. L. (eds) *Global Burden of Disease and Risk Factors*. New York: World Bank.

Fogelholm, M. (2010). Physical activity, fitness and fatness: relations to mortality, morbidity and disease risk factors. A Systematic review. *Obes Rev*, 11, 202–221.

Fogelholm, M. and Kukkonen-Harjula, K. (2000). Does physical activity prevent weight gain –a systematic review. *Obes Rev*, 1, 95–111.

Gallagher, D., Heymsfield, S. B., Heo, M., Jebb, S. A., Murgatroyd, P. R. and Sakamoto, Y. (2000). Healthy percentage body fat ranges: an approach for developing guidelines based on body mass index. *Am J Clin Nutr*, 72, 694–701.

Gallagher, D., Visser, M., Sepulveda, D., Pierson, R. N., Harris, T. and Heymsfield, S. B. (1996). How useful is body mass index for comparison of body fatness across age, sex, and ethnic groups? *Am J Epidemiol*, 143, 228–39.

Garrow, J. S. and Summerbell, C. D. (1995). Meta-analysis: effect of exercise, with or without dieting, on the body composition of overweight subjects. *Eur J Clin Nutr*, 49, 1–10.

Gregg, E. W., Cheng, Y. J., Cadwell, B. L., Imperatore, G., Williams, D. E., Flegal, K. M., Narayan, K. M. and Williamson, D. F. (2005). Secular trends in cardiovascular disease risk factors according to body mass index in US adults. *JAMA*, 293, 1868–74.

Haapanen-Niemi, N., Miilunpalo, S., Pasanen, M., Vuori, I., Oja, P. and Malmberg, J. (2000). Body mass index, physical inactivity and low level of physical fitness as determinants of all-cause and cardiovascular disease mortality--16 y follow-up of middle-aged and elderly men and women. *Int J Obes Relat Metab Disord*, 24, 1465–74.

Hassan, M. K., Joshi, A. V., Madhavan, S. S. and Amonkar, M. M. (2003). Obesity and health-related quality of life: a cross-sectional analysis of the US population. *Int J Obes Relat Metab Disord*, 27, 1227–32.

Hu, F. B. (2008a). Descriptive epidemiology of obesity trends. In: Hu, F. B. (ed.) *Obesity Epidemiology*. New York: Oxford.

Hu, F. B. (ed.) (2008b). *Obesity Epidemiology*, New York: Oxford.

Hu, F. B., Li, T. Y., Colditz, G. A., Willett, W. C. and Manson, J. E. (2003). Television watching and other sedentary behaviors in relation to risk of obesity and type 2 diabetes mellitus in women. *JAMA*, 289, 1785–91.

Jakicic, J. M., Marcus, B. H., Lang, W. and Janney, C. (2008). Effect of exercise on 24-month weight loss maintenance in overweight women. *Archives of Internal Medicine*, 168, 1550–59.

Janssen, I., Lam, M. and Katzmarzyk, P. T. (2009). Influence of overweight and obesity on physician costs in adolescents and adults in Ontario, Canada. *Obes Rev*, 10, 51–7.

Jebb, S. A. and Prentice, A. M. (1995). *Is Obesity an Eating Disorder? Proceedings of the Nutrition Society*, 54, 721–728.

Jeffery, R. W., Wing, R. R., Sherwood, N. E. and Tate, D. F. (2003). Physical activity and weight loss: does prescribing higher physical activity goals improve outcome? *Am J Clin Nutr*, 78, 684–9.

Johnstone, A. M., Faber, P., Gibney, E. R., Elia, M., Horgan, G., Golden, B. E. and Stubbs, R. J. (2002). Effect of an acute fast on energy compensation and feeding behaviour in lean men and women. *International Journal of Obesity*, 26, 1623–8.

Kay, S. J. and Fiatarone Singh, M. A. (2006). The influence of physical activity on abdominal fat: a systematic review of the literature. *Obes Rev*, 7, 183–200.

King, N., A., Caudwell, P., Hopkins, M., Byrne, N. M., Colley, R., Hills, A. P., Stubbs, J. R. and Blundell, J. E. (2007). Metabolic and behavioral compensatory responses to exercise interventions: barriers to weight loss. *Obesity*, 15, 1373–1383.

King, N. A., Caudwell, P. P., Hopkins, M., Stubbs, J. R., Naslund, E. and Blundell, J. E. (2009a). Dual-process action of exercise on appetite control: increase in orexigenic drive but improvement in meal-induced satiety. *Am J Clin Nutr*, 90, 921–7.

King, N. A., Hopkins, M., Caudwell, P., Stubbs, R. J. and Blundell, J. E. (2008). Individual variability following 12 weeks of supervised exercise: identification and characterization of compensation for exercise-induced weight loss. *Int J Obes (Lond)*, 32, 177–84.

King, N. A., Hopkins, M., Caudwell, P., Stubbs, R. J. and Blundell, J. E. (2009b). Beneficial effects of exercise: shifting the focus from body weight to other markers of health. *Br J Sports Med*, 43, 924–7.

Kissebah, A. H. and Krakower, G. R. (1994). Regional adiposity and morbidity. *Physiol Rev*, 74, 761–809.

Kraemer, W. J., Volek, J. S., Clark, K. L., Gordon, S. E., Puhl, S. M., Koziris, L. P., Mcbride, J. M., Triplett-Mcbride, N. T., Putukian, M., Newton, R. U., Hakkinen, K., Bush, J. A. and Sebastianelli, W. J. (1999). Influence of exercise training on physiological and performance changes with weight loss in men. *Med Sci Sports Exerc*, 31, 1320–9.

Kremers, S. P., De Bruijn, G. J., Schaalma, H. and Brug, J. (2004). Clustering of energy balance-related behaviours and their intrapersonal determinants. *Psychology and Health*, 19, 595–606.

Layman, D. K., Evans, E., Baum, J. I., Seyler, J., Erickson, D. J. and Boileau, R. A. (2005). Dietary protein and exercise have additive effects on body composition during weight loss in adult women. *J Nutr*, 135, 1903–10.

Lee, C. D. and Blair, S. N. (2002). Cardiorespiratory fitness and smoking-related and total cancer mortality in men. *Med Sci Sports Exerc*, 34, 735–9.

Lee, I. M., Djousse, L., Sesso, H. D., Wang, L. and Buring, J. E. (2010). Physical activity and weight gain prevention. *JAMA*, 303, 1173–9.

Levine, J. A., Eberhardt, N. L. and Jensen, M. D. (1999). Role of nonexercise activity thermogenesis in resistance to fat gain in humans. *Science*, 283, 212–4.

Long, S. J., Hart, K. and Morgan, L. M. (2002). The ability of habitual exercise to influence appetite and food intake in response to high- and low-energy preloads in man. *British Journal of Nutrition*, 87, 517–523.

Martins, C., Morgan, L. and Truby, H. (2008). A review of the effects of exercise on appetite regulation: an obesity perspective. *Int J Obes (Lond)*, 32, 1337–47.

Martins, C., Truby, H. and Morgan, L. M. (2007). Short-term appetite control in response to a 6-week exercise programme in sedentary volunteers. *Br J Nutr*, 98, 834–42.

Mata, J., Silva, M. N., Vieira, P. N., Carraca, E. V., Andrade, A. M., Coutinho, S. R., Sardinha, L. B. and Teixeira, P. J. (2009). Motivational 'spill-over' during weight control: increased self-determination and exercise intrinsic motivation predict eating self-regulation. *Health Psychol*, 28, 709–16.

May, A. M., Bueno-de-Mesquita, H. B., Boshuizen, H., Spijkerman, A. M., Peeters, P. H., Verschuren, W. M.. (2010). Effect of change in physical activity on body fatness over a 10-y period in the Doetinchem Cohort Study. *Am J Clin Nutr*.; 92(3):491–9.

Mayo, M. J., Grantham, J. R. and Balasekaran, G. (2003). Exercise-induced weight loss preferentially reduces abdominal fat. *Med Sci Sports Exerc*, 35, 207–13.

Meijer, E. P., Westerterp, K. R. and Verstappen, F. T. (1999). Effect of exercise training on total daily physical activity in elderly humans. *Eur J Appl Physiol Occup Physiol*, 80, 16–21.

Mekary, R. A., Feskanich, D., Hu, F. B., Willett, W. C. and Field, A. E. (2010). Physical activity in relation to long-term weight maintenance after intentional weight loss in premenopausal women. *Obesity (Silver Spring)*, 18, 167–74.

Miller, W. C., Koceja, D. M. and Hamilton, E. J. (1997). A meta-analysis of the past 25 years of weight loss research using diet, exercise or diet plus exercise intervention. *Int J Obes Relat Metab Disord*, 21, 941–7.

Must, A., Spadano, J., Coakley, E. H., Field, A. E., Colditz, G. and Dietz, W. H. (1999). The disease burden associated with overweight and obesity. *JAMA*, 282, 1523–9.

Ohkawara, K., Tanaka, S., Miyachi, M., Ishikawa-Takata, K. and Tabata, I. (2007). A dose-response relation between aerobic exercise and visceral fat reduction: systematic review of clinical trials. *Int J Obes (Lond)*, 31, 1786–97.

Physical Activity Guidelines Advisory Committee (2008). *Physical Activity Guidelines Advisory Committee Report*, Washington DC, U.S. Department of Health and Human Services.

Prentice, A. M., Black, A. E., Murgatroyd, P. R., Goldberg, G. R. and Coward, W. A. (1989). Metabolism or appetite: questions of energy balance with particular reference to obesity. *Journal of Human Nutrition and Dietetics*, 2, 95–104.

Prentice, A. M. and Jebb, S. A. (1995). Obesity in Britain: gluttony or sloth? *British Medical Journal*, 311, 437–439.

Puhl, R. M. and Heuer, C. A. (2009). The stigma of obesity: a review and update. *Obesity (Silver Spring)*, 17, 941–64.

Ross, R., Dagnone, D., Jones, P. J., Smith, H., Paddags, A., Hudson, R. and Janssen, I. (2000). Reduction in obesity and related comorbid conditions after diet-induced weight loss or exercise-induced weight loss in men. A randomized, controlled trial. *Ann Intern Med*, 133, 92–103.

Ross, R. and Janssen, I. (2001). Physical activity, total and regional obesity: dose-response considerations. *Med Sci Sports Exerc*, 33, S521–7; discussion S528–9.

Ross, R. and Katzmarzyk, P. T. (2003). Cardiorespiratory fitness is associated with diminished total and abdominal obesity independent of body mass index. *Int J Obes Relat Metab Disord*, 27, 204–10.

Sallis, J. F. and Glanz, K. (2009). Physical activity and food environments: solutions to the obesity epidemic. *Milbank Q*, 87, 123–154.

Sardinha, L. B. and Teixeira, P. J. (2005). Measuring adiposity and fat distribution in relation to health. In: Heymsfield, S. B., Lohman, T. G., Wang, Z. and Going, S. B. (eds) *Human Body Composition*. Champaign, IL: Human Kinetics.

Schoeller, D. A. (2009). The energy balance equation: looking back and looking forward are two very different views. *Nutr Rev*, 67, 249–54.

Shaw, K., Gennat, H., O'Rourke, P. And Del Mar, C. (2006). Exercise for overweight or obesity. *Cochrane Database System Reviews*, CD003817.

Silva, M. N., Markland, D., Minderico, C. S., Vieira, P. N., Castro, M. M., Coutinho, S. R., Santos, T. C., Matos, M. G., Sardinha, L. B. and Teixeira, P. J. (2008). A randomized controlled trial to evaluate Self-Determination Theory for exercise adherence and weight control: Rationale and intervention description. *BMC Public Health*, 8, 234.

Silva, M. N., Vieira, P. N., Coutinho S. R., Matos M. G., Sardinha L. B. and Teixeira, P. J. (2010a). Using self-determination theory to promote physical activity and weight contol: a randomized controlled trial in women. *J Behav Med*, 33, 110–22.

Silva M. N., Markland D., Vieira P. N., Coutinho S. R., Palmeira A. L., Carraça E. V., Minderico C. S., Matos M. G., Sardinha L. B. and Teixeira P. J. (2010b). Helping overweight women become more active: need support and motivational regulations for different forms of physical activity. *Psychology of Sport and Exercise*, 11, 591–601.

Silva M. N., Markland D., Carraça, E. V., Vieira P. N., Coutinho S. R., Minderico, C. S., Matos, M. G., Sardinha L. B., Teixeira P. J. (in press). Exercise autonomous motivation predicts 3-year weight loss in women. *Medicine and Science in Sports and Exercise*.

Smith, S. R., De Jonge, L., Zachwieja, J. J., Roy, H., Nguyen, T., Rood, J., Windhauser, M., Volaufova, J. and Bray, G. A. (2000). Concurrent physical activity increases fat oxidation during the shift to a high-fat diet. *Am J Clin Nutr*, 72, 131–8.

Stevens, J., Truesdale, K. P., Mcclain, J. E. and Cai, J. (2006). The definition of weight maintenance. *Int J Obes (Lond)*, 30, 391–9.

Stubbs, R. J. and Tolkamp, B. J. (2006). Control of energy balance in relation to energy intake and energy expenditure in animals and man: an ecological perspective. *British Journal of Nutrition*, 95, 657–676.

Stubbs, R. J., Hughes, D. A., Johnstone, A. M., Horgan, G. W., King, N., Elia, M. and Blundell, J. E. (2003). Interactions between energy intake and expenditure in the development and treatment of obesity. In: Medeiro-Neto, G., Halpern, A. and Bouchard, C. (eds) *Progress in Obesity Research 9*. Surrey, UK: John Libbey Eurotext Ltd.

Stubbs, R. J., Hughes, D. A., Johnstone, A. M., Whybrow, S., Horgan, G. W., King, N. and Blundell, J. (2004). Rate and extent of compensatory changes in energy intake and expenditure in response to altered exercise and diet composition in humans. *American Journal of Physiology-Regulatory Integrative and Comparative Physiology*, 286, R350–R358.

Stubbs, R. J., Whybrow S., King N., Blundell J. E. And Elia M. (2005). Effect of physical activity and other stressors on appetite: overcoming underconsumption of military operational rations, revisited. *Nutrient Composition of Rations for Short-Term, High-Intensity Combat Operations*. Washington DC: Food and Nutrition Board, Institute of Medicine of the National Academies Press.

Swinburn, B. A., Sacks, G., Lo, S. K., Westerterp, K. R., Rush, E. C., Rosenbaum, M., Luke, A., Schoeller, D. A., Delany, J. P., Butte, N. F. and Ravussin, E. (2009). Estimating the changes in energy flux that characterize the rise in obesity prevalence. *Am J Clin Nutr*, 89, 1723–8.

Teixeira, P. J., Going, S. B., Houtkooper, L. B., Cussler, E. C., Metcalfe, L. L., Blew, R. M., Sardinha, L. B. and Lohman, T. G. (2006). Exercise motivation, eating, and body image variables as predictors of weight control. *Med Sci Sports Exerc*, 38, 179–88.

Teixeira, P. J., Going, S. B., Sardinha, L. B. and Lohman, T. G. (2005). A review of psychosocial pre-treatment predictors of weight control. *Obes Rev*, 6, 43–65.

Teixeira, P. J., Silva, M. N., Coutinho, S. R., Palmeira, A. L., Mata, J., Vieira, P. N., Carraca, E. V., Santos, T. C. and Sardinha, L. B. (2010). Mediators of weight loss and weight loss maintenance in middle-aged women. *Obesity (Silver Spring)*, 18, 725–35.

Trogdon, J. G., Finkelstein, E. A., Hylands, T., Dellea, P. S. and Kamal-Bahl, S. J. (2008). Indirect costs of obesity: a review of the current literature. *Obes Rev*, 9, 489–500.

USDHHS (1998). *Clinical Guidelines on the Identification, Evaluation, and Treatment of Overweight and Obesity in Adults*. Bethesda, MD: NIH – National Heart, Lung and Blood Institute.

USDHHS (2000). *The Practical Guide to the Identification, Evaluation, and Treatment of Overweight and Obesity in Adults*. Bethesda, MD: NIH – National Heart, Lung, and Blood Institute.

Wang, Y., Beydoun, M. A., Liang, L., Caballero, B. and Kumanyika, S. K. (2008). Will all Americans become overweight or obese? estimating the progression and cost of the US obesity epidemic. *Obesity (Silver Spring)*, 16, 2323–30.

Wang, Y., Rimm, E. B., Stampfer, M. J., Willett, W. C. and Hu, F. B. (2005). Comparison of abdominal adiposity and overall obesity in predicting risk of type 2 diabetes among men. *Am J Clin Nutr*, 81, 555–63.

Wei, M. (2008). Cardiorespiratory fitness, adiposity, and mortality. *JAMA*, 299, 1013; author reply 1014.

Wei, M., Gibbons, L. W., Kampert, J. B., Nichaman, M. Z. And Blair, S. N. (2000). Low cardiorespiratory fitness and physical inactivity as predictors of mortality in men with type 2 diabetes. *Ann Intern Med*, 132, 605–11.

Wei, M., Kampert, J. B., Barlow, C. E., Nichaman, M. Z., Gibbons, L. W., Paffenbarger, R. S., Jr. and Blair, S. N. (1999). Relationship between low cardiorespiratory fitness and mortality in normal-weight, overweight, and obese men. *JAMA*, 282, 1547–53.

WHO (1998). Obesity – Preventing and Managing the Global Epidemic. Report of a WHO Consultation on Obesity. Geneva: World Health Organization.

Whybrow, S., Hughes, D. A., Ritz, P., Johnstone, A. M., Horgan, G. W., King, N., Blundell, J. E. and Stubbs, R. J. (2008). The effect of an incremental increase in exercise on appetite, eating behaviour and energy balance in lean men and women feeding ad libitum. *Br J Nutr*, 100, 1109–15.

Williams, G. C., Grow, V. M., Freedman, Z. R., Ryan, R. and Deci, E. (1996). Motivational predictors of weight loss and weight-loss maintenance. *Journal Personal Social Psychology*, 70, 115–26.

Williams, G. C., McGregor, H., Zeldman, A., Freedman, Z. R., Deci, E. and Elder, D. (2005). Promoting glycemic control through diabetes self-management: evaluating a patient activation intervention. *Patient Education Counsulting*, 56, 28–34.

Williams, G. C., McGregor, H. A., Sharp, D., Levesque, C., Kouides, R. W., Ryan, R. and Deci, E. (2006). Testing a self-determination theory intervention for motivating tobacco cessation: supporting autonomy and competence in a clinical trial. *Health Psychology*, 25, 91–101.

Wilson, P., Mack, D. and Grattan, K. (2008). Understanding motivation for exercise: a Self-Determination Theory perspective. *Canadian Psychology*, 49.

Wong, S. L., Katzmarzyk, P., Nichaman, M. Z., Church, T. S., Blair, S. N. and Ross, R. (2004). Cardiorespiratory fitness is associated with lower abdominal fat independent of body mass index. *Med Sci Sports Exerc*, 36, 286–91.

Wu, T., Gao, X., Chen, M. and Van Dam, R. M. (2009). Long-term effectiveness of diet-plus-exercise interventions vs. diet-only interventions for weight loss: a meta-analysis. *Obesity Reviews*, 10, 313–323.

Yan, L. L., Daviglus, M. L., Liu, K., Pirzada, A., Garside, D. B., Schiffer, L., Dyer, A. R. and Greenland, P. (2004). BMI and health-related quality of life in adults 65 years and older. *Obes Res*, 12, 69–76.

16

CHRONIC FATIGUE SYNDROME

Jo Nijs, Karen Wallman and Lorna Paul

Introduction

Chronic fatigue syndrome (CFS) describes a disorder that consists of chronic debilitating fatigue that cannot be explained by any known chronic medical or psychological condition (Holmes *et al.*, 1988). The most commonly used diagnostic criteria and definition of CFS for research and clinical purposes was published by the United States Centers for Disease Control and Prevention (Fukuda *et al.*, 1994). The core feature of a CFS diagnosis is the exclusion of any active medical condition which may explain the presence of the symptoms (e.g. primary sleep disorders, severe obesity, cancer hypothyroidism, Hepatitis B or C, major depressive disorders with psychotic or melancholic features, bipolar affective disorders, schizophrenia, dementia, alcohol abuse, etc.). In addition, the presence of a new onset (not lifelong), unexplained, persistent fatigue is required. The fatigue should be unrelated to exertion, is not substantially relieved by rest and should be severely disabling (i.e. causing substantial reductions in activity levels). Finally, four or more of the following symptoms should be present for six months or longer: impaired memory or concentration; post-exertional malaise, 'extreme, prolonged exhaustion and sickness' as a result of physical or mental exertion; unrefreshing sleep; muscle pain; pain in multiple joints; headaches of a new kind or greater severity; sore throat and tender lymph nodes (cervical or axillary). A large increase in pain and fatigue following too vigorous physical (or mental) activity is called post-exertional malaise, which is considered a key feature of the illness CFS. It remains a challenge for clinicians to deal with post-exertional malaise. This will be addressed in more detail below.

Over the years, attempts to develop an effective treatment therapy for CFS have been confounded by the evolution of various case definitions, lack of consensus regarding aetiology, as well as difficulty in defining and measuring the symptom of fatigue, the principal complaint in CFS. To date, no reliable laboratory markers have been identified, nor has a cure been discovered. In response to regular reports of exhaustion following previously tolerable levels of physical exertion, many earlier studies assessed muscle function and structure in patients with CFS. However, no consistent evidence has yet been found for muscular dysfunction and it is now generally accepted that the fatigue experienced in CFS has a central rather than a peripheral basis (Lloyd *et al.*, 1991; Sharpe *et al.*, 1996; Edwards *et al.*, 1994).

In previous years, a common treatment used in CFS was rest therapy, with the primary justification being that if one felt fatigued then one should rest (Wessely, 1991). However, while rest therapy is a sound short-term coping strategy, particularly during the acute phase of CFS (Deale and Davis, 1994) or when an inflammatory response is evident (Pheby, 1997*)*, prolonged inactivity has adverse physiological, psychological and social consequences (Sharpe and Wessely, 1998; Wessely and Edwards, 1993). Prolonged physical inactivity has been shown to result in muscle wasting and reduced muscle protein turnover (Booth, 1987); decreased muscular strength (Muller, 1970); compromised cardiovascular responses to exertion (Saltin *et al.*, 1968); as well as impaired neuropsychological performance, altered autonomic regulation and impaired thermoregulation (Greenleaf and Kozlowski, 1982; Haines, 1974; Zuber and Wilgosh, 1963). Additionally, prolonged physical inactivity has been reported by Duclos, Corcuff, Rashedi, Fougere and Manier (1997) to result in endocrine dysfunction as demonstrated by lower adrenocorticotrophic hormone responses to exercise in untrained men compared to trained men. Further to this, prolonged physical inactivity has been associated with psychological effects represented by increased feelings of fatigue, a reduced desire to perform activity (Zorbas and Matveyev, 1986), sleep disturbance (Ryback and Lewis, 1971) and depression (Martinsen, 1994). Thus, prolonged physical inactivity can have damaging effects in the general population, including patients with CFS.

Of particular importance to patients with CFS is that the consequences of prolonged physical inactivity are proposed by numerous researchers to perpetuate and promote symptoms in CFS, regardless of the initial trigger for this disorder (Sharpe *et al.*, 1997; Deale and Davis, 1994; Clark and Katon, 1994). While an initial response to this proposition is to advise patients with CFS to participate in regular exercise, a dilemma exists in that many sufferers describe extreme fatigue, or even relapse, following physical exertion and consequently avoid further exercise in an attempt to control symptoms (Chalder *et al.*, 1996; Sharpe *et al.*, 1992; Vercoulen *et al.*, 1997). Too vigorous exercise (Lapp, 1997, Sorensen *et al.*, 2003, Jammes *et al.*, 2005) or even a 30 per cent increase in activity (Black *et al.*, 2005) may trigger a relapse, which could in part explain the fluctuating symptom pattern commonly seen in CFS. This notion is supported by the following findings: 1) the lifestyle of patients with CFS is characterised by activity peaks followed by very long rest periods (van der Werf *et al.*, 2000); 2) a premorbid overactive lifestyle may play a predisposing and/or initiating role in CFS (Van Houdenhove *et al.*, 2001); and 3) continuing to be active despite increasing fatigue is likely to be a crucial step in the development of CFS (Harvey *et al.*, 2008). It is worthwhile mentioning that specific activities, expected to result in high fatigue levels, are less frequently performed by patients with CFS, and furthermore high fatigue expectations are related to low activity levels (Vercoulen *et al.*, 1997).

In accordance with this is the notion that on days that patients with CFS feel comparatively better, they often perform many more physical tasks (Deale and Davis, 1994; Sharpe and Wessely, 1998), most likely in an attempt to make up for all the days that they have been incapacitated. This may result in over-exertion followed by a relapse the next day (Deale and Davis, 1994; Sharpe and Wessely, 1998), which further cements the association between exercise and the exacerbation of symptoms. However, this negative scenario and association can be addressed by the employment of a formal, regulated aerobic exercise regime that is gentle, graded and flexible, as opposed to participation in activity that is erratic with no defined rules regarding duration or intensity.

From what is explained above, a dilemma becomes apparent. On the one hand, prolonged physical inactivity can be a detrimental consequence of CFS, while on the other hand, physical activity/exercise can trigger or exacerbate symptoms in patients with CFS. Consequently, these seemingly contradictory issues have inspired many researchers around the globe to study exercise physiology, exercise therapy, exercise psychology and physical activity interventions in patients with CFS. This chapter provides a balanced review of the scientific literature on exercise/physical activity in CFS. It will explain how scientific evidence provides a solution to the dilemma of combating the damaging consequences of prolonged physical inactivity versus symptom exacerbations in response to exercise. In addition, the chapter explains how science can be applied to clinical practice. An approach which considers the physiological and psychological rationale for exercise treatment in CFS is presented, and is discussed in relation to a comprehensive rehabilitation approach for CFS.

Evidence for the role of exercise/physical activity in the management of CFS

The benefits of graded aerobic exercise were first demonstrated in a 12-week randomised, controlled trial by Fulcher and White (1997) that compared the efficacy of graded aerobic exercise to flexibility exercises in patients with CFS. In this study, graded aerobic exercise therapy resulted in a significant reduction in the symptom of fatigue, as well as a significant improvement in aerobic capacity, as measured by $\dot{V}O_{2max}$ testing. Follow-up assessments held at 3 and 12 months after the completion of the trial revealed that of the 79 per cent of participants contacted, 74 per cent of those who had participated in the exercise treatment felt better and had returned to premorbid levels of physical activity. A later trial by Weardon *et al.* (1998) assessed the efficacy of fluoxetine and graded aerobic exercise in patients with CFS. This six-month, randomised, double-blind, placebo-controlled trial allocated participants to one of four treatments which consisted of exercise and fluoxetine, exercise and placebo drug, appointments and fluoxetine, and appointments and placebo drug. Assessments made before the trial and at the 12 and 26 week mark during the trial, indicated that graded aerobic exercise produced improvements in functional work capacity and fatigue. Reasons offered for attenuated improvements in this study, as compared to those recorded by Fulcher and White (1997), include recruitment of more impaired participants with psychiatric and/or sleep disorders, less face-to-face contact with participants and longer exercise periods that commenced at a higher intensity (Weardon *et al.*, 1998).

A further randomised, controlled trial by Powell, Bentall, Nye and Edwards (2001) compared a number of interventions that included graded aerobic exercise in conjunction with varying levels of an education programme designed to inform participants of the effects of deconditioning. After one year of therapy, participants involved in graded aerobic exercise and education therapy had significantly improved scores for physical function and reported reduced fatigue compared to participants in the control group, which consisted of standardised medical care (Powell *et al.*, 2001). On completion of the study, 61 (81 per cent) participants in the active intervention group believed that their condition was related to physical deconditioning, compared to a 15 per cent belief rate prior to treatment. Finally, a randomised controlled study by Wallman *et al.* (2004) reported significant improvement in numerous physiological, psychological and cognitive variables in patients with CFS after a 12-week graded aerobic exercise intervention that included pacing. Pacing involves a flexible graded aerobic exercise programme that varies in intensity and duration according to symptom severity (Shepherd, 2001). This approach allows exercise to be reduced or even abandoned on days when symptoms are worse.

The success of appropriate graded aerobic exercise therapy in CFS most likely relates initially to its ability to demonstrate to sufferers that exercise can be safely undertaken without the consequence of relapse, therefore assisting patients with CFS to abandon any avoidance behaviours to which they had have previously adhered to (Deale *et al.*, 1998a). Second, graded aerobic exercise can negate the physiological, psychological and social consequences of physical inactivity proposed earlier which can play a role in perpetuating and promoting symptoms in this condition. Success of graded aerobic exercise may also be associated with the multi-dimensional nature of CFS, where specific improvements in one area may result in generalised improvements in other related areas (Deale *et al.*, 1998b). Of relevance, graded aerobic exercise is a relatively inexpensive, simple and an easily applied therapy that needs only minimal professional involvement and can be performed either outdoors or indoors.

From the evidence summarised in the preceding paragraphs, it appears that all studies that investigated exercise/physical activity as a treatment for CFS have yielded positive results. Some patient support groups and other researchers in the field have argued that graded aerobic exercise can have detrimental effects and may explain the relatively high drop-out rates sometimes reported, although not explained in previous studies. However overall while not a cure for CFS, graded aerobic exercise can result in improved physical function, mood state, cognitive function and quality of life. This is underscored by a systematic literature review from the Cochrane Collaboration, concluding that graded aerobic exercise therapy is effective for CFS (Edmonds *et al.*, 2004). Of all the treatment interventions assessed to date in CFS, graded aerobic exercise is one of only two therapies (the other being cognitive behavioural therapy (Price and Couper, 1998) that has consistently resulted in improvements. Of relevance, graded aerobic exercise/graded physical activity is included in many, if not all, cognitive behavioural therapy programmes for CFS. Still, clinicians often struggle to implement graded aerobic exercise/graded physical activity in the treatment of patients with CFS. In this respect, the dilemma of how to apply graded aerobic exercise/graded physical activity to their patients with CFS without triggering or exacerbating symptoms remains.

Besides graded aerobic exercise therapy, other types of exercise cannot be recommended at this stage. There is insufficient evidence in support of other types of exercise for the management of CFS. However, strength training has shown its benefits for people with fibromyalgia syndrome, an illness that resembles CFS. Strength training starting at low loads and progressing to 60–80 per cent of the maximum voluntary contraction has shown to improve muscle strength (Busch *et al.*, 2008).

Balancing the physiological with the psychological rationale

Is there a physiological basis for symptom exacerbations in response to exercise or is it purely psychological? There is increasing evidence for a physiological basis to post-exertional malaise in CFS. Exercise or activity-induced symptom exacerbations in patients with CFS appear to be related to immune (dys)function in CFS. Compared to healthy controls, patients with CFS respond to an exercise challenge with enhanced complement activation (Sorensen *et al.*, 2003; Jammes *et al.*, 2005) and an exaggeration of resting differences in gene expression profile in peripheral blood mononuclear cells (Whistler *et al.*, 2005). Vigorous exercise, as well as inappropriate intensities of sub-maximal exercise, can result in increased oxidative stress and subsequent increased fatigue and musculoskeletal pain (post-exertional malaise) in patients with CFS (Figure 16.1) (Jammes *et al.*, 2005). In addition, exercise activates powerful descending pain inhibitory mechanisms in healthy participants and those with chronic low back pain. Of importance, in CFS, studies have demonstrated that exercise does not activate pain inhibition (Whiteside *et al.*, 2004; Meeus, 2008). The net result is a further decrease of the pain threshold during and immediately after exercise, making patients with CFS more vulnerable to various nociceptive and non-nociceptive stimuli (such as increased oxidative stress and the build-up of metabolic waste products that occurs during exercise). Thus, it becomes clear that the application of exercise or physical activity interventions should be applied to CFS patients with great caution, keeping in mind the physiological response to exercise in patients with CFS.

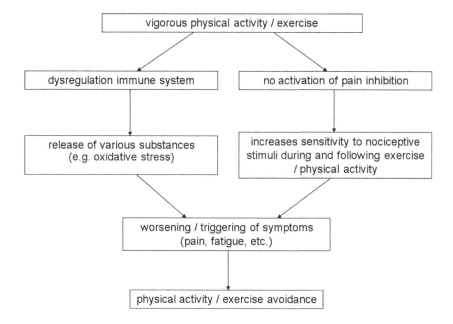

FIGURE 16.1 The physiology of post-exertional malaise in patients with CFS (reproduced with permission from Nijs, J., Van Oosterwijck, J. and Meeus, M. (2011) Myalgic encephalomyeltitis/chronic fatigue syndrome: Rehabilitation through activity management, stress management and exercise therapy. In Stone, J. H. and Blouin, M. (eds) *International Encyclopedia of Rehabilitation.* Available at: http://cirrie.buffalo.edu/encyclopedia/en/article/113/. [Accessed 15 August 2009]).

Besides physiological issues, psychological factors are known to perpetuate the illness and hence are crucial to treatment approaches, including those using exercise. The psychology of CFS has been studied at length, yet few studies have addressed the interactions between psychology and exercise performance (Nijs *et al.*, 2008c). Two psychological factors are known to interfere with physical activity or exercise performance in CFS. First, avoidance behaviour towards physical activity is likely to influence participation in exercise and compliance with exercise interventions in any chronic illness, including CFS. Specific activities, which are expected to result in high fatigue levels, are less frequently performed by patients with CFS, and furthermore, high fatigue expectations are related to low physical activity levels (Vercoulen *et al.*, 1997). On the other hand, irrational fear of movement (kinesiophobia) does not appear to be a determinant of exercise performance in CFS (Silver *et al.*, 2002; Nijs *et al.*, 2004a, 2004b). Second, in CFS patients with chronic widespread pain, pain catastrophising is strongly related to physiological variables of exercise performance (Nijs *et al.*, 2008c). Those patients catastrophising the consequences of pain showed the lowest exercise capacity.

Applying science to practice

Considering both the physiological and psychological rationale for exercise/physical activity interventions for patients with CFS, graded aerobic exercise therapy or graded activity is not suitable per se for *all* patients with CFS *at certain stages* of their illness. Rather, graded aerobic exercise therapy or graded physical activity (i.e. time spent gardening, housework, shopping, etc) can be one component of an overall rehabilitation approach to CFS. From the evidence summarised previously, it is clear that a number of patients with CFS will benefit from a graded aerobic exercise therapy programme. On the other hand, some patients with CFS are struggling to find enough energy to get through the day. These individuals are only able to perform a minimum amount of physical activity and are constantly at risk of triggering post-exertional malaise. Others ignore the physical boundaries of their body and continue to be active despite increasing symptoms. Both these types of CFS patients can be termed as 'overactive'. These patients will not benefit from a graded aerobic exercise/physical activity programme at this particular stage of their illness. Instead, they require other therapeutic strategies *prior to* commencing a graded aerobic exercise/physical activity programme. Therefore, we have divided rehabilitation for patients with CFS into two stages.

Stage I rehabilitation for those with CFS: stabilisation of the client's health status

Stage I consists of an individually tailored combination of conservative strategies, each aimed at stabilising the patients' health status (Figure 16.2). The ultimate goal of stage I is to reduce the fluctuating nature of symptoms in order to achieve a more stable health status, that is, a health status that the client feels able to control. Therefore, stage I of the rehabilitation programme targets those aspects of the illness such as: too vigorous exercise/physical activity, emotional stressors, poor sleep quality and quantity, localised musculoskeletal disorders, etc. which are known to trigger health status changes (i.e. worsening of symptoms and concomitant decreases in vitality and other aspects of quality of life). Patients with CFS who are inactive but have a reasonably stable health status at baseline may not require stage I and can immediately enter stage II. In this case, it can be decided on an individual basis whether some aspects of stage I should be combined with the graded aerobic exercise/physical activity programme of stage II (e.g. patient receives graded aerobic exercise therapy and a stress management programme simultaneously).

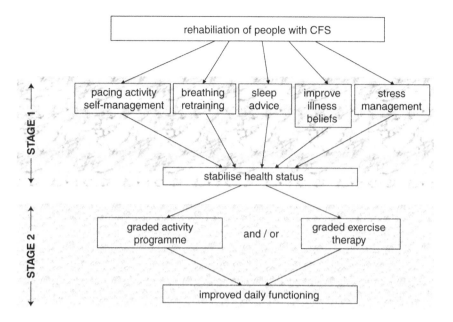

FIGURE 16.2 Content, goals and structure of rehabilitation patients with chronic fatigue syndrome (reproduced with permission from Nijs, J., Van Oosterwijck, J. and Meeus, M. (2011) Myalgic encephalomyeltitis/chronic fatigue syndrome: Rehabilitation through activity management, stress management and exercise therapy. In Stone, J. H. and Blouin, M. (eds) *International Encyclopedia of Rehabilitation.* Available at: http://cirrie. buffalo.edu/encyclopedia/en/article/113/. [Accessed 15 August 2009]).

Patients with CFS who have a fluctuating activity pattern and who are moderately active, as well as those who are rather active or pervasively active (van der Werf *et al.*, 2000), may benefit from a self-management programme which encompasses graded aerobic exercise therapy (Nijs *et al.*, 2008a). This self-management programme should focus on teaching the patient to estimate their current physical capabilities, then to commence an activity at this level, keeping in mind the regular fluctuating nature of their symptoms. The pacing self-management treatment is explained in detail elsewhere (Nijs *et al.*, 2008a). For very inactive or passive patients, a formal, regulated exercise regime that is gentle, graded, flexible and manageable according to each individual's capabilities is required. This is explained below.

Breathing retraining might benefit those patients with CFS complaining of hyperventilation and shortness of breath during exercise, and presenting with an asynchronous breathing pattern (Nijs *et al.*, 2008b). Some patients with CFS benefit from using breathing retraining as a relaxation/stress management technique. In addition, due to the possible role of hypofunction of the hypothalamic–pituitary–adrenal axis in a proportion of patients with CFS (Cleare, 2004; Crofford *et al.*, 2004; Van den Eede *et al.*, 2007), many patients with CFS struggle to cope with various kinds of stressors. Teaching them stress management techniques appears warranted.

Stage II rehabilitation for those with CFS: application of graded aerobic exercise therapy

Once the symptoms are stable, patients with CFS can enter a graded aerobic exercise/physical activity programme (stage II in Figure 16.2). Still, even at this stage of the rehabilitation process, one must remain cautious in not triggering an exacerbation of symptoms following physical exertion. At this stage, the client should be aware that the cause of an exacerbation of symptoms following physical exertion may be related to the intensity and duration of activities attempted.

Before exercise is undertaken in CFS, various factors need to be considered. As CFS is a heterogeneous condition, graded aerobic exercise therapy needs to be flexible, realistic and manageable according to each individual's needs and abilities, while graded physical activity (as opposed to exercise) should be introduced first for the more disabled participants (Deale and Davis, 1994). Introduction of exercise that is beyond a participant's capacity may not only promote relapse but can also result in feelings of demoralisation and pain, thus reinforcing avoidance behaviour (see Figure 16.1). Graded aerobic exercise therapy should also include the concept of pacing, as described earlier. Of further importance is the need to schedule rest periods in conjunction with the exercise periods, as this can help in establishing a manageable routine that can assist in promoting a sense of control over one's life (Pheby, 1997; Sharpe *et al.*, 1997).

This type of 'flexible' graded aerobic exercise therapy is based on the exercise prescription used in the study by Wallman *et al.* (2004). The exercise prescription is aimed at non-bedbound, sedentary patients with debilitating CFS, as well as patients who are moderately affected. The exercise prescription is home based and requires minimal specialist supervision. Once the exercise programme has commenced, specialist input can be performed over the phone on a fortnightly basis; however, occasional appointments may provide greater motivation and adherence to the exercise regime. After six months of exercise, contact can be minimised to a level that is negotiated between the healthcare professional/exercise specialist and the participant. Prior to commencing any exercise programme, participants should be screened by a medical doctor in order to assess for any condition that could be contraindicated.

Graded aerobic exercise therapy in CFS

Baseline assessment

While not necessary, assessment of individual aerobic capacity prior to the commencement of an exercise programme provides a benchmark for future comparison, which may inherently also provide motivation. Baseline assessment of aerobic capacity can be performed using the Aerobic Power Index, which is a sub-maximal cycle ergometer test that has established normative values and has previously been shown to be reliable (intraclass correlation coefficient = 0.97; Wallman *et al.*, 2003) and valid as a predictor for peak exercise capacity (Nijs *et al.*, 2007) in patients with CFS. Of importance is that this particular exercise test was previously used repeatedly (eight times each) in 61 patients with CFS without the consequence of relapse (Wallman *et al.*, 2003). The protocol for the Aerobic Power Index test can be found in Wallman *et al.* (2004). Follow-up testing should be performed at least three and six months later. It is important to note, however, that an improvement in exercise capacity in patients with CFS does not always accompany clinical improvements in quality of life and *vice versa* (Pardaens *et al.*, 2006). In addition to exercise testing, self-reported measures like the Checklist Individual Strength (Vercoulen *et al.* 1994), CFS Symptom List (Nijs and Thielemans, 2008), or the Chronic Fatigue Syndrome Activities and Participation Questionnaire (Nijs *et al.*, 2003) can generate valuable information.

Getting started

Prior to commencing the exercise programme, the participant should be informed that the exercise sessions are *in addition* to their normal activities and do not replace other therapeutic strategies that the client is currently adhering to (e.g. stress management programme and pacing activity self-management). Rather, graded aerobic exercise builds onto the previous accomplishments of rehabilitation. The participant should also be informed that some aches and pains are normal when commencing exercise and that these should resolve in a few days. Most individuals are able to differentiate between aches and pains associated with the commencement of exercise (e.g. delayed onset of muscle soreness) and abnormal feelings of pain and exhaustion. Additionally, where possible, the participant should purchase or hire a heart rate monitor, as the ability to monitor heart rate intensity will help to ensure that an appropriate exercise stimulus is being applied and will also provide data on relative effort from one session to another.

Intensity and duration of exercise

Patients with CFS should be given a copy of the Borg scale (Borg, 1982) as this is needed to rate the perceived exertion associated with each completed exercise session. Participants should be instructed on how to use the heart rate monitor and how to score their ratings of perceived exertion (RPE) using the Borg scale. A rating of perceived exertion score associated with the initial exercise session provides a benchmark for future comparisons, while the averaged RPE values recorded for each fortnight of the exercise programme forms the basis for determining the intensity and duration of future exercise sessions. An exercise diary is also necessary. This can be an exercise book, or a record kept on a computer database.

Information recorded in this diary should contain the date and time of the exercise session, the duration of the exercise session, the average heart rate intensity of the exercise session and the overall effort (i.e. RPE) associated with each exercise session. In addition, the participant should be encouraged to record how they felt during the exercise session and whether any event had occurred in the previous 48 hours that may have affected their performance. Keeping such a record not only allows a participant to monitor their progress over time (and see how much they have improved) but also helps to link poor performance with a possible event. An example of an entry in the exercise diary is shown in Table 16.1.

Exercise should be attempted once every second day, while the mode of exercise should be one that uses the major muscles of the body such as walking, jogging, swimming or cycling. The duration of each exercise session to be undertaken during the first fortnight should be negotiated with the participant and will ultimately depend upon their current physical capabilities. If severely deconditioned but not bed-bound, the time it takes to walk the length of a passageway in the home may be appropriate, while for more able participants, 5–10 minutes might represent a good starting point.

The intensity of the exercise should represent a pace that the participant can perform comfortably. Of importance is that this intensity be determined on a day when the severity of symptoms are similar to those experienced on a typical day, as opposed to a day when symptoms are either comparatively better or exacerbated. The average peak heart rate intensity (beats per minute: bpm) that occurs when exercising at a comfortable pace on a typical day should be recorded, with this intensity representing the participant's target heart rate (± 5 bpm) for future exercise sessions. The 'warm-up' time that it takes for the participant's heart rate to reach their target heart rate intensity should be included in the overall exercise duration. If the participant does not have a heart rate monitor then participants should attempt to equate their comfortable exercise pace with an RPE score from the Borg scale. It is presumed that this pace would not exceed a rating of '12' within the first few minutes of exercise.

TABLE 16.1 Example of an extract from an exercise diary

Date & time of exercise	Friday, 12 Feb, 10.00 am
Exercise duration	10 mins
HR intensity	135 bpm
Ratings of perceived exertion (RPE)	14
Comments	Struggled with the exercise today, felt very tired – however, did not sleep well last night.

After the first exercise session, the participant should contact the healthcare professional/exercise specialist on the following day to discuss how they coped with the session. If the participant felt that their initial exercise session was too easy (i.e. an RPE score of 9 or lower), a slight increase in duration could be considered. Conversely, if the initial exercise session elicited an RPE score greater than 14, then the duration of subsequent sessions for that fortnight should be reduced to a time period that elicits an RPE score between 11 and 14. It is important that the participant is eased gently into their new exercise programme.

At the end of each fortnight, the participant should contact the clinician/specialist in order to discuss any concerns, as well as to determine the following fortnight's exercise prescription. If the participant is coping with their exercise regime, has not experienced a major relapse and reported averaged fortnightly RPE values of 14 or less, then the exercise duration for the following fortnight should be increased by 2–5 minutes, based on negotiation between the specialist and the participant. If the averaged RPE score was 15 or higher, then the exercise duration should be reduced to a time period that elicits an averaged fortnightly RPE score between 11 and 14. The same procedure and recommendations for the first fortnight apply to the next and subsequent fortnights, in that individual target heart rate is kept constant and RPE scores are recorded after each exercise session and averaged at the end of each fortnight.

If the participant already performs aerobic exercise, then they should continue with their normal routine for a fortnight, making sure that they keep their exercise duration and intensity constant. They should then follow the same exercise guidelines as outlined earlier, noting that only the duration of exercise is manipulated in the initial stages of the programme.

Even in stage II of the rehabilitation programme, patients with CFS may still describe a limited fluctuating nature to their symptoms and capabilities. Consequently, on a day that the participant feels comparatively well they MUST ADHERE to their current exercise regimen and not perform any extra exercise above this level. As noted earlier, overdoing physical activity on days that patients with CFS feel comparatively better often results in a relapse the next day. Conversely, on a day when symptoms are worse, the participant should either reduce their exercise duration to a time that they consider manageable, or if feeling particularly unwell, the exercise session should be abandoned altogether. There may be times when the exercise session may need to be abandoned for a period of time due to exacerbated symptoms, other illnesses or relapse; however the participant should always endeavour to commence their exercise programme again when symptoms subside to a tolerable level. When recommencing exercise, the duration should be reduced to a time that the individual considers to be manageable and elicits an RPE score between 11 and 14, while the pace should be a comfortable one as determined previously. The return to exercise is more important than the duration of exercise performed. The participant should follow the same procedures and guidelines recommended earlier, in that they would continue at this new duration for a fortnight and only increase the duration of exercise for the subsequent fortnight if their averaged fortnightly RPE score was 14 or lower.

Where the duration of exercise reaches 30 minutes, the participant could consider increasing the intensity of sections of their exercise session, as is done when performing interval training. An example of this would be where the first minute of every tenth minute of the exercise session is performed at a pace that elicits an RPE score that is between 15 and 16. Extra short bouts of high intensity interval exercise can be added to the exercise regimen each fortnight if averaged fortnightly RPE scores fall within the guidelines described earlier. The inclusion of higher intensity intervals should be undertaken with caution, with the participant making sure that any increase in intensity is minimal and only performed when they are coping with the existing exercise routine. Of importance, patients with CFS should view their graded aerobic exercise programme as a long-term intervention with gradual increases in duration and intensity spread over weeks and possibly even months.

Summary of exercise recommendations for patients with CFS

Key points when prescribing exercise:

- Physical exercise/activity should be aerobic, gentle, incremental and matched to the individual's capability.
- Patients with CFS should take care not to overdo exercise/physical activity.
- On days when symptoms are less, exercise/physical activity should not be more than that prescribed in the programme. Participation in levels of exercise that are higher intensity or longer than recommended typically results in relapse.
- Physical exercise/physical activity should be paced, i.e. on days when symptoms are worse, physical activity should be reduced or even avoided.
- If exercise/physical activity is stopped due to the exacerbation of symptoms (or for any other reason), it should be recommenced when symptoms have abated, but at an intensity and duration that is achievable.
- Exercise should be undertaken under the direction/supervision of a trained professional with experience in CFS.

References

Black, C. D., O'Connor, P. J. and McCully, K. K. (2005) Increased daily physical activity and fatigue symptoms in chronic fatigue syndrome. *Dynamic Med*, 4: 3. doi:10.1186/1476-5918-4-3.

Booth, F. (1987) Physiologic and biochemical effects of immobilization on muscle. *Clinical Orthopedics*, 10: 15–20.

Borg, G. (1982) Psychophysical bases of perceived exertion. *Medicine and Science in Sports and Exercise*, 14(5): 377–381.

Busch, A. J., Barber, K. A., Overend, T. J., Peloso, P. M. and Schachter, C. L. (2008) Exercise for treating fibromyalgia syndrome. Review. *Cochrane Library*, Issue 4.

Chalder, A., Power, M. and Wessely, S. (1996) Chronic fatigue in the community: a question of attribution. *Psychological Medicine*, 26(4): 791–797.

Clark, M. and Katon, W. (1994) The relevance of psychiatric research on somatisation to the concept of chronic fatigue syndrome. In Straus, S. (ed.), *Chronic Fatigue Syndrome* (pp. 329–349). New York: Marcel Dekker Inc.

Cleare, A. J. (2004) The HPA axis and the genesis of chronic fatigue syndrome. *Trends Endocrinol Metab*, 15: 55–59.

Crofford, L. J., Young, E. A., Engleberg, C., Korszun, A., Brucksch, C. B., McClure, L. A., Brown, M. B. and Demitrack, M. A. (2004) Basal circadian and pulsatile ACTH and cortisol secretion in patients with fibromyalgia and/or chronic fatigue syndrome. *Brain Behaviour and Immunity*, 18: 314–325.

Deale, A., and Davis, A. (1994) Chronic fatigue syndrome: evaluation and management. *Journal of Neuropsychiatry*, 6: 189–194.

Deale, A., Chalder, T. and Wessely, S. (1998a) Illness beliefs and treatment outcome in chronic fatigue syndrome. *Journal of Psychosomatic Research*, 45(1): 77–83.

Deale, A., Chalder, T. and Wessely, S. (1998b) Commentary on: randomised, double-blind, placebo-controlled trial of fluoxetine and graded exercise for chronic fatigue syndrome. The British Journal of Psychiatry, 172: 491.

Duclos, M., Corcuff, J.B., Rashedi, M., Fougere, V. and Manier, G. (1997) Trained versus untrained men: different post exercise responses of pituitary adrenal axis: a preliminary study. *European Journal of Applied Physiology*, 75: 343–350.

Edmonds, M., McGuire, H. and Price, J. (2004) Exercise therapy for chronic fatigue syndrome. *Cochrane Database Syst Rev*, 3:CD003200.pub2. Doi: 10.1002/14651858. CD003200.pub2.

Edwards, R., Clague, J., Gibson, H. and Helliwell, T. (1994) Muscle metabolism, histopathology and physiology in chronic fatigue syndrome. In Straus, S. (ed.), *Chronic Fatigue Syndrome* (pp. 241–261). New York: Marcel Dekker Inc.

Fukuda, K., Straus, S., Hickie, I., Sharpe, M., Dobbins, J., Komaroff, A. and The International Chronic Fatigue Syndrome Study Group. (1994) The chronic fatigue syndrome: a comprehensive approach to its definition and study. Annals of Internal Medicine, 121(12): 953–959.

Fulcher, K. Y. and White, P. (1997) Randomised controlled trial of graded exercise in participants with the chronic fatigue syndrome. *British Medical Journal*, 314 (7095): 1647–1652.

Greenleaf, J., and Kozlowski, S. (1982) Physiological consequences of reduced physical activity during bed rest. *Exercise in Sport and Science Review*, 10: 84–119.

Haines, R. (1974) Effect of bed rest and exercise on body balance. *Journal of Applied Physiology*, 36: 323–327.

Harvey, S. B., Wadsworth, M., Wessely, S. and Hotopf, M. (2008) Etiology of chronic fatigue syndrome: testing popular hypotheses using a national birth study. *Psychosomatic Medicine*, doi: 10.1097/PSY.0b013e31816a8dbc.

Holmes, G., Kaplan, J., Gantz, N., Komaroff, A., Schonberger, L., Straus, S., Jones, J., Dubois, R., Cunningham-Rundles, C., Pahwa, S., Tosato, G., Zegans, I., Purtilo, D., Brown, N., Schooley, R. and Brus, I. (1988) Chronic fatigue syndrome: a working case definition. *Annals of Internal Medicine*, 108: 387–389.

Jammes, Y., Steinberg, J. G., Mambrini, O., Brégeon, F. and Delliaux, S. (2005) Chronic fatigue syndrome: assessment of increased oxidative stress and altered muscle excitability in response to incremental exercise. *J Intern Med*, 257: 299–310.

Lapp, C. W. (1997) Exercise limits in chronic fatigue syndrome. *Am J Med*, 103: 83–84.

Lloyd, A. R., Gandevia, S. and Hales, J. (1991) Muscle performance, voluntary activation, twitch properties and perceived effort in normal subjects and participants with the chronic fatigue syndrome. *Brain*, 114(1): 85–98.

Martinsen E.W. (1994) Physical activity and depression: clinical experience. *Acta Psychiatrica Scandinavica*, (Suppl 377): 23–27.

Meeus, M. (2008) Chronic musculoskeletal pain in chronic fatigue syndrome: A biopsychological approach. PhD theses. Vrije Universiteit Brussel.

Muller, E. (1970) Influence of training and inactivity on muscle strength. *Archives of Physical and Medical Rehabilitation*, 51: 449–452.

Nijs, J., Demol, S. and Wallman, K. (2007) Can submaximal exercise variables predict peak exercise performance in women with chronic fatigue syndrome? *Archives of Medical Research*, 38: 350–353.

Nijs, J., Paul, L. and Wallman, K. (2008a) Chronic fatigue syndrome: an approach combining self-management with graded exercise to avoid exacerbations. *J Rehabil Med*, 40: 241–247.

Nijs, J., Adriaens, J., Schuermans, D., Buyl, R. and Vincken, W. (2008b) Breathing retraining in patients with chronic fatigue syndrome: a pilot study. *Physiotherapy Theory and Practice*, 24: 83–94.

Nijs, J., Van de Putte, K., Louckx, F., Truijen, S. and De Meirleir, K. (2008c) Exercise performance and chronic pain in chronic fatigue syndrome: The role of pain catastrophizing. *Pain Med*, 9: 1164–1172.

Nijs, J., Vanherberghen, K., Duquet, W. and De Meirleir, K. (2004a) Chronic fatigue syndrome: lack of association between pain-related fear of movement and exercise capacity and disability. *Phys Ther*, 84: 696–705.

Nijs, J., De Meirleir, K. and Duquet, W. (2004b) Kinesiophobia in chronic fatigue syndrome: assessment and associations with disability. *Arch Phys Med Rehabil*, 85: 1586–1592.

Nijs, J., Vaes, P., McGregor, N., Van Hoof, E. and De Meirleir, K. (2003) Psychometric properties of the Dutch Chronic Fatigue Syndrome Activities and Participation Questionnaire (CFS-APQ). *Phys Ther*, 83: 444–454.

Nijs, J. and Thielemans, A. (2008) Kinesiophobia and symptomatology in chronic fatigue syndrome: A psychometric study of two questionnaires. *Psychol Psychother*, 81: 273–83.

Pardaens, K., Haagdorens, L., Van Wambeke, P., Van den Broeck, A. and Van Houdenhove, B. (2006) How relevant are exercise capacity measures for evaluating treatment effects in chronic fatigue syndrome? Results from a prospective, multidisciplinary outcome study. *Clin Rehabil*, 20: 56–66.

Pheby, D. (1997) Chronic fatigue syndrome: a challenge to the clinical professions. *Physiotherapy*, 83(2): 53–56.

Powell, R., Bentall, R., Nye, F. J. and Edwards, R. H. (2001) Randomised controlled trial of participant education to encourage graded exercise in chronic fatigue syndrome. *British Medical Journal*, 322(7283): 387–390.

Price, J. R. and Couper, J. (1998) Cognitive behaviour therapy for chronic fatigue syndrome in adults. *Cochrane Database Syst Rev*, 4:CD001027. Doi:10.1002/14651858. CD001027.

Ryback, R. S. and Lewis, O. F. (1971) Effects of prolonged bed rest on EEG sleep patterns in young healthy volunteers. *Electroencephalogy Clinical Neurophysiology*, 31: 395–399.

Saltin, B., Blomquist, G., Mitchell, J., Johnson, R., Wildenthal, K. and Chapman, C. (1968) Responses to exercise after bed rest and training: a longitudinal study of adaptive changes in oxygen transport and body composition. *Circulation*, 38(Suppl 7): 1–55.

Sharpe, M., and Wessely, S. (1998) Putting the rest cure to rest again: rest has no place in treating chronic fatigue. *British Medical Journal*, 316(7134): 796.

Sharpe, M., Hawton, K.E., Seagroatt, V. and Pasvol, G. (1992) Participants who present with fatigue; a follow up of referrals to an infectious diseases clinic. *British Medical Journal*, 305: 147–152.

Sharpe, M., Clements, A., Hawton, K., Young, A., Sargent, P. and Cowen, P. (1996) Increased prolactin response to buspirone in chronic fatigue syndrome. *Journal of Affective Disorders*, 41: 71–76.

Sharpe, M., Chalder, T., Palmer. I. and Wessely, S. (1997) Chronic fatigue syndrome: a practical guide to assessment and management. *General Hospital Psychiatry*, 19(3): 185–199.

Shepherd, C. (2001) Pacing and exercise in chronic fatigue. *Physiotherapy*, 87(8): 395–396.

Silver, A., Haeney, M., Vijayadurai, P., Wilks, D., Pattrick, M. and Main, C. J. (2002) The role of fear of physical movement and activity in chronic fatigue syndrome. *J Psychosom Res*, 52: 485–493.

Sorensen, B., Streib, J. E., Strand, M., Make, B., Giclas, P. C., Fleshner, M. and Jones, J. F. (2003) Complement activation in a model of chronic fatigue syndrome. *J Allergy Clin Immunol*, 12: 397–403.

Van den Eede, F., Moorkens, G., Van Houdenhove, B., Cosyns, P. and Claes, S. J. (2007) Hypothalamic-pituitary-adrenal axis function in chronic fatigue syndrome. *Neuropsychobiology*, 55: 112–120.

van der Werf, S. P., Prins, J. B., Vercoulen, J. H. M. M., van der Meer, J. W. M. and Bleijenberg, G. (2000) Identifying physical activity patterns in chronic fatigue syndrome using actigraph assessment. *J Psychosom Res*, 49: 373–379.

Van Houdenhove, B., Neerinckx, E., Onghena, P., Lysens, R. and Vertommen, H. (2001) Premorbid 'overactive' lifestyle in chronic fatigue syndrome and fibromyalgia. An etiological factor or proof of good citizenship? *J Psychosom Res*, 51: 571–576.

Vercoulen, J. H. M. M., Bazelmans, E., Swanink, C. M. A., Fennis, J. F. M., Galama, J. M. D., Jongen, P. J. H., Hommes, O., Van der Meer, J. W. M. and Bleijenberg, G. (1997) Physical activity in chronic fatigue syndrome: assessment and its role in fatigue. *J Psychiat Res*, 31: 661–673.

Vercoulen, J. H. M. M., Swanink, C. M. A., Fennis, J. F. M., Galama, J. M. D., van der Meer, J. W. M, and Bleijenberg, G. (1994) Dimensional assessment of chronic fatigue syndrome. *J Psychosom Res*, 38: 383–392.

Wallman, K. Morton, A. R., Goodman, C., Grove, R. and Dawson, B. (2003) Reliability studies of the aerobic power index submaximal exercise test in a CFS population. *J Chronic Fatigue Syndrome*, 11(4): 19–32.

Wallman, K., Morton, A. R., Goodman, C. and Grove R. (2004) Randomised controlled trial of graded exercise in chronic fatigue syndrome. *Medical Journal of Australia*, 180(9): 444–448.

Weardon, A., Morriss, R., Mullis, R., Strickland, P., Pearson, D., Appleby, L., Campbell, I. and Morris, J. (1998) Randomised, double-blind, placebo-controlled treatment trial of fluoxetine and graded exercise for chronic fatigue syndrome. *The British Journal of Psychiatry*, 172: 485–490.

Wessely, S. (1991) History of postviral fatigue syndrome. *British Medical Bulletin*, 47(4): 919–941.

Wessely, S., and Edwards, R. (1993) Chronic fatigue. In Greenwood, R., Barnes, M., McMillan, T. and Ward, C. (eds), *Neurological Rehabilitation* (pp. 311–325). London: Churchill Livingstone.

Whistler, T., Jones, J. F., Unger, E. R. and Vernon, S. D. (2005) Exercise responsive genes measured in peripheral blood of women with chronic fatigue syndrome and matched control subjects. *BMC Physiol*, 5: 5. doi:10.1186/1472–6793–5–5.

Whiteside, A., Hansen, S. and Chaudhuri, A. (2004) Exercise lowers pain threshold in chronic fatigue syndrome. *Pain*, 109: 497–499.

Zorbas, Y. G. and Matveyev, I. O. (1986) Man's desirability in performing physical exercise under hypokinesia. *International Journal of Rehabilitation Research*, 9: 170–174.

Zuber, J. and Wilgosh, L. (1963) Prolonged immobilization of the body changes in performances and electroencephalogram. *Science*, 140: 306–308.

17

FIBROMYALGIA SYNDROME

Borja Sañudo Corrales

Introduction

Fibromyalgia syndrome (FMS) is a chronic widespread pain condition with characteristic tender points (TP) on physical examination, often associated with a constellation of other symptoms such as fatigue, sleep disturbance, stiffness and mood disorders (Wolfe *et al.*, 1990). The etiology of FMS is not completely understood, but the syndrome is thought to arise from a number of possible influencing factors, including genetic disposition and dysfunction of the central and autonomous nervous system (resulting in amplification of pain transmission and interpretation), although various other mechanisms could be involved.

Most patients with FMS are sedentary females with low physical fitness (Bennett *et al.*, 1989; Sañudo and Galiano, 2008). This can be compounded by pain, fatigue or depression, which limits daily living activities and affects quality of life and employability. Although there are several treatment options available, optimal management of FMS is unknown (Busch *et al.*, 2008). Clinical guidance, which is based on current scientific evidence, recommends a broad range of pharmacological and non-pharmacological therapies but such treatments cannot reliably resolve the functional limitations and the deterioration in quality of life of patients. Nevertheless, it has been suggested that non-pharmacological interventions can have a greater impact on physical function than drug treatments (Rossy *et al.*, 1999). In this respect, physical exercise is considered to be the main non-pharmacological strategy in the management of FMS. The number of published studies, particularly randomized controlled trials, has risen steadily over the past decade (Rooks, 2008; Carville *et al.*, 2008; Busch *et al.*, 2008; Brosseau *et al.*, 2008a, 2008b). Despite this, many clinically relevant and practically important questions remain in relation to the most effective method of implementing exercise therapy for FMS. For the exercise to be effective, it has to be carefully prescribed and controlled. Exercise intensity has to be such that it can induce beneficial effects but not so high that it will increase symptoms. Getting patients with FMS to initiate and maintain an exercise programme remains challenging.

Scientific evidence supports the use of physical exercise programmes for the overall management of FMS (Busch *et al.*, 2008; Brosseau *et al.*, 2008a, 2008b; Carville *et al.*, 2008). Improvements have been reported in:

- Cardiorespiratory capacity (Wigers *et al.*, 1996; Verstappen *et al.*, 1997; Meiworm *et al.*, 2000; Gowans *et al.*, 2001; Jentoft *et al.*, 2001; van Santen *et al.*, 2002a, 2002b; Schachter *et al.*, 2003; Valim *et al.*, 2003; Assis *et al.*, 2006; Gusi *et al.*, 2006)
- Muscular strength (Jentoft *et al.*, 2001; Häkkinen *et al.*, 2002; Valkeinen *et al.*, 2004; Valkeinen *et al.*, 2005; Gusi *et al.*, 2006; Valkeinen *et al.*, 2006; Bircan *et al.*, 2008; Valkeinen *et al.*, 2008), and flexibility (Verstappen *et al.*, 1997; Gowans *et al.*, 2001; Jones *et al.*, 2002; Gandhi *et al.*, 2002; Valim *et al.*, 2003).
- Pain relief (Wigers *et al.*, 1996; Meiworm *et al.*, 2000; Jentoft *et al.*, 2001; van Santen *et al.*, 2002b; Valim *et al.*, 2003; Schachter *et al.*, 2003; Altan *et al.*, 2004; Sencan *et al.*, 2004; Valkeinen *et al.*, 2004; Da Costa *et al.*, 2005; Gusi *et al.*, 2006; Tomas-Carus *et al.*, 2008; Valkeinen *et al.*, 2008).
- Sleep quality (McCain *et al.*, 1988; Wigers *et al.*, 1996; Verstappen *et al.*, 1997; Schachter *et al.*, 2003; Valkeinen *et al.*, 2004).
- Psychological wellbeing (Gowans *et al.*, 2001; van Santen *et al.*, 2002b; Sencan *et al.*, 2004; Redondo *et al.*, 2004; Da Costa *et al.*, 2005; Tomas-Carus *et al.*, 2008), such as improvements in mood and well-being (Ramsay *et al.*, 2000) or self-efficacy (Gowans *et al.*, 2001; Redondo *et al.*, 2004).
- Anxiety (McCain *et al.*, 1988; Clark *et al.*, 2001; Gowans *et al.*, 2001; Gusi *et al.*, 2006; Bircan *et al.*, 2008; Tomas-Carus *et al.*, 2008),
- Depression (McCain *et al.*, 1988; Wigers *et al.*, 1996; Clark *et al.*, 2001; Gowans *et al.*, 2001; Valim *et al.*, 2003; Valkeinen *et al.*, 2004; Assis *et al.*, 2006; Gusi *et al.*, 2006; Bircan *et al.*, 2008; Tomas-Carus *et al.*, 2008).
- Quality of life (QoL) (Wigers *et al.*, 1996; Jentoft *et al.*, 2001; van Santen *et al.*, 2002a, 2002b; Valim *et al.*, 2003; Schachter *et al.*, 2003; Gusi *et al.*, 2006; Assis *et al.*, 2006; Bircan *et al.*, 2008; Tomas-Carus *et al.*, 2008).

Evidence for the benefits of exercise training

Aerobic exercise

The first study to evaluate the effects of aerobic exercise at a moderate-high intensity was performed by McCain *et al.* (1988), who compared the effects of an aerobic exercise programme (cycle ergometry), three times a week for 20 weeks, with a flexibility programme, showing improvements in the aerobic exercise group versus the flexibility group in pain threshold, cardiovascular capacity and tender points count but no change in pain intensity, sleep disturbance or psychological function. Since that original study, other research groups have reported benefits. For example, Meiworm *et al.* (2000) evaluated a 12-week aerobic exercise programme using an intensity of 50 per cent $\dot{V}O_{2max}$ and a frequency of three times a week and reported improvements in aerobic capacity and bodily pain. In addition, Ramsay *et al.* (2000) compared the effects of supervised aerobic exercise (60 minutes per week for 12 weeks) and unsupervised home exercises and reported improvements in anxiety and well-being in the supervised group. Meyer and Lemley (2000) evaluated the effects of a walking programme of low and high intensity for 24 weeks. Although no significant changes in physical function or symptoms between groups were found, improvements were somewhat greater in the low intensity group, with low intensity exercise reducing the impact of the disease in a greater proportion of patients. Van Santen *et al.* (2002b) also compared low-intensity aerobic exercise with a high intensity programme for 20 weeks (2–3 days a week depending on intensity) and reported increased pain in the high intensity group.

Although evidence from the latter two studies supports the use of low intensity exercise for patients with FMS, aerobic exercise programmes that start at low intensity and short duration and which are progressed gradually, in terms of intensity and duration, can also bring benefits (Richards and Scott, 2002). Aerobic 'interval training' is another approach which can bring benefits to patients with FMS. Schachter *et al.* (2003) compared the effects of interval training based on two aerobic sessions of 15 minutes each, with a continuous exercise session of 30 minutes, for 16 weeks. Although no significant differences were found between the programmes, both were useful for improving self-efficacy and severity of symptoms.

Not all studies have reported positive results after programmes of aerobic exercise training. Nichols and Glenn (1994) allocated patients to either an aerobic exercise programme, based on 20 minutes walking at an intensity of 60–70 per cent predicted maximum heart rate (HR_{max}), three times a week for eight weeks, or a control group without treatment. No differences were found between groups in pain and even patients in the aerobic group showed a decrement in their functional capacity after the study. Neither were improvements in pain, muscle strength, aerobic capacity and fatigue observed in groups of patients allocated to dance or aerobic exercise, 2–3 times per week, for 12 weeks (Norregaard *et al.*, 1997).

TABLE 17.1 Aerobic exercise programmes in FMS patients

Authors	Participants	Duration and frequency	Intervention	Type of exercise	Outcomes
Mengshoel et al., (1992)	A (n=18); B(n=17)♀FM	60min 2×/wk. (20 wks.)	A. Supervise aerobic dance (120–150 bpm); B: control group	Aerobic	Handgrip strength, aerobic capacity, VAS pain, sleep disturbance, fatigue

Results: Handgrip strength improvement in aerobic exercise group when comparing with control group

Authors	Participants	Duration and frequency	Intervention	Type of exercise	Outcomes
Nichols and Glenn, (1994)	A(n=10); B(n=9): (17♀,2♂)FM	20min 3×/wk. (8 wks.)	A. walking (60–70% HR_{max}); B= control group	Aerobic	MPQ, psychological function, physical function

Results: Walking did not produce significant improvements in pain or psychological well-being, but control group had a greater impact of the disease

Authors	Participants	Duration and frequency	Intervention	Type of exercise	Outcomes
Wigers et al., (1996)	3 groups(n=20 × group, 55♀,5♂) FM	45 min. 3×/wk. (14 wks.) + 4.5 years follow-up	A. Aerobic Ex. (60–70% HR_{max} × 20 min.); B. Stress control; C. usual care	Aerobic	VAS pain, TP, fatigue, sleep disturbance, physical function, psychological function

Results: short-term improvements in TP were found in A and B groups, although greater improvements were found in group A in pain and aerobic capacity. Long-term significant improvements were not found

Authors	Participants	Duration and frequency	Intervention	Type of exercise	Outcomes
Norregaard et al., (1997)	A(n=5); B(n=11); C(n=7)♀FM	A. 50 min – 3×/w (B–C 2×/wk.) (12 wks.)	A. Dance (aerobic exercise); B. mixed exercise; C. hot packs control	Aerobic	VAS pain and fatigue, TP, FIQ, BDI, aerobic capacity, physical function

Results: After 12 weeks there were no improvements in pain, fatigue, strength or aerobic capacity in all groups

Authors	Participants	Duration and frequency	Intervention	Type of exercise	Outcomes
Meyer and Lemley, (2000)	A(n=8); B(n=8); C(n=5)♀FM	10–30 min. – 3×/wk. (24 wks.)	A. high intensity walking; B. low intensity walking; C. Control group	Aerobic	TP, BDI, BAI, VAS pain, FIQ

Results: Low-intensity exercise group reduce FMS impact (35% improvements in FIQ) and symptomatology, while high-intensity exercise group increased pain when FIQ improved just 8%

Meiworm et al., (2000)	A(n=27); B(n=12), 36♀ and 3♂ FM	25 min. – 3×/wk (12 wks.)	A. Aerobic exercise (walking, cycling, swimming) at 50% $\dot{V}O_{2max}$; B. Control group	Aerobic	Aerobic capacity, TP, VAS pain

Results: Aerobic capacity, TP count and pain were better in aerobic capacity group when comparing with control group

Jentoft et al., (2001)	A(n=18); B(n=16) ♀FM	60 min. – 2×/wk. (20 wks.)	A. Aerobic exercise (60–80% HR_{max}); B. Pool-based exercise	Aerobic	FIQ, handgrip strength, distance walked, fatigue, VAS pain

Results: Both groups increases their aerobic capacity and improved their symptomatology by exercise, although group A improvements were greater in handgrip strength than group B

Gowans et al., (2001)	A(n=27); B(n=23) ♀FM	30 min. – 3×/wk. (23 wks) – 1° one pool × wk.	A. Aerobic exercise + flexibility; B. Control group	Aerobic	TP, muscular capacity, FIQ, anxiety, depression and 6MWT

Results: Group A patients showed significant improvements in 6MWT, anxiety, depression, mental health and self-efficacy

Continued

TABLE 17.1 *continued*

Authors	*Participants*	*Intervention*	*Duration and frequency*	*Type of exercise*	*Outcomes*
van Santen *et al.*, (2002a)	A(n=18); B(n=15) ♀FM	A. High intensity aerobic exercise (70% HR$_{max}$); B. Low intensity aerobic exercise	A. 1h. – 3×/wk. B. 1h. – 2×/wk. (20 wks.)	Aerobic	Pain, TP count, general health, anxiety, depression, psychological function

Results: Group A patients slightly improved their aerobic capacity and general well-being, although psychological function and general health remained unchanged

van Santen *et al.*, (2002b)	A(n=47); B(n=43); C(n=28)♀FM	A. Aerobic exercise; B. Biofeedback; C. Control group; D. 50% of treatment A and B, 6 education sessions	A. 1h. – 2 – 3×/wk. (24 wks.); B. 30min. – 2×/wk.(8 wks.)	Aerobic	Pain, TP count, fatigue, aerobic capacity, SIP

Results: There were no significant differences between groups

Schachter *et al.* (2003)	A(n=56); B(n=51); C(n=36) ♀FM	A. Short bouts of aerobic exercise; B. Long bouts of A. exercise; C. Control group	10 to 30 min. 3 – 5×/ wk (16 wks.)	Aerobic	Pain, TP count, sleep disturbances, stiffness, functional disturbances

Results: Low impact aerobic exercises improved physical function and symptomatology. Interval-training did not show significant improvements

Sencan *et al.*, (2004)	A-B-C (n=20) ♀FM	A. Aerobic exercise; B. Paroxetine; C. Placebo	(6 wk.) + 6 weeks follow-up	Aerobic	Self-efficacy, VAS pain, BDI, TP count, psychological disturbances

Results: VAS and BDI decreased in A and B groups when comparing with group C patients, even at follow-up period. Group A also reduced analgesic intake

Authors	Participants	Duration and frequency	Intervention	Type of exercise	Outcomes
Redondo et al., (2004)	A(n=19); B(n=21) ♀FM	(8 wks.) + 6 and 12 months follow-up	A. Aerobic exercise; B. CBT	Aerobic	Pain, TP count, FIQ, SF-36, physical function, self-efficacy, psychological function

Results: A and B groups improved most outcomes, however, improvements in self-efficacy and aerobic capacity were not correlated with the clinical manifestation

Authors	Participants	Duration and frequency	Intervention	Type of exercise	Outcomes
Altan et al., (2004)	A(n=24); B(n=22) ♀FM	(12 wks.) + 1 year follow-up	A. warm pool exercises; B. Balneotherapy	Aerobic	Pain, TP count, fatigue, sleep disturbances, FIQ, muscular endurance,

Results: Pool based exercises has some positive effects on FM symptoms but those has not been shown to be superior to balneotherapy

Authors	Participants	Duration and frequency	Intervention	Type of exercise	Outcomes
Assis et al., (2006)	A(n=26), B(n=26), ♀FM	1h. – 3×/wk. (15 wks.)	A. Deep pool exercises; B. Land based aerobic exercises	Aerobic	VAS pain, FIQ, BDI, SF-36

Results: Both treatments were effective in improving pain and function in women with FM, although patients allocated in group A obtained further improvements in emotional well-being

Authors	Participants	Duration and frequency	Intervention	Type of exercise	Outcomes
Tomas-Carus et al., (2008)	A(n=15); B(n=15) ♀FM	1h. – 3×/wk. (8 months)	A. Pool-based exerc. (10'warm up, 2×10'aerobic ex. at 65–75% HR$_{max}$, 20' Strength – 4×10reps, 10' cool down. B. Control	Aerobic	FIQ, VAS pain, aerobic capacity, physical function, balance, anxiety and depression

Results: Treatment was effective in improving functional capacity, pain, stiffness, anxiety, depression, FIQ, aerobic capacity, and balance

Key VAS: Visual analogue scale; TP: Tender Points; BDI: Beck Depression Inventory; BAI: Beck Anxiety Inventory; MPQ: McGill Pain Questionnaire; FIQ: Fibromylagia Impact Questionnaire; 6MWT: Six Minute Walk Test Distance.

Pool-based aerobic exercise

The first evidence of the benefits to be gained from pool-based aerobic exercise training was reported by Jentoft *et al.* (2001), who compared the relative effects of 20-week programmes of land-based and pool-based exercise. Both groups showed an improvement in aerobic capacity and symptoms, although changes in hand-grip strength were greater in the land-based group. In this line, Gowans *et al.* (2001) examined the impact of a 23-weeks aerobic exercise programme, incorporating both land-based and pool-based exercises, on physical function and mood. Exercise consisted of 30-minute sessions with 10 minutes of stretching and 20 minutes of aerobic exercise (60–75 per cent HR_{max}), three times per week. Aerobic capacity (6 minutes walk time), depression, anxiety, mental health and self-efficacy improved in exercise group versus controls. Similarly, Assis *et al.* (2006) also showed improvements in pain, mood, physical ability, QoL and physical function in 60 sedentary women with a high level of impairment (Fibromyalgia Impact Questionnaire (FIQ) score > 60) after 15 weeks of moderate intensity land-based and pool-based aerobic exercise. A summary of aerobic exercise programmes in FMS patients is presented in Table 17.1.

Altan *et al.* (2004) allocated 50 FMS patients to either pool-based exercise (aerobic, strengthening and flexibility exercises), using 3×35 minute sessions per week for 12 weeks, or balneotherapy. Both groups reported improved symptoms, including pain severity, stiffness or fatigue, and inter-group analysis showed significant improvements in the exercise group for depression compared to the spa treatment. These improvements were similar to those reported by Cedraschi *et al.* (2004), which were maintained for at least six months. Zijlstra *et al.* (2005) combined exercise and balneotherapy in a 2.5-week treatment programme, achieving symptomatic improvements, but these improvements were not maintained at six months of follow-up. Recently, several long-term interventions have evaluated the benefits of exercise in a waist-pool with positive results in terms of symptomatic improvements, functional capacity and QoL (e.g. Gusi *et al.*, 2006; Tomas-Carus *et al.*, 2008).

In summary, there is moderate evidence that aerobic exercise produces improvements in pain, psychological well-being, anxiety, depression and global impact in patients with FMS, which positively contribute to QoL improvements. Aerobic exercise might also have positive effects on TP counts, but these improvements have been inconsistent or statistically insignificant (Goldenberg *et al.*, 2004).

Frequency, duration and intensity of aerobic exercise

The optimum frequency, intensity and duration of aerobic exercise for patients with FMS are currently unknown but most studies have used a frequency of 2–3 times per week. However, to minimize pain and enhance adherence, a starting frequency of two days per week can be recommended. Many studies have used exercise durations of 30–60 minutes, with the average length of aerobic exercise programmes being approximately 12 weeks, although some studies were maintained for more than 20 weeks. Given that FMS is a pain syndrome that limits physical activity and can cause severe decrements in physical capacity, performance of continuous exercise is often a problem. For this reason, the effect of shorter intermittent sets of aerobic exercise has been assessed with promising results (Kesaniemi *et al.*, 2001; Schachter *et al.*, 2003). Regarding intensity, aerobic exercise performed at 60–75 per cent HR_{max} can be tolerated, although some authors have shown that this intensity might be unattainable (Norregaard *et al.*, 1997). Most studies suggest intensity between 40 and 80 per cent HR_{max}, although studies using 50 per cent HR_{max} have reported the lowest rates of attrition and, therefore, seem to be better tolerated than those with a higher intensity (Jones *et al.*, 2006). Nevertheless, some studies have even reported difficulties with low intensity exercise (Busch *et al.*, 2008). Pool-based aerobic exercise studies have successfully used intensities of between 55 and 75 per cent HR_{max} (Gowans *et al.*, 1999; 2001; Jentoff *et al.*, 2001; Altan *et al.*, 2004; Gusi *et al.*, 2006).

Strength training programmes

Häkkinen *et al.* (2001) investigated the effects of 21 weeks of progressive strength (resistance exercise) training on neuromuscular function and symptomatic perception in women with FMS compared to healthy women. The intervention group exercised twice weekly, starting at 40–60 per cent of the one-repetition maximum (1RM) strength, increasing to 60–80 per cent of the 1RM over time. Improvements in muscle strength, mood, fatigue and neck pain were observed but there was no change in overall pain or TP count. In a subsequent strength training study, these authors analyzed strength and neuromuscular function in a group of women with FMS compared to healthy controls (Häkkinen *et al.*, 2002). After 21 weeks of strength training, the patients achieved improvements in maximum force and neuromuscular function (assessed using electromyography (EMG)) that were comparable to healthy women. Jones *et al.* (2002) studied the impact of a 12-week programme of progressive strength training versus flexibility exercises. The strength training programme evoked significant improvements in muscle strength, pain and global FIQ score. Pain was not exacerbated by participation in either group. Other studies have also reported improvements in strength, neuromuscular function, pain, functional capacity and sleep disturbance after programmes of strength training exercise (using intensities of 40–80 per cent of the 1RM strength) in FMS patients, with no reported exacerbation of symptoms (e.g. Geel and Robergs, 2002; Valkeinen *et al.*, 2005; Kingsley *et al.*, 2005). A summary of strength training intervention studies is presented in Table 17.2.

TABLE 17.2 Exercise programmes to improve muscle strength in patients with FM

Authors	Participants	Duration and frequency	Intervention	Type of exercise	Outcomes
Häkkinen et al., (2001)	A(n=11); B(n=10); C(n=12) ♀FM	2×/wk. (21 wks.)	A. Strength training, 1°.40–60% – 2°.60–80% 1RM; B. Control group; C. Healthy subjects	Strength	TP count, Strength, EMG signal, VAS pain and sleep disturbances, BDI, fatigue

Results: Muscle Strength, EMG signal and depression improved in group A patients when comparing with group B patients. This training can be used safely in FM, diminishing the impact of the syndrome and the symptoms

| Häkkinen et al., (2002) | A(n=11); B(n=10); C(n=12) ♀FM | 2×/wk. – (21 wks) | A. Strength training; B. FM patients without training; C. Control group | Strength | Muscle strength, Anthropometry, hormonal response |

Results: Patients in training group increase their maximum force, EMG signal and neuromuscular adaptation comparable to healthy women

| Valkeinen et al., (2004) | A(n=13); B(n=13); C(n=10) ♀FM | 2×/wk. – (21 wks) | A. Strength training; B. FM control; C. Strength training in healthy subjects | Strength | Pain, TP count, fatigue, sleep disturbance, muscle strength, physical function, depression |

Results: Strength training has positive effects on perceived symptoms and improves functional capacity without complications. FM patients have normal neuromuscular function

Authors	Participants	Duration and frequency	Intervention	Type of exercise	Outcomes
Kingsley et al., (2005)	A(n=15); B(n=14) ♀FM	2×/wk. – (21 wks)	A. Strength training (1 set 8–12 reps. 1° 40–60% and 2° 60–80%RM). B. Control group	Strength	Muscle strength, TP count, FIQ, physical function

Results: Muscular capacity and functional capacity in upper limb improved in group A patients, but improvements in FIQ and TP count were not significant

Valkeinen et al., (2006)	A(n=13); B(n=13)♀FM	2×/wk. – (21 wks)	A. Strength training (6–7 exercises at 40–80%RM); B. Control group	Strength	Muscle strength, EMG signal, VAS pain, Hormonal response

Results: Strength training improved isometric strength (36%), concentric strength (33%) and EMG activity but did not alter hormone concentrations

VAS: Visual analogue scale; TP: Tender Points; BDI: Beck Depression Inventory; FIQ: Fibromyalgia Impact Questionnaire; EMG: electromyography; RM: one repetition maximum.

Flexibility programmes

Studies that have compared the benefits of flexibility exercises compared to a control group are not available, as flexibility exercises have only been studied as part of combined exercise programmes or as the control group (McCain et al., 1988; Mannerkorpi et al., 2000; Gowans et al., 2001; Jones et al., 2002; Richards and Scott, 2002; Valim et al., 2003). The first study to compare aerobic exercise with flexibility exercises (McCain et al., 1988), showed non-significant improvements in pain and sleep disturbance after an intervention of 20 weeks (60 minutes, three times per week). In another study that compared strengthening with flexibility exercises, Jones et al. (2002) allocated 56 women with FMS to either a strengthening or flexibility group and they exercised twice weekly (1 hour per session) for 12 weeks. Women allocated to the flexibility group showed improvements in strength, flexibility, self-efficacy and symptom severity, confirming that patients can get significant benefits from this type of exercise intervention, although to a lesser degree than a programme of muscle strengthening exercises.

Richards and Scott (2002) compared aerobic exercise with flexibility exercises of the upper- and lower-limbs, in combination with relaxation techniques. The programme duration was 12 weeks and patients exercised twice weekly. After the intervention, both groups had a decreased TP count and these changes were maintained one year later. No changes were observed in FIQ score, bodily pain or physical components of SF-36 generic QoL instrument, although fatigue levels decreased in both groups. Finally, Valim et al. (2003) compared flexibility exercises as a control therapy with the responses to an aerobic exercise intervention. Sessions of 45 minutes were performed three times weekly for 20 weeks, including 17 exercises that held the stretched position for 30 seconds. While the aerobic exercise group achieved superior changes in most outcomes versus the flexibility group, benefits in range of motion, anxiety and pain were observed in the latter. Depression and mental health outcomes were unchanged.

These studies suggest that flexibility exercises could be beneficial for increasing range of motion and, to a lesser extent, improving other key health outcomes without evoking adverse effects (Table 17.3). More studies are needed to confirm the efficacy of flexibility exercises as a treatment for FMS (Brosseau et al., 2008b).

TABLE 17.3 Flexibility exercise programmes in fibromyalgia patients

Authors	Participants	Duration and frequency	Intervention	Type of exercise	Outcomes
McCain et al., (1988)	A (n=18); B(n=20)♀♂FM	60min 3×/wk. (20 wks.)	A: Cicloergometer (150–170bpm) or B: flexibility training	Aerobic Vs Flexibility	Physical function, VAS pain, TP count, fatigue and sleep disturbances
Results: Aerobic capacity, pain threshold and number of TP were greater in aerobic exercise group than in the flexibility one. No adverse effects were found in either groups					
Jones et al., (2002)	A(n=28); B(n=28) ♀FM	1h. – 2×/wk. (12 wks.)	A. Strength training; B. Flexibility training	Strength Vs Flexibility	VAS pain, TP count, FIQ, muscle strength, range of motion, QoL, BDI, anxiety and self-efficacy
Results: Significant improvements in muscle strength were found in both groups although slightly better in strength training group. Pain did not worsen and improvements were maintained after one year follow-up					
Richards and Scott, (2002)	A(n=69); B(n=67) ♀FM	A. 60min. – 2×/wk. (12 wks.)	A. Aerobic exercise (walking or cicloergometer); B. Flexibility-relaxation	Aerobic Vs Flexibility	Painr, TP count, FIQ, SF-36, fatigue
Results: 35% of those in group A reported improvements compared with 18% in group B. Improvements in number of TP were maintained after one year follow-up					
Valim et al., (2003)	A(n=32); B(n=28) ♀FM	45 min; 3×/wk. – (20 wks.)	A. Aerobic exercise; B. Flexibility training	Aerobic Vs Flexibility	VAS pain, TP count, FIQ, SF-36, range of motion, anxiety, BDI
Results: Significant improvements in most outcomes were found in both programs, although those improvements were greater in the aerobic exercise group					

VAS: Visual analogue scale; TP: Tender Points; BDI: Beck Depression Inventory; FIQ: Fibromyalgia Impact Questionnaire; QoL: Quality of life.

Combined exercise programmes

One of the first studies to investigate the effects of combined exercise interventions in FMS was designed by Burckhardt *et al.* (1994). One group attended an education programme for six weeks, based on coping strategies and relaxation, and another group received the education programme with physical training, including stretching exercises, two sessions of pool-based exercises and a single period of aerobic exercise. A control group was also included in the study design. Both treatment groups showed improvements in QoL, pain, function and other symptoms compared with control group. Martin *et al.* (1996) then evaluated the effects of a six-week programme of aerobic, strength and flexibility exercise compared to a relaxation group. Improvements in TP count and aerobic capacity were observed in the exercise group. However, the authors concluded that although this practice could be advised (due to the absence of any adverse effects), the duration of the programme was too short to evoke meaningful benefits. Verstappen *et al.* (1997) studied the effects of a six-month programme of aerobic, strength and flexibility exercises and, although no differences on the main outcomes measured were observed, 80 per cent of patients reported feeling better following exercise and stiffness and QoL were slightly improved. A similar study was performed by Buckelew *et al.* (1998), who compared the effects of aerobic exercise (walking at moderate-high intensity), flexibility and strength training, with another group who were engaged in biofeedback/relaxation therapy and a third group receiving both therapies together. All treatment strategies evoked improvements in physical fitness, TP count and self-efficacy, which were maintained a year after the intervention. Improvements in physical capacity and pain were also maintained for two years. Many other studies, which have included combined programmes of exercise training (some including pool-based exercise and the addition of an educational package), have reported improvements in key health outcomes in patients with FMS (Table 17.4).

TABLE 17.4 Combined exercise programmes in patients with fibromyalgia

Authors	Participants	Duration and frequency	Intervention	Type of exercise	Outcomes
Burckhardt et al., (1994)	A(n=30); B(n=28); C(n=28) ♀FM	A= 1h, 1×/wk. (6 wks.). B=1.5h, 1×/wk. (6 wks.)	A. Education; B. Education + Aerobic exercise + Flexibility exercise; C. Control group without treatment	Mixed	Pain, TP count, FIQ, self-efficacy, fatigue, sleep disturbance, psychological function.

Results: QoL, pain, psychological function and other symptoms improved in both experimental groups compared with control group. FIQ, pain, fatigue and stiffness improved in group B after 11 months follow-up

Martin et al., (1996)	A(n=18); B(n=20) ♀♂FM	A. 1h – 3×/wk. (6 wks.); B. 1h – 1×/wk. (6 wks.)	A. Aerobic exercise (60–80% HR_{max}) + Strengthening + Flexibility exercises; B. Relaxation	Combined	Aerobic capacity, Isokinetic dynamometry, Sit and Reach, TP count, VAS pain, FIQ, ASES

Results: Aerobic capacity, number of TP and pain were significantly better in group A compared with group B

Gowans et al., (1999)	A(n=20), B(n=21) ♀FM	Ej. 30min – 2×/wk + Education. 1h – 2×/ wk. (6 wks.)	A. aquaerobic + strengthening + Flexibility.+ Educacion; B. waiting list	Mixed	6MWT, FIQ, fatigue, sleep disturbance, psychological function

Results: Group A patients improved aerobic capacity, well-being, fatigue and self-efficacy compared to control group. After 3 months follow-up benefits in aerobic capacity and well-being were maintained

Rooks et al., (2002)	n=15 ♀FM	1h – 3×/wk. (20 wks.)	Aerobic exercise + Strengthening + flexibility. No control group	Combined	6MWT, muscle capacity, FIQ

Results: Exercise programme significantly improved muscle strength, aerobic capacity and FIQ

Continued

TABLE 17.4 continued

Authors	Participants	Duration and frequency	Intervention	Type of exercise	Outcomes
Ramsay et al., (2000)	A(n=37); B(n=37) ♀FM	1h. 1×/wk. (12 wks.)	A. Aerobic exercise + flexibility exercises + relaxation; B. home exercises	Combined	Pain, TP count, HAQ, sleep disturbance, anxiety and depression
Results: Improvements in anxiety were found in combined exercise group. After 24 and 48 weeks follow-up improvements were not maintained					
Mannerkorpi et al., (2000)	A(n=28); B(n=29) ♀FM	35 min. – 1×/wk. (6 months) + 6 wks. Education	A. Low intensity pool exercises.+ aerobic exercises + Flexibility + Education; B. Control group	Mixed	FIQ, 6MWT, SF-36, psychological function, fatigue, sleep disturbance, handgrip strength
Results: Group A patients improved FIQ, handgrip strength, aerobic capacity and QoL compared with group B. Improvements were mantained after 6 months follow-up					
King et al., (2002)	A(n=42); B(n=41); C(n=35); D(n=34) ♀FM	(12 wks.) + 3 months follow-up	A. Aerobic exercise; B. Education; C. Aerobic exercise + Education; D. Control group	Aerobic or Mixed	TP, FIQ, functional capacity, self-efficacy
Results: The combination of exercise + education improves the ability to control symptoms. Aerobic exercise increases walking distance that remained after the follow-up only in this group					
Cedraschi et al., (2004)	A(n=84); B(n=80) ♀FM	(6 wks.) + 6 months follow-up	A. multidisciplinar treatment with aerobic exercise; B. Control group	Combined	Pain, TP count, SF-36, FIQ
Results: Multidisciplinary treatment based on exercise training and education can improve patients QoL and these benefits can be maintained 6 months after treatment					

Authors	Participants	Duration and frequency	Intervention	Type of exercise	Outcomes
Da Costa et al., (2005)	A(n=39); B(n=40) ♀FM	(12 wks.) + 9 months follow-up	A. Home exercises; B. Control group	Mixed	FIQ, Pain

Results: Moderate intensity home exercises significantly improved health status and pain in women with FM (mainly in severe affected patients), which were maintained during the follow-up period

Zijlstra et al., (2005)	A(n=58); B(n=76) ♀FM	(2.5 wks.) + 12 months follow-up	A. Spa; B. Control group	Mixed	Pain, TP count, FIQ, fatigue, sleep disturbance, general health, depression

Results: The combination of aerobic exercise and talasotherapy improved symptoms and QoL in FMS patients, although improvements were not significant after 6 months follow-up

Gusi et al., (2006)	A(n=17); B(n=17)♀FM	1h. – 3×/wks. (12 wks.)	A. Pool exer. (10′ warm up, 2×10′ aerobic exerc. at 65–75% HR$_{max}$, 20′ strengthening- 4×10reps, 10′ cool down	Aerobic + strength	Muscle strength, functional capacity, QoL, VAS pain, anxiety and depression

Results: Increase of muscle strength in the lower limbs (20%) that were maintained during follow-up. QoL (93%) and pain (29%) also improved during training but the pain returned to initial levels after the intervention

Bircan et al., (2008)	A(n=13); B.(n=13)	3×/wk. – (8 wks.)	A. Aerobic exercise (20–30′at 60–70% HR$_{max}$. B. Strengthening (5–12reps)	Aerobic vs Strength	VAS pain, 6MWT, SF-36, anxiety, depression

Results: A and B treatments were similarly effective in all outcomes examined

Continued

TABLE 17.4 *continued*

Authors	Participants	Duration and frequency	Intervention	Type of exercise	Outcomes
Valkeinen *et al.*, (2008)	A(n=13); B(n=11)♀FM	1h. – 3×/wks. (21 wks.)	A. strength and endurance (40–80%, 2–6 sets, 30–60 min). B. Control group	Aerobic + strength	Muscle strength, aerobic and functional performance, HAQ, VAS pain, fatigue, sleep quality and well-being

Results: W_{max}, work time, concentric leg extension force, walking and stair climbing time and fatigue were significantly better in group A patients. Concurrent strength and endurance training in low to moderate volume improves the muscle strength, endurance and symptomatology in women with FMS

Key VAS: Visual analogue scale; TP: Tender Points; BDI: Beck Depression Inventory; ASES: Arthritis Self-Efficacy Scale; HAQ: Health Assessment Questionnaire; FIQ: Fibromyalgia Impact Questionnaire; 6MWT: Six Minute Walk Test Distance; QoL: Quality of life.

Recommendations for exercise prescription

Patients with FMS have different initial levels of physical ability and while some are capable of exercising at moderate-high intensity, for others this may increase the pain that they experience (van Santen *et al.*, 2002b). Hence, individual capability and baseline fitness level needs to be assessed before starting any exercise programme. Initially, exercise programmes should include 5–10 minutes each of light aerobic exercise (e.g. walking, cycle ergometry, etc.), light resistance exercises (strength-training) and stretching. The duration of an exercise session should not extend beyond 60 minutes. Patients must first warm up for 5–10 minutes using muscles of the entire body and including multi-joint movements. Warm-up is particularly beneficial for FMS patients because it can help reduce feelings of stiffness before exercise and may help to reduce exercise-induced injury (Rooks, 2008).

Following warm-up activities, aerobic exercise can then be performed. In general, aerobic exercise intensities between 60 and 75 per cent HR_{max} are well tolerated by many patients (Clark *et al.*, 2001; Rooks *et al.*, 2002), although they should take frequent rest (or lighter exercise) breaks between short bouts of aerobic exercise to enable a greater total volume of exercise without undue fatigue. Higher intensity aerobic exercise must be avoided initially as this can exacerbate symptoms in some patients (Meyer and Lemley, 2000; van Santen *et al.*, 2002a). Most FMS patients can engage in low-intensity aerobic exercise or aerobic exercise performed at self-selected intensity by adjusting the load and pausing during the programme (Rooks, 2008). Treadmill walking is a good form of aerobic exercise for FMS patients but the level of effort must be controlled by holding people back during the first 5–6 weeks, before progressing the speed of walking or the incline within the individual's level of capability. It is important to inform patients that they can always return to a lower level of intensity but that they should not be afraid to try and increase their level of effort. Because of the risk of exercise causing an exacerbation of symptoms and prolonged pain, appropriate but effective exercise intensity has to be carefully determined. This can be achieved using a heart rate monitor, together with perceived exertion scales (e.g. Borg RPE scale). The rate of exercise progression of exercise intensity will vary between patients and it is not uncommon to go back and forth with progression as patients suffer flares of symptoms. A heart rate monitor and perceived exertion scale (together with a good knowledge of the patient's symptoms and level of overall fatigue) are good tools for establishing appropriate exercise intensities at any time-point. After several months, the frequency of aerobic exercise training should be 2–3 days per week, being mindful that higher exercise training frequencies can be harmful for some women with FMS (Mengshoel *et al.*, 1992; Wigers *et al.*, 1996; Meyer and Lemley, 2000). Any type of aerobic exercise can be prescribed and should be maintained for a period of at least 30 minutes (or an accumulated amount of intermittent aerobic exercise should be aimed for). For patients with more severe physical limitations, stationary cycling, arm-cranking, elliptical devices and other exercise ergometers are good alternatives.

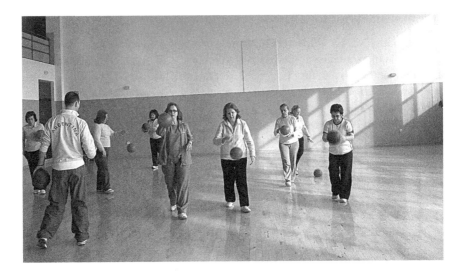

FIGURE 17.1 Group aerobic exercise in FMS patients.

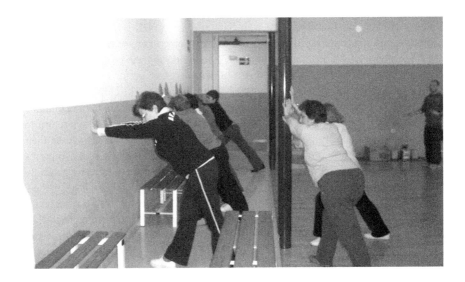

FIGURE 17.2 Stretching exercises in FMS patients.

Group-based aerobic exercise can improve adherence and bring psychosocial benefits (Figure 17.1) (Mannerkorpi, 2005). If 'circuit exercise' sessions are performed in a gymnasium setting, three sets of 1–2 minutes on a treadmill, and a further three sets on a rowing machine or stationary bike, resting for 1–1.5 minutes after each set is sufficient, always keeping within the prescribed intensity thresholds using heart rate and perceived exertion (Borg RPE scale rating of 13–15). Alternatively, other group-based activities can be performed, e.g. ball games of 1–2 minutes (to accumulate at least 10 minutes of exercise), with inter-polated rest periods of 1–1.5 min between sets (Figure 17.2).

Resistance (muscle strengthening) exercises should also be included in any exercise programme. Resistance exercises can be performed for 15–20 minutes and should involve the major skeletal muscle groups of the body and multi-joints movements. Intense muscle contractions or extreme muscle fatigue should be avoided (Rooks, 2008). In general, body resistance exercises are adequate in patients with FMS, although elastic (Thera-) bands or small weights (1–5 kg) can also be used. Pool-based exercises offer an alternative for patients who have problems supporting and mobilizing their body weight. As a general rule, 1–2 sets of 8 repetitions, using one's own body weight, and gradually progressing this until 3–4 sets of 10–12 repetitions (perhaps also using small weights) and always including active recovery between sets is recommended. Patients should not experience pain or excessive joint stress during or after resistance exercise. Eccentric muscle actions that could aggravate certain symptoms and evoke muscle micro-trauma, and isometric exercises that can elevate blood pressure and restrict blood flow in skeletal muscle, should be avoided. As for aerobic exercise training, progression should be individually tailored, taking into account flares of symptoms and current overall levels of fatigue.

Finally, 10 minutes of flexibility exercise, using 8–9 different exercises (1–3 sets of 3 repetitions, holding the stretched position for 15–25 seconds, and resting between each set) is recommended. Exercises should be performed close to the maximum range of motion but doing this gradually to reduce the risk of exercise-induced muscle soreness and injury.

Summary and conclusions

There is strong evidence to support the use of aerobic exercise training and an increasing body of evidence supports the use of muscle strengthening and flexibility exercises as part of the overall management of FMS. All forms of aerobic exercise training can be recommended: aerobic exercise on land and in the water demonstrates physical, emotional and functional benefits. Strength and flexibility exercises are beneficial for symptom control and fitness improvements. Individualized programmes are recommended and a multidisciplinary approach, combining these exercise modalities, may be the most beneficial. Exercise prescriptions should begin with low intensity, short duration exercise bouts, with the intensity and duration of exercise being gradually increased. Progression should be individually tailored, taking into account flares of symptoms and current levels of fatigue.

References

Altan, L., Bingol, U., Aykac, M., Koc, Z. and Yurtkuran, M. (2004). Investigation of the effects of pool-based exercise on fibromyalgia syndrome. *Rheumatol Int*, 24, 272–7.

Assis, M. R., Silva, L. E., Alves, A. M., Pessanha, A. P., Valim, V., Feldman, D., Neto, T. L. and Natour, J. (2006). A randomized controlled trial of deep water running: clinical effectiveness of aquatic exercise to treat fibromyalgia. *Arthritis Rheum*, 55, 57–65.

Bennett, R. M., Clark, S. R., Goldberg, L., Nelson, D., Bonafede, R. P., Porter, J., Specht, D. (1989). Aerobic fitness in patients with fibrositis. A controlled study of respiratory gas exchange and 133xenon clearance from exercising muscle. *Arthritis Rheum*, 32(4), 454–60.

Bircan, C., Karasel, S.A., Akgün, B., El, O. and Alper, S. (2008). Effects of muscle strengthening versus aerobic exercise program in fibromyalgia. *Rheumatol Int*, 28(6), 527–32.

Brosseau, L., Wells, G. A., Tugwell, P., Egan, M., Wilson, K. G., Dubouloz, C. J., Casimiro, L., Robinson, V. A., McGowan, J., Busch, A., Poitras, S., Moldofsky, H., Harth, M., Finestone, H. M., Nielson, W., Haines-Wangda, A., Russell-Doreleyers, M., Lambert, K., Marshall, A .D. and Veilleux, L. (2008a). Ottawa Panel Members. Ottawa Panel evidence-based clinical practice guidelines for aerobic fitness exercises in the management of fibromyalgia: part 1. *Phys Ther*, 88(7), 857–71.

Brosseau, L., Wells, G. A., Tugwell, P., Egan, M., Wilson, K. G., Dubouloz, C. J., Casimiro, L., Robinson, V. A., McGowan, J., Busch, A., Poitras, S., Moldofsky, H., Harth, M., Finestone, H. M., Nielson, W., Haines-Wangda, A., Russell-Doreleyers, M., Lambert, K., Marshall, A. D. and Veilleux, L. (2008b). Ottawa Panel Members. Ottawa Panel evidence-based clinical practice guidelines for strengthening exercises in the management of fibromyalgia: part 2. *Phys Ther*, 88(7), 873–86.

Buckelew, S. P., Conway, R., Parker, J., Deuser, W. E., Read, J., Witty, T. E., Hewett, J. E., Minor, M., Johnson, J. C., Van Male, L., McIntosh, M. J., Nigh, M. and Kay, D. R. (1998). Biofeedback/relaxation training and excerise interventions for fibromyalgia: a prospective trial. *Arthritis Care Res*, 11, 196–209.

Burckhardt, C. S., Mannerkorpi, K., Hedenberg, L.and Bjelle, A. (1994). A randomized, controlled clinical trial of education and physical training for women with fibromyalgia. *J Rheumatol*, 21, 714–20.

Busch, A. J., Schachter, C. L., Overend, T. J., Peloso, P. M. and y Barber, K. A. (2008). Exercise for fibromyalgia: a systematic review. *J Rheumatol*, 35(6), 1130–44.

Carville, S. F., Arendt-Nielsen, S., Bliddal, H., Blotman, F., Branco, J. C., Buskila, D., Da Silva, J. A., Danneskiold-Samsøe, B., Dincer, F., Henriksson, C., Henriksson, K. G., Kosek, E., Longley, K., McCarthy, G. M., Perrot, S., Puszczewicz, M., Sarzi-Puttini, P., Silman, A., Späth, M. and Choy, E. H. (2008). EULAR. EULAR evidence-based recommendations for the management of fibromyalgia syndrome. *Ann Rheum Dis*, 67(4), 536–41.

Cedraschi, C., Desmeules, J., Rapiti, E., Baumgartner, E., Cohen, P., Finckh, A., Allaz, A. F. and Vischer, T. L. (2004). Fibromyalgia: a randomised, controlled trial of a treatment programme based on self management. *Ann Rheum Dis*, 63, 290–6.

Clark, S. R., Jones, K. D., Burckhardt, C. S. and Bennett, R. M. (2001). Exercise for patients with fibromyalgia: risks versus benefits. *Curr Rheumatol Rep*, 3, 135–46.

Da Costa, D., Abrahamowicz, M., Lowensteyn, I., Bernatsky, S., Dritsa, M., Fitzcharles, M. A. and Dobkin, P. L. (2005). A randomized clinical trial and individualized home-based exercise programme for women with fibromyalgia. *Rheumatol* (Oxford), 44, 1422–7.

Gandhi, N., DePauw, K. P., Dolny, D. G. and Freson, T. (2002). Effect of an exercise program on quality of life of women with fibromyalgia. *Women Ther*, 25, 91–103.

Geel, S. E. and Robergs, R. A. (2002). The effect of graded resistance exercise on fibromyalgia symptoms and muscle bioenergetics: a pilot study. *Arthritis Care Res*, 47, 82–6.

Goldenberg, D. L., Burckhardt, C. and Crofford, L. (2004). Management of fibromyalgia syndrome. *JAMA*, 292(19), 2388–95.

Gowans, S. E., deHueck, A., Voss, S., Silaj, A., Abbey, S. E. and Reynolds, W. J. (2001). Effect of a randomized, controlled trial of exercise on mood and physical function in individuals with fibromyalgia. *Arthritis Rheum*, 45, 519–29.

Gowans, S. E., deHueck, A., Voss, S. and Richardson, M. (1999). A randomized, controlled trial of exercise and education for individuals with fibromyalgia. *Arthritis Care Res*, 12, 120–8.

Gusi, N., Tomas-Carus, P., Häkkinen, A., Häkkinen, K. and Ortega-Alonso, A. (2006). Exercise in waist-high warm water decreases pain and improves health-related quality of life and strength in the lower extremities in women with fibromyalgia. *Arthritis Rheum*, 55(1), 66–73.

Häkkinen, A., Häkkinen, K., Hannonen, P. and Alén, M. (2001). Strength training induced adaptations in neuromuscular function of premenopausal women with fibromyalgia: comparison with healthy women. *Ann Rheum Dis*, 60, 21–6.

Häkkinen, K., Pakarinen, A., Hannonen, P., Häkkinen, A., Airaksinen, O., Valkeinen, H. and Alen, M. (2002). Effects of strength training on muscle strength, cross-sectional area, maximal electromyographic activity, and serum hormones in premenopausal women with fibromyalgia. *J Rheumatol*, 29(6), 1287–95.

Jentoft, E. S., Kvalvik, A. G. and Mengshoel, A. M. (2001). Effects of pool-based and land-based aerobic exercise on women with fibromyalgia/chronic widespread muscle pain. *Arthritis Rheum*, 45, 42–47.

Jones, K. D., Adams, D., Winters-Stone, K. and Burckhardt, C. S. (2006). A comprehensive review of 46 exercise treatment studies in fibromyalgia (1988–2005). *Health Qual Life Outcomes*, 25, 4–67.

Jones, K. D., Burckhardt, C. S., Clark, S. R., Bennett, R. M., Potempa. K. M. (2002). A randomized controlled trial of muscle strengthening versus flexibility training in fibromyalgia. *J Rheumatol*, 29, 1041–8.

Kesaniemi, Y. A., Danforth, E. Jr., Jensen, M. D., Kopelman, P. G., Lefebvre, P. and Reeder, B. A. (2001). Dose-response issues concerning physical activity and health: an evidence-based symposium. *Med Sci Sports Exerc*, 33, S351–8.

King, S. J., Wessel, J., Bhambhani, Y., Sholter, D. and Maksymowych, W. (2002). The effects of exercise and education, individually or combined, in women with fibromyalgia. *J Rheumatol*, 29, 2620–7.

Kingsley, J. D., Panton, L. B., Toole, T., Sirithienthad, P., Mathis, R. and McMillan, V. (2005). The effects of a 12-week strength-training program on strength and functionality in women with fibromyalgia. *Arch Phys Med Rehabil*, 86, 1713–21.

Mannerkorpi, K. (2005). Exercise in fibromyalgia. *Curr Opin Rheumatol*, 17,190–4.

Mannerkorpi, K., Nyberg, B., Ahlme'n, M. and Ekdahl, C. (2000). Pool exercise combined with an education program for patients with fibromyalgia syndrome: a prospective, randomized study. *J Rheumatol*, 27, 2473–81.

Martin, L., Nutting, A., MacIntosh, B. R., Edworthy, S. M., Butterwick, D. and Cook, J. (1996). An exercise programme in the treatment of fibromyalgia. *J Rheumatol*, 23, 1050–3.

McCain, G. A., Bell, D. A., Mai, F. M. and Halliday, P. D. (1988). A controlled study of the effects of a supervised cardiovascular fitness training program on the manifestations of primary fibromyalgia. *Arthritis Rheum*, 31, 1135–41.

Meiworm, L., Jakob, E., Walker, U. A. and Peter, H. H. (2000). Patients with flbromyalgia benefit from aerobic endurance exercise. *Clin Rheumatol*, 19, 253–7.

Mengshoel, A. M., Komnaes, H. B. and Førre, Ø. (1992). The effects of 20 weeks of physical fitness training in female patients with fibromyalgia. *Clin Exp Rheumatol*, 10(4), 345–9.

Meyer, B. B. and Lemley, K. J. (2000). Utilizing exercise to affect the symptomology of fibromyalgia: a pilot study. *Med Sci Sports Exerc*, 32, 1691–7.

Nichols, D. S. and Glenn, T. M. (1994). Effects of aerobic exercise on pain perception, affect, and level of disability in individuals with fibromyalgia. *Phys Ther*, 74, 327–32.

Norregaard, J., Lykkegaard, J. J., Mehlsen, J. and Danneskiold-Samsoe, B. (1997). Exercise training in treatment of fibromyalgia. *J Musculoskel Pain*, 5, 71–9.

Ramsay, C., Moreland, J., Ho, M., Joyce, S., Walker, S. and Pullar, T. (2000). An observer-blinded comparison of supervised and unsupervised aerobic exercise regimens in fibromyalgia. *Rheumatology* (Oxford), 39(5), 501–5.

Redondo, J. R., Justo, C. M., Moraleda, F. V., Velayos, Y. G., Puche, J. J., Zubero, J. R., Hernández, T. G., Ortells, L. C. and Pareja, M. A. (2004). Long-term efficacy of therapy in patients with fibromyalgia: a physical exercise-based program and a cognitive behavioral approach. *Arthritis Rheum*, 51, 184–92.

Richards, S. C. and Scott, D. L. (2002). Prescribed exercise in people with fibromyalgia: parallel group randomised controlled trial. *BMJ*, 325, 185.

Rooks, D. S. (2008). Talking to patients with fibromyalgia about physical activity and exercise. *Curr Opin Rheumatol*, 20(2), 208–12.

Rooks, D. S., Silverman, C. B. and Kantrowitz, F.G. (2002). The effects of progressive strength training and aerobic exercise on muscle strength and cardiovascular fitness in women with fibromyalgia: a pilot study. *Arthritis Rheum*, 47, 22–8.

Rossy, L. A., Buckelew, S. P., Dorr, N., Hagglund, K. J., Thayer, J. F., McIntosh, M. J., Hewett, J. E. and Johnson, J. C. (1999). A meta-analysis of fibromyalgia treatment interventions. *Ann Behav Med*, 21, 180–191.

Sañudo, B. and Galiano, D. (2008). Relación entre capacidad cardiorrespiratoria y fibromialgia en mujeres. *Rheum Clin*, 4(1), 8–12.

Schachter, C. L., Busch, A. J., Peloso, P. M. and Sheppard, M. S. (2003). Effects of short versus long bouts of aerobic exercise in sedentary women with fibromyalgia: a randomized controlled trial. *Phys Ther*, 83, 340–358.

Sencan, S., Ak, S., Karan, A., Muslumanoglu, L., Ozcan, E. and Berker, E. (2004). A study to compare the therapeutic efficacy of aerobic exercise and paroxetine in fibromyalgia syndrome. *J Back Musculoskeletal Rehabil*, 17(2), 57–61.

Tomas-Carus, P., Gusi, N., Häkkinen, A., Häkkinen, K., Leal, A. and Ortega-Alonso, A. (2008). Eight months of physical training in warm water improves physical and mental health in women with fibromyalgia: a randomized controlled trial. *J Rehabil Med*, 40(4), 248–52.

Valim, V., Oliveira, L., Suda, A., Silva, L., de Assis, M., Barros, T., Feldman, D. and Natour, J. (2003). Aerobic fitness effects in fibromyalgia. *J Rheumatol*, 30(5), 1060–9.

Valkeinen, H., Alén, M., Häkkinen, A., Hannonen, P., Kukkonen-Harjula, K. and Häkkinen, K. (2008). Effects of concurrent strength and endurance training on physical fitness and symptoms in postmenopausal women with fibromyalgia: a randomized controlled trial. *Arch Phys Med Rehabil*, 89(9), 1660–6.

Valkeinen, H., Alen, M., Hannonen, P., Häkkinen, A., Airaksinen, O. and Häkkinen, K. (2004). Changes in knee extension and flexion force, EMG and functional capacity during strength training in older females with fibromyalgia and healthy controls. *Rheumatology* (Oxford), 43, 225–8.

Valkeinen, H., Häkkinen, A., Hannonen, P., Häkkinen, K., Alén, M. (2006). Acute heavy resistance exercise induced pain and neuromuscular fatigue in elderly women with fibromyalgia and in healthy controls: effects of strength training. *Arthritis Rheum*, 54, 1334–9.

Valkeinen, H., Häkkinen, K., Pakarinen, A., Hannonen, P., Häkkinen, A., Airaksinen, O., Niemitukia, L., Kraemer, W. J. and Alén, M. (2005). Muscle hypertrophy, strength development, and serum hormones during strength training in elderly women with fibromyalgia. *Scand J Rheumatol*, 34, 309–14.

van Santen, M., Bolwijn, P., Landewé, R., Verstappen, F., Bakker, C., Hidding, A., van der Kemp, D., Houben, H. and van der Linden, S. (2002a). High or low intensity aerobic fitness training in fibromyalgia: does it matter? *J Rheumatol*, 29, 582–587.

van Santen, M., Bolwijn, P., Verstappen, F., Bakker, C., Hidding, A., Houben, H., van der Heijde, D., Landewé, R. and van der Linden, S. (2002b). A randomized clinical trial comparing fitness and biofeedback training versus basic treatment in patients with fibromyalgia. *J Rheumatol*, 29, 575–81.

Verstappen, F. T. J., van Santen-Houefft, H. M. S., Bolwijn, P. H., Linden, S. and Kuipers, H. (1997). Effects of a group activity program for fibromyalgia patients on physical fitness and well being. *J Musculoskel Pain*, 5, 17–29.

Wigers, G. H., Stiles, T. C. and Vogel, P. A. (1996). Effects of aerobic exercise versus stress management treatment in fibromyalgia: a 4.5 year prospective study. *Scand J Rheumatol*, 25, 77–86.

Wolfe, F., Smythe, H. A, Yunus, M. B., Bennett, R. M., Bombardier, C., Goldenberg, D. L., Tugwell, P., Campbell, S. M., Abeles, M, Clark, P., Fam, A. G., Farber, S. J., Fiechtner, J. J., Franklin, C. M., Gatter, R. A., Hamaty, D., Lessard, J., Lichtbroun, A. S., Masi, A. T., Mccain, G. A., Reynolds, W. J., Romano, T. J, Russell, I. J. and Sheon, R. P. (1990). The American College of Rheumatology 1990 criteria for the classification of fibromyalgia. Report of the multicenter criteria committee. *Arthritis Rheum*, 33, 160–72.

Zijlstra, T. R., van de Laar, M. A., Bernelot, H. J., Taal, E., Zakraoui, L. and Rasker, J. J. (2005). Spa treatment for primary fibromyalgia syndrome: a combination of thalassotherapy, exercise and patient education improves symptoms and quality of life. *Rheumatology* (Oxford), 44, 539–46.

18

COLORECTAL, BREAST AND PROSTATE CANCER

Liam Bourke and John M. Saxton

Introduction

The global burden of cancer has more than doubled during the last 30 years and with the continued growth and ageing of the world's population, it is expected to double again by 2020 (Boyle and Lewin, 2008). Worldwide, there were 12.4 million new cancer diagnoses in 2008, 7.6 million cancer deaths and 25 million people living with cancer (Boyle and Lewin, 2008). Continued advances in early detection and effective treatments have resulted in the hope of longer survival and even cure for many cancer patients. However, older individuals diagnosed with cancer are at increased risk of other cancers and chronic age-related conditions and are susceptible to functional losses that can threaten independent living (Aziz, 2002; Hewitt *et al.*, 2003).

Studies have shown that regular exercise participation during and after cancer treatment is associated with higher levels of physical functioning and cardiovascular fitness, reduced feelings of fatigue and improved health-related quality of life (Demark-Wahnefried *et al.*, 2004; Knols *et al.*, 2005; Schmitz *et al.*, 2005; McNeely *et al.*, 2006). Nevertheless, the specific beneficial effects of exercise may vary as a function of disease stage, treatment approach and current lifestyle of the patient (Knols *et al.*, 2005). However, the full range of positive benefits resulting from habitual physical activity are as yet, unknown (Schmitz *et al.*, 2005). This chapter considers the evidence for exercise therapy in cancer patients and cancer survivors in relation to key health outcomes. As cancer is an 'umbrella-term' for a group of over 200 different diseases, the focus of attention has been limited to three of the most common cancers affecting men and women: colorectal cancer, breast cancer and prostate cancer.

Introduction to colorectal cancer

Colorectal cancer is the third most common cancer in the UK after breast and lung cancer, with 38,600 cases being diagnosed each year (Cancer Research UK, 2010). Surgery with curative intent is the primary treatment for localised colorectal cancer. Chemotherapy is administered as an adjuvant to surgery in a minority of patients, usually those whose tumour has spread to lymph nodes (Dukes' stage C). The standard treatment has been a course of 5-fluorouracil and folinic acid (FUFA), given intravenously over six months. The absolute increase in five-year survival rates achieved by FUFA chemotherapy in patients with stage III colon cancer is between 4 per cent and 13 per cent (NICE, 2004).

Exercise interventions in colorectal cancer survivors

There is a paucity of exercise intervention studies in this patient population; however preliminary evidence supports the potential health benefits of prescribed exercise. One of the few randomised controlled trials (RCTs) was undertaken by Courneya *et al.* (2003a). In this study, 103 colorectal cancer survivors were randomised (ratio of 2:1) to an exercise intervention or control group. The exercise intervention consisted of home-based aerobic exercise for 20–30 minutes, at 65–75 per cent predicted maximum heart rate, 3–5 times per week, for 16 weeks. An intention-to-treat analysis did not reveal any significant difference in QoL in the exercise group compared to controls. A large proportion of the control group (52 per cent), however, were also undertaking more than 60 minutes of moderate/strenuous exercise per week. In a subsequent ancillary analysis, significant differences were elucidated in terms of improved QoL and anxiety for the patients who demonstrated an increase in cardiovascular fitness.

Since the Courneya *et al.* (2003a) study, there has been one further RCT conducted in this cancer population. Houborg *et al.* (2006) investigated (hospital/home based) physical training in the post-operative period immediately following surgery in 119 colorectal cancer patients. Individuals were either randomised to an exercise training programme that included 45 minutes of mobilisation, upper- and lower-body resistance exercise six days per week or control group. Baseline physical performance and fatigue outcomes were compared with 30-day post-operative performance. No significant changes were observed in physical function between groups, but fatigue increased significantly less seven days post-operatively in the exercise group. This finding should be interpreted with caution however, as intervention group patients were more fatigued pre-operatively than controls. Indeed, no difference was observed between groups at day 30 or 90 in terms of change in fatigue. The above evidence, whilst not substantial, indicates that there could be health benefits for colorectal cancer patients from participating in exercise interventions.

Epidemiological evidence of secondary prevention in colon cancer survivors

Meyerhardt *et al.* (2006a) investigated physical activity and colorectal cancer specific survival/mortality in the context of pre-/post-diagnosis exercise. Using a prospective observational study design, the physical activity levels of 573 women with stage I–III colorectal cancer were assessed via a Nurses' Health Study mail questionnaire in the six months prior to and at least one year but no longer than four years (median 22 months) post-diagnosis. Compared with women who engaged in less than 3 MET-hours.week^{-1} of physical activity post-diagnosis, those engaging in at least 18 MET-hours.week^{-1} had a 61 per cent reduced risk of colorectal cancer-specific and 57 per cent reduced risk of overall mortality. In addition, women who increased their physical activity levels (comparing pre-diagnosis to post-diagnosis) had a 52 per cent reduced risk of colorectal cancer-specific mortality and 49 per cent reduced risk of all cause mortality compared with those with no change in physical activity level. Notably, pre-diagnosis physical activity was not predictive of mortality. Meyerhardt *et al.* (2006b) also reported similar effects in women with stage III colon cancer enrolled in a randomised chemotherapy trial. Compared with patients engaged in less than 3 MET-hours.week^{-1} of physical activity, patients engaging in 18 to 26.9 MET-hours.week^{-1} or over 27 MET-hours.week^{-1} had a 49 per cent reduced risk of cancer recurrence and 45 per cent reduced risk of death from any cause. This research is highly encouraging in terms of survivorship, as it suggests that increasing physical activity levels post-diagnosis can be beneficial, despite activity levels prior to diagnosis.

A suggested exercise prescription for colon cancer

Data from Courneya *et al.* (2003a) suggest that an exercise prescription which is based on UK and USA physical activity recommendations (Department of Health, 2004; Haskell *et al.*, 2007), i.e. a minimum of 30 minutes a day of at least moderate intensity physical activity (60–75 per cent of predicted maximum heart rate) on five or more days of the week, could be sufficient to evoke improvements in QoL and anxiety in colorectal cancer survivors. However, on the basis of the observational evidence presented by Meyerherdt *et al.* (2006a), colon cancer survivors should aim to accrue at least 18 MET-hours.week^{-1} of physical activity to reduce their risk of cancer specific mortality. This equates to 6 hours per week of brisk walking (3 METs intensity), 2.25 hours of cycling or 4.5 hours of water aerobics (Ainsworth *et al.*, 2000). Colon cancer patients should avoid strenuous exercise of the abdominal region up to six months post surgery as colon resection is a major surgical procedure and the trauma takes time to heal properly. This could take longer if there are post-surgical complications (e.g. secondary infections, breach of sutures etc). It is recommended that in the initial stages, individuals perform exercises that only indirectly require core activation (e.g. upright exercise) and then only when the surgical wounds have fully healed, move onto direct core activation exercise (e.g. prone/supine activities).

Introduction to breast cancer

Breast cancer is the most prevalent form of cancer diagnosed in females in the UK with 45,700 women diagnosed in 2007 (Cancer Research UK, 2010). Incidence rates of breast cancer have increased by approximately 50 per cent over the last 25 years but this should be interpreted in the context of increased breast cancer screening. In the majority of cases, treatment for breast cancer begins with surgery. Although the type of procedure undertaken depends on the size and location of the tumour, this can entail removal of the tumour with some surrounding breast tissue (lumpectomy) plus several weeks of radiotherapy. Alternatively, the whole breast might be removed (mastectomy) followed by reconstructive surgery. Alongside surgery/radiotherapy, in the instance of large or locally advanced cancer, chemotherapy or hormone therapy might be employed as adjuvant treatment to reduce the mass of the cancer to make the tumour easier to remove, and/or reduce the probability of disease recurrence. The side effects of breast cancer treatment include fatigue (Servaes *et al.*, 2002), anxiety/depression (Spiegel, 1997), lymphedema, cardiac and pulmonary toxicity (Truong *et al.*, 2004), changes in body composition (Rooney and Wald, 2007), reduced body strength, fitness and function (Hack *et al.*, 1999; Collins *et al.*, 2004).

Exercise in breast cancer

Physical fitness and body composition

Impairments in various physiological systems, including cardiovascular, pulmonary, musculoskeletal, endocrine, immune, neurological and lymphatic system functioning are commonly observed after breast cancer treatments (Schmitz and Speck, 2010). Hence, exercise therapy could have a major role to play in reversing such physiological decrements in women recovering from breast cancer. Studies have reported improvements in many different fitness parameters following programmes of exercise training in breast cancer patients and survivors (for comprehensive review refer to McNeely *et al.*, 2006). For example, studies have reported improvements in 12-minute walk distance (Cambell *et al.*, 2005; Mutrie *et al.*, 2007) and aerobic capacity (MacVicar *et al.*, 1989; Segal *et al.*, 2001; Courneya *et al.*, 2003b) in breast cancer patients and survivors using combined programmes of aerobic and resistance exercise or aerobic exercise alone. In addition to gains in aerobic capacity, improvements in upper- and lower-body strength have also been observed using progressive resistance exercise training (Schmitz *et al.*, 2005; Courneya *et al.*, 2007).

Weight gain is a particular concern in breast cancer patients (Irwin *et al.*, 2005) as it is associated with poorer long-term prognosis (Hede, 2008), as well as increased likelihood of associated co-morbidities such as cardiovascular disease (Rooney and Wald, 2007). However, emerging evidence suggests that exercise training can have beneficial effects on body composition in breast cancer survivors. Segal *et al.* (2001) reported evidence of reduced body weight (–4.8 kg) following a programme of aerobic exercise training at 50–60 per cent of $\dot{V}O_{2max}$ five times per week for 26 weeks in breast cancer survivors receiving hormone therapy, chemotherapy or radiotherapy compared to controls. Furthermore reductions in body fat (–1.15 per cent) (Schmitz et al., 2005) and increases in lean body mass (1.0 kg) (Courneya et al., 2007) have been observed through progressive resistance exercise training over 26 and 17 weeks, respectively. Evidence also suggests that ~2 h per week of moderate intensity walking exercise over 26 weeks can evoke reductions in body fat (–1.9 per cent) (Irwin et al., 2009). Hence, available studies suggest that aerobic and resistance exercise training could be effective adjuvant/adjunctive treatments for helping to reverse the declines in physiological function and body composition commonly occurring after breast cancer diagnosis and treatment.

Fatigue

Cancer-related fatigue, defined as 'a distressing, persistent, subjective sense of physical, emotional and/or cognitive tiredness or exhaustion related to cancer or cancer-related treatment that is not proportional to recent activity and interferes with usual functioning' (Velthuis et al., 2010), is commonly reported by breast cancer survivors. The evidence for exercise as a therapy for combating fatigue in this patient group is currently equivocal. Supervised, combined aerobic and resistance exercise training for two (Campbell et al., 2005) or three times (Mutrie et al., 2007) per week has proved to have no significant effect on symptoms of fatigue in two previous RCTs. Conversely, trials that have used exercise prescriptions requiring moderate intensity walking exercise four to five (Mock et al., 1997) or five to six times per week (Mock et al., 2004) have reportedly been more successful in mitigating fatigue. Accordingly, this would suggest more frequent physical activity might evoke a greater improvement of symptoms. However, additional exercise studies are required to draw firmer conclusions.

QoL and psychosocial health status

Ohira et al. (2006) reported improvements in global physical and psychological QoL in 86 breast cancer survivors after twice-weekly progressive resistance exercise training over six months. This evidence was supported by Campbell et al. (2005), who demonstrated improvements in general QoL (FACT-G questionnaire) with twice-weekly combined aerobic and resistance training but the FACT-B (breast cancer specific) QoL measure did not reach significance in the between group comparison (P=0.094). This small-scale trial however (n=22) was unlikely to have sufficient statistical power to detect between group differences. In contrast, evidence from larger-scale RCTs indicates that three exercise training sessions per week has more potential to evoke improvements in the FACT-B score (Courneya et al., 2003b; Daley et al., 2007; Mutrie et al., 2007). These results were not corroborated by another RCT, which reported no effect on cancer specific QoL as a result of supervised aerobic and resistance exercise (Courneya *et al.*, 2007) or separate home-based and supervised exercise interventions (Cadmus *et al.*, 2009). Moreover, trials that have investigated the effect of exercise training on feelings of anxiety and depression have failed to produce evidence of any beneficial effect (Ohira *et al.*, 2006; Mutrie *et al.*, 2007; Cadmus *et al.*, 2009). McNeely *et al.* (2006) following a meta-analysis that identified 14 studies (only four of which were deemed to be of high quality) cautiously concluded that exercise is an affective intervention for improving QoL in breast cancer patients/survivors, but highlighted the need for larger trials of high methodological quality and longer-term follow-up.

Lymphoedema

Lymphoedema can become a chronic and lifelong condition, characterised by swelling and recurring skin infections in breast cancer survivors as a result of insufficient lymph transport caused by the surgery (Rockson, 2008). Clinicians have traditionally recommended limiting physical activity to help prevent lymphoedema (particularly in the arms) in breast cancer survivors. However, in a multi-centre RCT, Courneya *et al.* (2007) reported that supervised resistance and aerobic exercise did not cause lymphoedema-related adverse events. In addition, another large RCT (n=204) which specifically investigated the difference in arm volume between breast cancer survivors after undergoing mastectomy or breast-conserving surgery with axillary node dissection, reported no significant difference in arm volume between an experimental group encouraged to exercise freely and a control group who had their physical activity restricted up to two years post-surgery (Sagen *et al.*, 2009).

Epidemiological evidence of secondary prevention in breast cancer survivors

The first study to report an association between post-diagnosis physical activity levels and mortality in breast cancer survivors was published by Holmes *et al.* (2005). In this study, physical activity data from the Nurses' Health Study in the USA was examined in women diagnosed with stages I, II or III invasive breast cancer between 1984 and 1998. Participants were asked to estimate the average time per week spent on a range of recreational activities, including walking, jogging, running, cycling, swimming and sports activities and the total MET-hours per week of leisure-time activity was determined. Compared with the women who were least active, the risk of overall mortality during the follow-up period was reduced by 41 per cent for women achieving the equivalent of 3–5 hours per week of average-pace walking. The risk of breast cancer recurrence was also reduced by 43 per cent for women in this physical activity category and the risk of breast cancer-specific mortality was reduced by 50 per cent. A particularly interesting finding of this study was that obese women who are physically active can gain similar benefits from engaging in a physically active lifestyle as their slimmer counterparts. Further analysis based on a small number of deaths suggested that the beneficial effects of physical activity (equivalent to at least 3–5 hours of average-pace walking) could be limited to women with hormone receptor positive tumours (consistent with a hormonal mechanism) and might be more pronounced in women with stage III disease (in comparison to stages I and II disease).

The findings of this study have since been consolidated by three other cohort studies of breast cancer survivors. Pierce *et al.* (2007) assessed post-diagnosis physical activity levels in addition to vegetable-fruit intake in a cohort of 1490 women from the Women's Healthy Eating and Living (WHEL) Study. The women were all aged 70 years at diagnosis of early stage breast cancer. All had completed primary therapy, although the majority were still taking tamoxifen. A nine-item questionnaire was used to record the frequency, duration and speed of walking outside the home, in addition to details of the frequency, intensity and duration of other physical exercise. Vegetable and fruit consumption was determined via a telephone-based dietary assessment (24-hour dietary recall) on random days. In comparison to women with the lowest physical activity levels (average 3.7 MET-hours.week^{-1}) and lowest vegetable-fruit consumption (average 3.1 servings per day), women with the highest physical activity levels (mean of 25 MET-hours.week^{-1}) who were consuming an average of 7.2 vegetable-fruit portions per day had a 44 per cent reduced risk of mortality. This level of physical activity equates to 4 hours per week of brisk walking (6 METs) or 6–8 hours per week of average-pace walking (3–4 METs).

Holick *et al.* (2008) reported associations between post-diagnosis physical activity levels and mortality in breast cancer survivors from the Collaborative Women's Longevity Study (CWLS). The women were mailed a questionnaire that assessed recreational physical activity within the last year a median of 5.6 years after breast cancer diagnosis. In addition, physical activity before diagnosis was available from a previous case control study on the same cohort of women. Should be replaced with: Using the least active women as the reference, total recreational physical activity in the range of 2.8 to 21 MET-hours.week^{-1} was associated with risk reductions of 35–49 per cent for breast cancer mortality (42–56 per cent risk reductions for all-cause mortality). Further analysis revealed that only women who participated in moderate intensity physical activity had a lower risk of breast cancer mortality, whereas there was no association with vigorous physical activity. Furthermore, the benefits associated with moderate intensity physical activity were independent of the time interval since breast cancer diagnosis. A physical activity level of 10.5 MET-hours.week^{-1} equates to a daily half-hour walk at average-pace. There was a dose-response relationship for moderate intensity physical activity, such that an increment of 5 MET-hours.week^{-1} was associated with 15 per cent lower risk of breast cancer death. Similar inverse associations between physical activity and breast cancer mortality were observed for young and older women at diagnosis, normal weight and overweight women and women diagnosed with local and regional stage disease.

In the most recent study, Irwin *et al.* (2008) reported inverse associations between post-diagnosis physical activity and mortality in breast cancer survivors enrolled onto the Health, Eating, Activity and Lifestyle (HEAL) Study, a multicentre, multiethnic prospective cohort study in the USA. All women had been diagnosed with *in situ* to regional breast cancer and physical activity was assessed using in-person interviews. In this study, associations with both pre-diagnosis and post-diagnosis physical activity levels were investigated in samples of 933 and 688 breast cancer survivors, respectively. A strong trend for a 31 per cent risk reduction in total mortality was observed in women who were achieving the equivalent of 150 minutes per week (30 minutes on at least 5 days of the week) of moderate intensity exercise in the year prior to breast cancer diagnosis in comparison to sedentary women. After diagnosis, any recreational physical activity and the equivalent of 150 minutes per week of moderate intensity physical activity were associated with risk reductions of 64 per cent and 67 per cent, respectively. Interestingly, women who decreased their physical activity levels by >3 MET-hours.week^{-1} after the breast cancer diagnosis had a four-fold increased risk of death in comparison to inactive women. No significant risk reduction for total mortality was observed in women who increased their physical activity levels by >3 MET-hours.week^{-1} after being diagnosed with breast cancer.

Considered together, these studies show good evidence of an inverse association between post-diagnosis physical activity and mortality in breast cancer survivors. Three of the four cohort studies show that women who are achieving the equivalent of the recommended 30 minutes of moderate intensity physical activity on at least five days of the week can halve their risk of mortality in up to eight years of follow-up. A particular strength of the HEAL study is (Irwin *et al.*, 2008) that it provided evidence of physical activity benefits in a multi-ethnic cohort, consistent with associations observed in the other cohort studies of mainly Caucasian women.

A suggested exercise prescription for breast cancer

Evidence suggests that an exercise prescription which is based on UK and USA physical activity recommendations (Department of Health, 2004; Haskell *et al.*, 2007), i.e. a minimum of 30 minutes a day of at least moderate intensity physical activity (60–75 per cent of predicted maximum heart rate) on five or more days of the week, is likely to elicit moderate benefits in breast cancer survivors, in terms of physical fitness, fatigue, body composition/weight management and QoL. The weight of epidemiological evidence also suggests that this level of physical activity is associated with positive effects on survival. Where patients are taking prescription medicine for other co-morbidities which might alter age predicted heart rate maximum (e.g. Beta-blockers), Borg RPE scale intensities of 11–14 should be aimed for. Where joint health permits and it can be tolerated, resistance exercise around 3–5 sets of 8–12 repetitions of moderate intensity (50–70 per cent of the one repetition maximum (1RM) strength), engaging major skeletal muscle groups can also be recommended to help reverse any reductions in lean body mass following breast cancer treatment. Programme frequency, duration and intensity should be reviewed every 6–8 weeks.

Introduction to prostate cancer

Prostate cancer is a major health burden throughout the world, and is the most frequent cancer among men in many developed countries (Schaid, 2004). In 2007, there were 36,000 new cases of prostate cancer in the UK and just over 10,000 deaths were recorded that year due to the disease (Cancer Research UK, 2010). A number of different treatment strategies are used for prostate cancer and the impact of exercise as and adjuvant/adjunctive therapy has to be considered in the context of the treatment being administered. Active surveillance avoids starting any potentially unnecessary treatment in men with indolent cancers until the disease shows any signs of progression. Radical prostatectomy for localised disease involves surgical removal of the entire prostate and seminal vesicles. External beam radiotherapy (EBRT) offers an alternative to surgery for men with localised disease, with an efficacy that is analogous to surgery. Surgical castration via orchidectomy is a relatively uncomplicated surgical procedure with minor risks (Loblaw *et al.*, 2004) but an unfavourable treatment for many patients. Finally, androgen deprivation therapy (ADT) is the cornerstone of modern treatment for advanced prostate cancer. The goal of ADT is to reduce the circulating levels of male sex steroid hormones (androgens) which stimulate prostate cancer cells to grow. ADT is commonly associated with compromised sexual function, bone mineral density degeneration, fatigue, central adiposity, increased risk of metabolic syndrome and elevated cardiovascular disease risk.

Evidence for the benefits of exercise in prostate cancer patients

During active surveillance

To date, no study has presented evidence of the effects of exercise in men undergoing active surveillance. However, studies have reported benefits of an intensive combined exercise and vegan diet intervention in relation to circulating prostate specific antigen (PSA) levels and inhibition of prostate (LNCaP) cell growth *in vitro* (Ornish *et al.*, 2005), as well as gene expression associated with tumorigenesis (Ornish *et al.*, 2008).

After surgery

Exercise interventions following radical prostatectomy have focused on the restoration of pelvic floor/bladder function. This form of exercise rehabilitation trains patients to isolate and repeatedly contract the pelvic floor muscles to improve urinary control (Bo, 2004). A systematic review undertaken by

MacDonald *et al.* (2007) concluded that this type of exercise rehabilitation hastens the return to continence in men following radical prostatectomy in comparison to no pelvic floor exercise training. The beneficial effects of this tend to take effect after 1–2 months with no further improvements seen after 3–4 months. Whilst this evidence is encouraging, men need to be motivated to undergo this treatment and the muscles involved must not be neurologically compromised by surgery (Dorey, 2007). More evidence is needed to assess whether pelvic floor training before radical prostatectomy helps prevent urinary incontinence post-surgery.

Men undergoing external beam radiotherapy

Exercise as adjuvant therapy for prostate cancer patients with localised disease undergoing radical radiotherapy has yielded some positive results. A home-based walking programme at 60–70 per cent of predicted maximum heart rate, three times a week, for four weeks successfully improved shuttle walk test scores and attenuated self-reported fatigue compared to controls (Windsor *et al.*, 2004). Furthermore, a supervised aerobic exercise intervention (30 minutes of treadmill walking three times per week for eight weeks) elicited an improvement in cardio-vascular fitness, timed sit-to-stand test, flexibility, strength, self-reported fatigue and QoL (Monga *et al.*, 2007). These results support the utility of aerobic exercise training in prostate cancer patients; however this study was limited by small groups sizes (exercise: n=11; control: n=10). To date the most scientifically robust evidence in support of the beneficial effects of exercise in prostate cancer patients undergoing radiotherapy has been presented by Segal *et al.* (2009) in a recent RCT (n=121). Patients were randomised to resistance exercise (n=40), aerobic exercise (n=40), or usual care (n=41). Men in the resistance exercise arm exercised three times per week performing two sets of 8–12 repetitions of 10 difference upper- and lower-body exercises at 60–70 per cent of one 1RM strength. Aerobic exercise consisted of three sessions per week, at 50–75 per cent $\dot{V}O_{2peak}$, for up to 45 minutes on treadmills, cycle ergometers and elliptical trainers. Resistance training improved aerobic fitness, upper- and lower-body strength after 24 weeks and also reduced body fat after 12 weeks compared to controls. In the aerobic group, only upper-body strength was improved after 24 weeks, although a strong trend was observed for an improvement in aerobic fitness. Resistance exercise improved QoL over 12 and 24 weeks but similar benefits were not seen in the aerobic exercise intervention. The authors also cited significant ameliorations in self-reported fatigue at 12 weeks in the aerobic exercise group, and at 12 and 24 weeks in the resistance exercise group compared to controls. Hence this trial indicates that resistance and aerobic training can be considered as supportive care therapies in prostate cancer patients undergoing radiotherapy.

Men undergoing androgen deprivation therapy

Two small-scale studies have investigated the effects of combined programmes of aerobic and resistance exercise in prostate cancer patients receiving ADT (Galvão et al., 2006; Culos-Reed et al., 2007) but both were single group design (excluding a control arm), and failed to show any increase in aerobic capacity. This research did, however, yield preliminary evidence of improvements in exercise behaviour, functional capacity and QoL.

To date, three RCTs have been successful in presenting evidence in support of the positive effects of exercise in prostate cancer patients receiving ADT. The first of these studies was conducted by Segal et al. (2003). In a multi-site trial, 155 prostate cancer patients who had been receiving ADT for > 3 months were randomised to 12 weeks of resistance exercise consisting of nine upper- and lower-body exercises performed at 60–70 per cent of the 1RM strength, three times per week or waiting list control group. The results demonstrated improved upper- and lower-body endurance in the exercise group, alongside a significant but modest change in fatigue perception. In addition, a significant improvement in disease specific QoL was observed. No effect was observed in body composition, circulating PSA or testosterone levels as a result of the intervention. This study reported a good attendance rate (75 per cent of prescribed sessions) and was the first to implement such an exercise regime in prostate cancer patients and demonstrate its effects on health-related QoL.

Culos-Reed et al. (2009) conducted a RCT in 100 prostate cancer patients (any stage) who may or may not have had previous treatment and were expected to receive ADT for at least 6 months. Patients were randomised to a 16-week individually tailored home-based aerobic and light resistance training programme (with one weekly booster session) or a control arm. As a result of the intervention, improvements were reported in exercise behaviour, neck and waist girth relative to controls. No significant interaction effect was reported in any other fitness, anthropometric or biochemistry outcomes. However, due to the high rate of dropout and the effect this would have on the statistical power to detect changes between groups, these results must be interpreted with caution.

Finally, Galvão et al. (2009) investigated the effects of a supervised programme of combined aerobic and resistance exercise training. Fifty-seven prostate cancer patients undergoing ADT (for longer than 2 months) were randomised to either the combined exercise programme or usual care. Resistance exercise was designed to progress from 12 to 6 repetition maximum strength, for 2–4 sets of upper- and lower-body exercises. Aerobic conditioning included 15–20 minutes of 65–80 per cent of predicted maximum heart rate exercise (Borg RPE scale 11–13). Exercise sessions were performed twice weekly for 12 weeks. The results demonstrated improvements in lean muscle mass, upper- and lower-body 1RM strength, QoL and perceptions of fatigue. The authors also reported improvements in 6-minute walk time but no improvement in 400 metres walking performance. Whilst this study corroborated the improvements in muscle strength and QoL demonstrated in previous studies, no evidence was presented to demonstrate that the aerobic component of the exercise prescription had any impact on the patient's aerobic capacity, or whether changes in physical function were linked to the observed improvements in fatigue/QoL.

A suggested evidence-based exercise prescription for prostate cancer

In accordance with the UK and USA physical activity recommendations (Department of Health, 2004; Haskell *et al.*, 2007), the evidence suggests that a minimum of 30 minutes a day of at least moderate intensity physical activity (60–75 per cent of predicted maximum heart rate) on five or more days of the week, is likely to elicit moderate health benefits in prostate cancer survivors. Where patients are taking prescription medicine for other co-morbidities which might alter age predicted maximum heart rate (e.g. Beta-blockers), Borg RPE scale intensities of 11–14 should be aimed for. Where joint health permits and it can be tolerated, resistance exercise based on 3–5 sets of 8–12 repetitions of moderate intensity (50–70 per cent of the 1RM strength), engaging major skeletal muscle groups, can also be recommended. Programme frequency, duration and intensity should be reviewed every 6–8 weeks.

Summary and conclusions

The role of exercise therapy for promoting improvements in key cancer health outcomes is increasingly being studied by research groups around the world. At present, we still have much to learn about the health impacts of regular exercise in different groups of cancer patients, during different phases of the cancer experience and after different treatment regimens. In particular, most of the data has been gleaned from middle-aged to older cancer patients and there is little available evidence for younger individuals. Nevertheless, the weight of current evidence supports the assertion that a physically active lifestyle can have a positive impact on a wide range of physical and psychological outcomes, with little evidence of adverse effects. Additional randomised controlled trials are needed to provide more robust data on the frequency, intensity, duration and type of physical activity which confers the greatest health benefits and risk reduction in relation to disease-free survival in patients recovering from different forms of cancer and associated treatments.

References

Ainsworth, B. E., Haskell, W. L., Whitt, M. C., Irwin, M. L., Swartz, A. M., Strath, S. J., O'Brien, W. L., Bassett, D. R., Schmitz, K. H., Emplaincourt, P. O., Jacobs, D. R. and Leon, A. S. (2000). Compendium of physical activities: an update of activity codes and MET intensities. *Medicine and Science in Sports and Exercise*, 32, 498–504.

Aziz, N. M. (2002). Cancer survivorship research: challenge and opportunity. *Journal of Nutrition* 132, 3494S–3503S.

Bo, K. (2004). Pelvic floor muscle training is effective in treatment of female stress urinary incontinence, but how does it work. *International Urogynecology Journal and Pelvic Floor Dysfunction*, 15, 76–84.

Boyle, P. and Lewin, B. (2008). *World Cancer Report 2008*. France, International Agency for Research on Cancer.

Campbell, A., Mutrie, N., White, F., McGuire, F. and Kearney, N. (2005). A pilot study of a supervised group exercise programme as a rehabilitation treatment for women with breast cancer receiving adjuvant treatment. *European Journal of Oncology Nursing*, 9, 56–63.

Cadmus, L. A., Salovey, P., Yu, H., Chung, G., Kasl, S. and Irwin, M. L. (2009). Exercise and quality of life during and after treatment for breast cancer: results of two randomized controlled trials. *Psychooncology*, 18, 343–352.

Cancer Research UK (2010). Cancer stats report – latest UK cancer incidence and mortality summary – numbers. London: Cancer Research UK.

Collins, L., Nash, R., Round, T. and Newman, B. (2004). Perceptions of upper-body problems during recovery from breast cancer treatment. *Support Care Cancer*, 12, 106–113.

Courneya, K. S., Friedenreich, C. M., Quinney, H. A., Fields, A. L., Jones, L. W. and Fairey, A. S. (2003a). A randomized trial of exercise and quality of life in colorectal cancer survivors. *European Journal of Cancer Care*, 12, 347–357.

Courneya, K. S., Mackey, J. R., Bell, G. J., Jones, L. W., Field, C. J. and Fairey, A. S. (2003b). Randomized controlled trial of exercise training in postmenopausal breast cancer survivors: cardiopulmonary and quality of life outcomes. *Journal of Clinical Oncology*, 21,1660–1668.

Courneya, K. S., Segal, R. J., Mackey, J. R., Gelmon, K., Reid, R. D., Friedenreich, C. M., Ladha, A. B., Proulx, C., Vallance, J. K., Lane, K., Yasui, Y. and McKenzie, D. C. (2007). Effects of aerobic and resistance exercise in breast cancer patients receiving adjuvant chemotherapy: a multicenter randomized controlled trial. *Journal of Clinical Oncology*, 25, 4396–4404.

Culos-Reed, S. N., Robinson, J. L., Lau, H., O'Connor, K. and Keats, M. R. (2007). Benefits of a physical activity intervention for men with prostate cancer. *Journal of Sport and Exercise Psychology*, 29, 118–127.

Culos-Reed, S. N., Robinson, J. W., Lau, H., Stephenson, L., Keats, M., Norris, S., Kline, G. and Faris, P. (2009). Physical activity for men receiving androgen deprivation therapy for prostate cancer: benefits from a 16-week intervention. *Supportive Care Cancer*, 18, 591–599.

Daley, A. J., Crank, H., Saxton, J. M., Mutrie, N., Coleman, R. and Roalfe, A. (2007). Randomized trial of exercise therapy in women treated for breast cancer. *Journal of Clinical Oncology*, 25, 1713–1721.

Demark-Wahnefried, W., Clipp, E. C., Morey, M. C., Pieper, C. F., Sloane, R., Snyder, D. C. and Cohen, H. J. (2004). Physical function and associations with diet and exercise: Results of a cross-sectional survey among elders with breast or prostate cancer. *Int J Behav Nutr Phys* 1, 16.

Department of Health (2004). *Chief Medical Officer's Report: Evidence on the Impact of Physical Activity and its Relationship to Health*. London, HSMO.

Dorey, G. (2007). A clinical overview of the treatment of post-prostatectomy incontinence. *British Journal of Nursing*, 16, 1194–1199.

Galvão, D. A., Nosaka, K., Taaffe, D. R., Spry, N., Kristjanson, L. J., McGuigan, M. R., Suzuki, K., Yamaya, K. and Newton, R.U. (2006). Resistance training and reduction of treatment side effects in prostate cancer patients. *Medicine and Science in Sport and Exercise*, 38, 2045–2052.

Galvão, D. A., Taaffe, D. R., Spry, N., Joseph, D. and Newton, R. (2009). Combined resistance and aerobic exercise training program reverses muscle loss in men undergoing androgen suppression therapy in prostate cancer without bone metastases: A randomised control trial. *Journal of Clinical Oncology*, November 30 (Epub only).

Hack, T. F., Cohen, L., Katz, J., Robson, L. S. and Goss, P. (1999). Physical and psychological morbidity after axillary lymph node dissection for breast cancer. *Journal of Clinical Oncology*, 17, 143–149.

Haskell, W. L., Lee, I. M., Pate, R. R., Powell, K. E., Blair, S. N., Franklin, B. A., Macera, C. A., Heath, G. W., Thompson, P. D. and Bauman, A. (2007). Physical activity and public health: updated recommendation for adults from the American College of Sports Medicine and the American Heart Association. Med.Sci.Sports Exerc 39, 1423–1434.

Hede K (2008). Fat may fuel breast cancer growth. *J Natl Cancer Inst* 100, 298–299.

Hewitt, M., Rowland, J. H. and Yancik, R. (2003). Cancer survivors in the United States: age, health, and disability. *Journals of Gerontology. Series A, Biological Sciences and Medical Sciences* 58, 82–91.

Holick, C. N., Newcomb, P. A., Trentham-Dietz, A., Titus-Ernstoff, L., Bersch, A. J., Stampfer, M. J., Baron, J. A., Egan, K. M. and Willett, W. C. (2008). Physical activity and survival after diagnosis of invasive breast cancer. *Cancer Epidemiol.Biomarkers Prev.* 17, 379–386.

Holmes, M. D., Chen, W. Y., Feskanich, D., Kroenke, C. H. and Colditz, G. A. (2005). Physical activity and survival after breast cancer diagnosis. *JAMA* 293, 2479–2486.

Houborg, K. B., Jensen, M. B., Rasmussen, P., Gandrup, P., Schroll, M. and Laurberg, S. (2006). Postoperative physical training following colorectal surgery: a randomised, placebo-controlled study. *Scandinavian Journal of Surgery*, 95, 17–22.

Irwin, M. L., Alvarez-Reeves, M., Cadmus, L., Mierzejewski, E., Mayne, S. T., Yu, H., Chung G. G., Jones, B., Knobf, M. T. and DiPietro, L. (2009). Exercise improves body fat, lean mass and bone mass in breast cancer survivors. *Obesity*, 17, 1534–1541.

Irwin, M. L., McTiernan, A., Baumgartner, R. N., Baumgartner, K. B., Bernstein, L., Gilliland, F. D. and Ballard-Barbash, R. (2005). Changes in body fat and weight after a breast cancer diagnosis: influence of demographic, prognostic, and lifestyle factors. *J Clin Oncol* 23, 774–782.

Irwin, M. L., Smith, A. W., McTiernan, A., Ballard-Barbash, R., Cronin, K., Gilliland, F. D., Baumgartner, R. N., Baumgartner, K. B. and Bernstein, L. (2008). Influence of pre- and postdiagnosis physical activity on mortality in breast cancer survivors: the health, eating, activity, and lifestyle study. *J.Clin.Oncol.* 26, 3958–3964.

Knols, R., Aaronson, N. K., Uebelhart, D., Fransen, J. and Aufdemkampe, G. (2005). Physical exercise in cancer patients during and after medical treatment: a systematic review of randomized and controlled clinical trials. *J Clin Oncol* 23, 3830–3842.

Loblaw, D. A., Mendelson, D. S., Talcott, J. A., Virgo K. S., Somerfield, M. R., Ben-Josef, E., Middleton, R., Porterfield, H., Sharp, S. A., Smith, T. J., Taplin, M. E., Vogelzang, N. J., Wade Jr, J. L., Bennett, C. L. and Scher, H. I. (2004). American Society of Clinical Oncology Recommendations for the Initial Hormonal Management of Androgen-Sensitive Metastatic, Recurrent, or Progressive Prostate Cancer. *Journal of Clinical Oncology*, 22, 2927–2941.

MacDonald, R., Fink, H. A., Huckabay, C., Monga, M. and Wilt, T. J. (2007). Pelvic floor muscle training to improve urinary incontinence after radical prostatectomy: a systematic review of effectiveness. *BJU International*, 100, 76–81.

MacVicar, M. G., Winningham, M. L. and Nickel, J. L. (1989). Effects of aerobic interval training on cancer patients' functional capacity. *Nursing Research*, 38, 348–351.

McNeely, M. L., Campbell, K. L., Rowe, B. H., Klassen, T. P., Mackey, J. R. and Courneya, K. S. (2006). Effects of exercise on breast cancer patients and survivors: a systematic review and meta-analysis. *CMAJ* 175, 34–41.

Meyerhardt, J. A., Giovannucci, E. L., Holmes, M. D., Chan, A. T., Chan, J. A., Colditz, G. A. and Fuchs, C. S. (2006a). Physical activity and survival after colorectal cancer diagnosis. *Journal of Clinical Oncology*, 24, 3527–3533.

Meyerhardt, J. A., Heseltine, D., Niedzwiecki, D., Hollis, D., Saltz, L. B., Mayer, R. J., Thomas, J., Nelson, H., Whittom, R., Hantel, A., Schilsky, R. L. and Fuchs, C. S. (2006b). Impact of physical activity on cancer recurrence and survival in patients with stage III colon cancer: findings from CALGB 89803. *Journal of Clinical Oncology*, 24, 3535–3541.

Mock, V., Dow, K. H., Meares, C. J., Grimm, P. M., Dienemann, J. A., Haisfield-Wolfe, M. E. (1997). Effects of exercise on fatigue, physical functioning, and emotional distress during radiation therapy for breast cancer. *Oncology Nursing Forum*, 24, 991–1000.

Mock, V., Frangakis, C., Davidson, N. E., Ropka, M. E., Pickett, M. and Poniatowski, B. (2004). Exercise manages fatigue during breast cancer treatment: A randomized controlled trial. *Psychooncology*, 14, 14.

Monga, U., Garber, S. L., Thornby, J., Vallbona, C., Kerrigan, A. J., Monga, T. N. and Zimmermann, K. P. (2007). Exercise prevents fatigue and improves quality of life in prostate cancer patients undergoing radiotherapy. *Archives of Physical Medicine Rehabilitation*, 88, 1416–1422.

Mutrie, N., Campbell, A. M., Whyte, F., McConnachie, A., Emslie, C., Lee, L., Kearney, N., Walker, A. and Ritchie, D. (2007). Benefits of supervised group exercise programme for women being treated for early stage breast cancer: pragmatic randomised controlled trial. *BMJ*, 334, 517.

National Institute for Clinical Excellence (NICE) (2004). *Guidance on Cancer Services – Improving Outcomes in Colorectal Cancers: Manual Update*. National Institute for Clinical Excellence. London, UK.

Ohira, T., Schmitz, K. H., Ahmed, R. L. and Yee, D. (2006). Effects of weight training on quality of life in recent breast cancer survivors: the Weight Training for Breast Cancer Survivors (WTBS) study. *Cancer*, 106, 2076–2083.

Ornish, D., Weidner, G., Fair, W. R., Marlin, R., Pettengill, E. B., Raisin, C. J., Dunn-Emke, S., Cruthfield, L., Jacobs, F. N., Barnard, R. J., Aronson, W. J., McCormac, P., McKnight, D., Fein, J. D., Dnistrian, A. M., Weinstein, J., Ngo, T. H., Mendell, N. R. and Carrole, P. E. (2005). Intensive lifestyle changes may affect the progression of prostate cancer. *The Journal of Urology*, 174, 1065–1070.

Ornish, D., Magbanua, M. J., Weidner, G., Weinberg, V., Kemp, C., Green, C., Mattie, M. D., Marlin, R., Simko, J., Shinohara, K., Haqq, C. M. and Carroll, P. R. (2008). Changes in prostate gene expression in men undergoing an intensive nutrition and lifestyle intervention. *Proceedings of the National Academy of Sciences of the United States of America*, 105, 8369–8374.

Pierce, J. P., Stefanick, M. L., Flatt, S. W., Natarajan, L., Sternfeld, B., Madlensky, L., Al-Delaimy, W. K., Thomson, C. A., Kealey, S., Hajek, R., Parker, B. A., Newman, V. A., Caan, B. and Rock, C. L. (2007). Greater survival after breast cancer in physically active women with high vegetable-fruit intake regardless of obesity. *J.Clin.Oncol.* 25, 2345–2351.

Rockson, S. G. (2008). Diagnosis and management of lymphatic vascular disease. *Journal of the American College of Cardiology*, 52, 799–806.

Rooney, M. and Wald, A. (2007). Interventions for the management of weight and body composition changes in women with breast cancer. *Clinical Journal of Oncology Nursing*, 11, 41–52.

Sagen, A., Kåresen, R. and Risberg, M. A. (2009). Physical activity for the affected limb and arm lymphedema after breast cancer surgery. A prospective, randomized controlled trial with two years follow-up. *Acta Oncologica*, 48, 1102–1110.

Servaes, P., Verhagen, S. and Bleijenberg, G. (2002). Determinants of chronic fatigue in disease-free breast cancer patients: a cross-sectional study. *Annals of Oncology*, 13, 589–598

Schaid, D. J. (2004). The complex genetic epidemiology of prostate cancer. *Human Molecular Genetics*, 13,103–121.

Schmitz, K. H., Holtzman, J., Courneya, K. S., Masse, L. C., Duval, S. and Kane, R. (2005). Controlled physical activity trials in cancer survivors: a systematic review and meta-analysis. *Cancer Epidemiol Biomarkers Prev* 14, 1588–1595.

Schmitz, K. H. and Speck, R. M. (2010). Risk and benefits of physical activity among breast cancer survivors who have completed treatment. *Women's Health* 6, 221–238.

Segal, R., Evans, W., Johnson, D., Smith, J., Colletta, S. and Gayton, J. (2001). Structured exercise improves physical functioning in women with stages I and II breast cancer: results of a randomized controlled trial. *Journal of Clinical Oncology*, 19, 657–665.

Segal, R. J., Reid, R. D., Courneya, K. S., Malone, S. C., Parliament, M. B. and Scott, C. G. (2003). Resistance exercise in men receiving androgen deprivation therapy for prostate cancer. *Journal of Clinical Oncology*, 21, 1653–1659.

Segal, R. J., Reid, R. D., Courneya, K. S., Sigal, R. J., Kenny, G. P., Prud'Homme, D. G., Malone, S. C., Wells, G. A., Scott, C. G. and D'Angelo M. E. (2009). Randomized controlled trial of resistance or aerobic exercise in men receiving radiation therapy for prostate cancer. *Journal of Clinical Oncology*, 27, 344–351.

Spiegel, D. (1997). Psychosocial aspects of breast cancer treatment. *Seminars in Oncology*, 24, 1–47.

Truong, P. T., Olivotto, I. A., Whelan, T. J. and Levine, M. (2004). Clinical practice guidelines for the care and treatment of breast cancer: 16. Locoregional post-mastectomy radiotherapy. *Canadian Medical Association Journal*, 170, 1263–1273.

Velthuis, M. J., Agasi-Idenburg S. C., Aufdemkampe, G. and Wittink H. M. (2010). The effect of physical exercise on cancer-related fatigue during cancer treatment: a meta-analysis of randomised controlled trials. *Clinical Oncology*, 22, 208–221.

Windsor, P. M., Nicol, K. F. and Potter, J. (2004). A randomized, controlled trial of aerobic exercise for treatment-related fatigue in men receiving radical external beam radiotherapy for localized prostate carcinoma. *Cancer*, 101, 550–557.

INDEX

Printed and bound by CPI Group (UK) Ltd, Croydon, CR0 4YY

01/11/2024

01782626-0016